Freak Show

Freak Show

Presenting Human Oddities
for Amusement and Profit

Robert Bogdan

The University of Chicago Press
Chicago and London

ROBERT BOGDAN is professor of special education, sociology, and cultural foundations of education at Syracuse University. He is the author of *Being Different: The Autobiography of Jane Fry* and *Inside Out: The Social Meaning of Retardation.*

THE UNIVERSITY OF CHICAGO PRESS, CHICAGO 60637
THE UNIVERSITY OF CHICAGO PRESS, LTD., LONDON

© 1988 by The University of Chicago
All rights reserved. Published 1988
Printed in the United States of America
97 96 95 94 93 92 91 90 89 88   54321

Library of Congress Cataloging in Publication Data

Bogdan, Robert.
  Freak show.

  Bibliography: p.
  Includes index.
  1. Carnivals—History. 2. Abnormalities, Human.
I. Title
GV1835.B64 1988   791'.1   87-35808
ISBN 0-226-06311-9

Contents

Preface

THE MEANING THAT DISABILITY has in our culture has been
an interest of mine for a long time. This book on "freak shows"
flows directly from a project in which I examined villains in horror and adventure movies. The idea of studying these mass media favorites came to me one night while I was watching television with my ten-year-old son and his friend. The film was a
Disney remake of the classic *Treasure Island*. Near the beginning of the film my son's friend, Jeremy, who was confused about
the plot, asked: "Who's the bad guy?" My son replied: "If they
look bad, they are bad."

I was struck by my son's insight. In the film, part of being bad
was looking bad, and villains were marked by various disfigure-
ments and disabilities, such as missing limbs and eyes. Disney
and other film producers use disability with great effect to con-
jure up fear in their audiences. The beautiful queen in *Snow
White and the Seven Dwarfs* had to be transformed into a wart-
nosed hunchback before she could set out to accomplish her
hideous scheme. The pattern was exemplified by Captain Hook
in *Peter Pan*. Disability is the black hat of these adventure
stories.

In horror films the association of evil with disability is even
more common, indeed ubiquitous. Horror film "monsters" are
scarred, deformed, disproportionately built, hunched over, exceptionally large, exceptionally small, deaf, speech impaired,
visually impaired, mentally ill, or mentally subnormal. In fact,
the word *monster* is standard medical terminology for infants
born with blatant "defects."

I soon discovered the film classic *Freaks*, produced and directed by a legend in filmmaking, Tod Browning. A box-office
flop when it was first issued in 1932, *Freaks* was re-issued in the

1960s for a limited "camp" audience. *Freaks* employed Ringling Brothers, Barnum and Bailey Circus sideshow exhibits as perpetrators of violence. After a beautiful aerial artist and her strongman lover wrong one of "their kind" one stormy night, the "monsters" get them. The sideshow attractions—a dwarf, three people with microcephaly, an armless woman, and a limbless man creep and crawl through the mud to carry out their revenge. They kill and disembowel the lover and turn the aerial artist into an exhibit like themselves. In the final scene, a freak show lecturer is coaxing people to step right up and feast their eyes on this oddest of anatomical wonders, who is the transformed protagonist.

The film was my invitation to journey into the world of freak shows. I started my work thinking that using human beings for such a purpose was exploitive and demeaning to the exhibits, and therefore despicable. I thought I could use the project to extend my work in the disability rights movement: yet another case of inhumanity.

At the outset my approach to the topic of "freaks" was simple, involving a clear and limited agenda. By studying the practice of exhibiting human beings with physical, mental, and behavioral anomalies I hoped to contribute to our present understanding of disability. I expected to organize my findings around two ideas: the association of disability with evil and the fact that disabled people are often mistreated. But as I began to study the archival material, I saw that the empirical world could not be confined by my preconceptions. Certainly, I found degradation, but I also found fame and fortune. People with disabilities were presented in demeaning ways, in ways to promote fear and contempt, but they were also presented in ways that positively enhanced their status.

Although freak shows contributed to the imagery of disability, there were other objects of study besides the exhibits themselves. In my original thinking I had forgotten the managers, the promoters, the audience, and a host of others who belonged to that world. In addition, I soon discovered that there were other human "freaks" on exhibit who would not now be considered disabled. Non-Western people were commonly exhibited in sideshows, as were large numbers of people who feigned physical and mental abnormalities to qualify for the business. A considerable portion of the sideshow performers were novelty acts as well, sword swallowers or knife throwers, whose talents were unusual but not the product of any condition with which they were born.

I remained true to my original concern with disability, but when I discovered non-Western exhibits and phony freaks I pursued them also. In order to place some limit on my work, however, I treated novelty acts only tangentially. My interest in exploring audience reaction to exhibits, moreover, was curtailed by a lack of primary material. A final point involves my original intention to include extensive research on the modern-day sideshow. Although modern exhibits are mentioned in the first and last chapters, in the end I decided to make this a historical study; I therefore confined myself to the period of the sideshow's greatest popularity, approximately 1840 to 1940.

In pursuing my topic I visited major depositories of circus, carnival, and other amusement world memorabilia and documents. It is important, however, in dealing with a topic so loaded with affect as freak shows, to document more than just the sources and formal procedures of the inquiry. Research is often more than an intellectual journey; it can be an emotional odyssey in which you confront who you are and what you carry with you as a member of your culture.

A few years ago I visited the New York State Fair. It was a family affair, a day in late August to take the kids to see the agricultural and other educational exhibits. My children insisted on visiting the rides and games of chance. My wife and I reluctantly agreed. In the center of the midway was a sideshow, "Sutton's Land of Wonders." Outside, on the bally platform, was an elderly dwarf wearing a suit and smoking a large cigar. The scene caught my interest. I suggested to the rest of the family that they try a ride a little farther down the strip—there was something I wanted to see. My teenage daughter asked where I was going and I reluctantly told her. She asked to come with me.

The only other time I remember seeing humans on exhibit was in New York City. I was about ten years old, and it was a day similar to the one I was now spending with my family. My parents had taken my sister and me on the long subway ride downtown from the Bronx to see the Ringling Brothers, Barnum and Bailey Circus in Madison Square Garden. We arrived a little early so we could see the elephants and other animals which were kept in a special section for exhibit prior to the main show. Right next to the menagerie was the freak show. I vaguely recollect sneaking a peek and seeing an immense woman sitting on a chair, but my parents scooted me off. I was left with a sense of my parents' disapproval, and a feeling that those people's sitting there to be stared at was lewd, something parents should not let their children be part of.

I felt the same when my daughter asked if she could accompany me into the contemporary New York State Fair version of the freak show, but my liberal self prevailed—the self that says that, with discussion, it might turn out to be an educational experience. We bought our tickets and hastily went in—I did not want to be seen entering such an establishment. The show was disappointing, though. It did not live up to the expectations created outside by the blaring taped pitch and the large banners on the facade telling of the wonders to behold.

The cigar-smoking dwarf, who went by the name "Prince Arthur," a person who pushed spikes up his nose and who doubled as the announcer, a magician and a contortionist, a sword swallower and a person with poorly formed arms and legs, were the attractions. The show made little impression on me. I remember feeling I had been cheated, that there should have been more to the show. But at the same time I felt guilty for staring at the few human beings with anomalies that were onstage. One thing I remember clearly, though. As my daughter and I turned to go, there, walking in, was a graduate student I knew from the semester before. We smiled and greeted each other, but we were both caught in deep embarrassment. Nice people don't go to, are not interested in, freak shows. We both felt a desperate need to "explain" our presence there—to separate ourselves from the motives that "other people" presumably had for entering the display.

I soon overcame my initial shame, however, and began to pursue the limited material that was available on the topic. The pictures and stories of the human oddities I encountered provoked feelings of distress; I felt uncomfortable being associated with them. We are carriers of our culture, but our feelings are not so ingrained that a deep intellectual and personal encounter with the empirical world cannot wear away the shell of fear and repulsion that first foils the pursuit of understanding.

Despite the occasional rejection of silence I encounter when I tell strangers what I am studying, I feel quite comfortable with my subject now. Ultimately, I reached the state of mind that allowed me to see the phenomenon as it was experienced by those who took part—not those who comdemn it.

My emotional and intellectual journey has left me with this thesis: Our reaction to freaks is not a function of some deep-seated fear or some "energy" that they give off; it is, rather, the result of our socialization, and of the way our social institutions managed these people's identities. Freak shows are not about isolated individuals, either on platforms or in an audience. They are about organizations and patterned relationships between them and us. "Freak" is not a quality that belongs to the person on display. It is something that we created: a perspective, a set of practices—a social construction.

The word *freak* offends most people. Disability rights activists find words such as *midget, giant,* and *pinhead* degrading. I use them here because individuals in the business used them. ·

In studying this relatively unexplored topic I made friends and built a network of acquaintances from many disciplines and walks of life. I corresponded with and interviewed freak show old-timers; academics in such diverse fields as popular culture, the sociology of deviance, medicine, special education, history, and photography; collectors of antique photographs and circus and carnival memorabilia; and museum and archive curators and their assistants. All spoke openly with me about my topic and gave freely of their time and resources. While some people hoard information and artifacts for themselves, others collect to share. This project was made possible by those people.

Richard Flint shared his extensive knowledge of amusement world research resources with me and pointed me in the right directions. Others who helped include: Gordon Brown, M.D.; Melvin Burkhart, "The Anatomical Wonder"; Ward Hall, sideshow operator; Betty King, Hertzberg Circus Collection, San Antonio Public Library; Craig Koste, collector of rare photographs; John Lentz and Nan Fisher, Ringling Circus Museum, Sarasota, Florida; Joe McKennon, internationally known circus and carnival trouper; Robert Parkinson and Bill McCarthy, Circus World Museum, Baraboo, Wisconsin; Kathy Peiss, University of Maryland; Fred Pfening, Jr., and Fred Pfening III, collectors; Warren Raymond, collector; Hy Roth, collector; Arthur Saxon, author; Ann Shumard and Will Stapp, National Portrait Gallery, Smithsonian Institution; and Don Wilmeth, Brown University. Ron Becker, a collector of Eisenmann photographs, deserves separate thanks. Because he donated a collection of over one thousand rare photographs to the Syracuse University George Arents Library, I had, within walking distance of my home, the archival resources needed to accomplish this work.

Other colleagues, although they did not have direct knowledge of the topic, were generous enough to critique my ideas and in other ways provided invaluable help. All scholarly writing is lonely and personal, but the enterprise can be made part of a community of scholarship when people understand—as the people listed below do—that to take a colleague's work seriously improves all academic endeavors. My supporters include Doug and Sari Biklen, Peter Conrad, Amy Doherty, Gunnar Dybwad, Michael Freedman, Barry Glassner, Sue Granai, Jerry Grant, Tom Green, Jim Knoll, Sally Kohlstedt, Will Provine, Alphonse Sallet, Joe Schneider, Dave Smith, Steve Taylor, Vince Tinto, and Wolf Wolfensberger.

Andrejs Ozolins read early drafts as editor and critic. Janet Bogdan, Faye Dudden, Margaret Hanousek, Julia Loughlin, and Lydia Miner performed similar duties on a later draft. David Broda contributed his photographic skills and knowledge. Thanks also are due Dorcus McDonald and her staff at interlibrary loan, Bird Library, Syracuse University, and Helen Anderson and Rosemary Alibrandi, who helped in many ways.

Great institutions of higher learning, by supporting and encouraging their faculty in the pursuit of scholarship, make them feel that their work is important. Syracuse University has done that for me throughout my academic career and particularly in the research reported here, the great bulk of which was accomplished while on a university-supported sabbatical. In addition, Senate Research Committee funds made possible much of the travel to the various repositories of freak show material.

A final word about a person who is not alive to read this book but who was its inspiration. Burton Blatt was a remarkable person. Although I met him after completing my graduate studies, Burt was my teacher. He taught me that what might appear to be offbeat was often central to understanding the human experience, that those whom others might shun were reflections of our own experience, and much, much more. A few weeks before his death I visited him in the hospital and we discussed the ideas, people, and photographs in this book. For a few hours there was no clock on life—just two friends lost in the joy of exploring subjects that had perhaps never before been discussed. Burton participated in such conversations often and taught a generation of us who knew him well the spirituality of such encounters. There is joy in this work because he helped me experience the pleasure of scholarship. If there is compassion in it, it is because he taught me that scholarship had to touch human experience. If there is courage, it is because he taught that to write one must be brave. I dedicate this book to him because I owe him so much.

Sections of Chapter 4, in modified form, first appeared in 1987 as

"Freakshow," *Policy Studies Journal* 15 (3). Chapter 5 is a much expanded and significantly revised version of a paper that was first published in the *American Journal of Mental Deficiency* 91 (2) as "Exhibition of Mentally Retarded People for Amusement and Profit, 1850–1940." Part of Chapter 9 was previously published in 1986 in *Bandwagon* 30 (3), as "Circassian Beauties." I thank these journals for permission to use this material here.

1

Introduction
In Search of Freaks

OTIS JORDAN, a man with poorly functioning and underformed limbs who is better known in the carnival world as "Otis the Frog Man," was banned in 1984 from appearing as part of the Sutton Sideshow at the New York State Fair. A vocal citizen had objected, calling the exhibition of people with deformities an "intolerable anachronism." The protester contended that handicapped people were being exploited and that the state's fair funds could be put to better use by helping people with disabilities instead of making them freaks.

As a result of the complaint, and in spite of Jordan's objections, Sutton's "Incredible Wonders of the World" was moved from the heart of the midway, where business and visibility were best, to the back of the fair. The showmen were asked not to use the term *freak* or allow performances of people like Otis Jordan, people the public would consider disabled (Kaleina 1984).[1]

On September 8, 1984, the Associated Press released a story ("City to Cite" 1984) about a committee formed in Alton, Illinois, to erect a statue in honor of Robert Wadlow, a local boy who had reached the height of eight feet eleven inches before his death in 1940 at the age of twenty-two. Wadlow had appeared in the circus in the 1930s and, using the novelty of his height, had gotten a job promoting shoes at stores throughout the United States (Fadner 1944). But a committee spokesperson wanted to clarify: "He was not a circus freak as a lot of people might think. He was an intelligent, caring man."

During the past twenty years numerous intellectuals and artists have confronted us with freaks.[2] Yet the frequent mention and coffee-table display of art-photography books, which include pictures taken at freak shows, are no indication that freak shows are now accepted. Rather, as the work of Diane Arbus

1

personifies, "freak" has become a metaphor for estrangement, aliena-
tion, marginality, the dark side of the human experience (Arbus 1972;
Sontag 1977). Indeed, Arbus's biographer suggests that her flirtation
with freaks was but one dimension of her odyssey through the bowels
of society—her suicide being the last stop on the trip (Bosworth 1984).

Otis Jordan and the spokesperson for Robert Wadlow's statue committee remind us of what we all sense when we hear the word *freak*
and think of "freak shows." Seen by many as crude, rude, and exploitive, the freak show is despicable, a practice on the margin, limited to a class with poor taste, representing, as one disability rights
activist put it, the "pornography of disability."[3]

Although freak shows are now on the contemptible fringe, from approximately 1840 through 1940 the formally organized exhibition for
amusement and profit of people with physical, mental, or behavioral
anomalies, both alleged and real, was an accepted part of American
life. Hundreds of freak shows traversed America in the last quarter of
the nineteenth and first quarter of the twentieth centuries. Yet only
five exist today,[4] and their continued existence is precarious. Personnel, plagued by low-priced admissions, poor attendance, and attacks from indignant activitists, cannot tell from week to week whether
they can last the season. Barely alive, the freak show is approaching
its finale.

Given the tradition of the study of deviance and abnormality, one
would expect a large body of social scientific literature on freak
shows. There is none.[5] The low status of the convention, combined
with the decline in the number of such businesses, may explain this
lack in part. In addition, until the relatively recent interest in the
natural history of social problems (Conrad and Schneider 1980; Spector and Kitsuse 1977), social scientists interested in deviance seldom
turned to the past for their data (see Erikson 1966 and Mizruchi 1983
for exceptions). Thus freak shows have remained in the hands of circus buffs and a few nonconformists in the humanities. I believe, however, that these displays of human beings present an exciting opportunity to develop understanding of past practices and changing
conceptions of abnormality, as well as the beginnings of a grounded
theory in the management of human differences.

The Social Construction of Freaks

In the mid 1920s, Jack Earle, a very tall University of Texas student,
visited the Ringling Brothers circus sideshow.[6] Clyde Ingalls, the

show's famous manager, spotted Earle in the audience; after the show he approached the young man to ask, "How would you like to be a giant?" (Fig. 1).

While it is uncertain how much of this story changed on becoming incorporated into circus lore, it clarifies a point that freak show personnel understood but outside observers neglect: being extremely tall is a matter of physiology—being a giant involves something more. Similarly, being a freak is not a personal matter, a physical condition that some people have (Goffman 1963; Becker 1963). The onstage freak is something else off stage. "Freak" is a frame of mind, a set of practices, a way of thinking about and presenting people.[7] It is the enactment of a tradition, the performance of a stylized presentation.

While people called "freaks" will be included in this discussion, the people themselves are not of primary concern. Rather, the focus is on the social arrangements in which they found themselves, the place and meaning of the freak show in the world of which they were a part, and the way the resulting exhibits were presented to the public. The social construction—the manufacture of freaks—is the main attraction.

But don't leave! There will be exhibits (and it will be okay to look!). For we need examples—flesh on the bones of institutional analysis. We need to understand what it was like to participate in the freak show and what meanings emerged to make the enterprise coherent to the exhibits, the promoters, and the audience alike.

VOCABULARY

Many terms have been used to refer to the practice of exhibiting people for money and to the various forms that such exhibits took. "Raree Show" and "Hall of Human Curiosities" were early-nineteenth-century terms. "Sideshow," "Ten in One," "Kid Show," "Pitshow," "Odditorium," "Congress of Oddities," "Congress of Human Wonders," "Museum of Nature's Mistakes," "Freak Show," and a host of variations on these titles were late-nineteenth- and twentieth-century designations.

A broad range of terms were applied to the people exhibited, the freaks. Because natural scientists and physicians were interested in many exhibits, and because showmen exploited scientific interest in constructing freaks, the lexicon is a complex hodgepodge of medical terminology and show-world hype. The more recent proliferation of euphemisms generated by the freak show's decline in popularity and

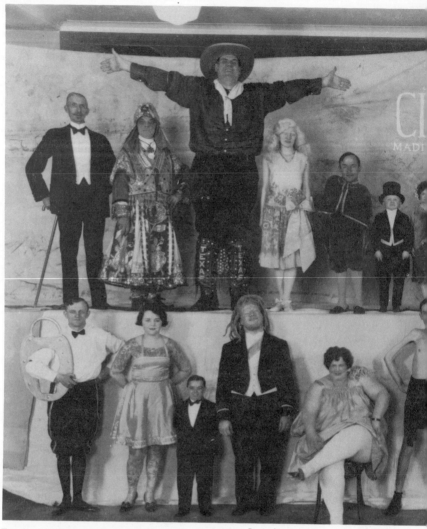

FIG. 1. Jack Earle in the Ringling Brothers, Barnum and Bailey Sideshow. Earle is in the top row, third from the right, wearing a tall hat and military outfit. Other well-known exhibits in the picture include the Doll Family, Koo-Koo the Bird Girl, Clicko the Bushman, and Iko and Eko. Photo by Century, c. 1934. (Hertzberg Coll., San Antonio Public Library.)

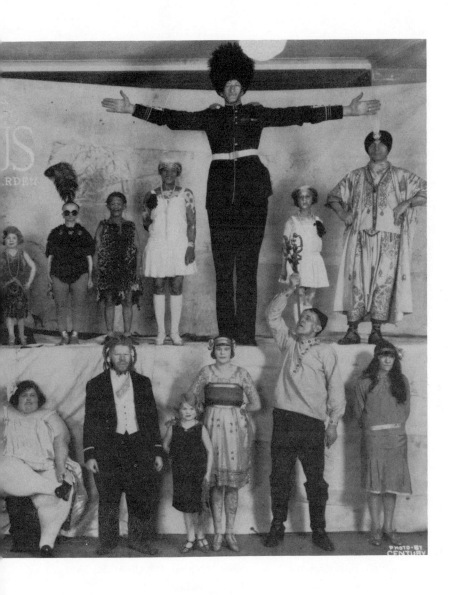

the moral indignation surrounding the exhibition of human anomalies creates a long list of imprecise terms.[8] "Curiosities," "lusus naturae," "freaks of nature," "rarities," "oddities," "eccentrics," "wonders," "marvels," "nature's mistakes," "strange people," "prodigies," "monsters,"[9] "very special people," and "freaks" form a partial list. The exact use and definition of these words varies from user to user and from time to time. They do not, however, all mean the same thing; indeed, some have very exact meanings when used by particular people. The terminology will be clarified as this discussion proceeds.

TYPES OF FREAKS

What were the various kinds of human freaks? In discussions of human oddities in the eighteenth and nineteenth centuries, there developed an important and revealing, albeit blurry and noninclusive, distinction between two types of exhibits. The distinction is revealing because it illustrates the connection between science and freak shows, a connection that showmen profited by and tried to maintain well into the twentieth century. The distinction was between so-called examples of new and unknown "races" and "lusus naturae" or nature's jokes or mistakes.

The first type is related to the exploration of the non-Western world then in progress. As explorers and natural scientists traversed the world, they brought back not only tales of unfamiliar cultures but also specimens of the distant wonders. Tribal people, brought to the United States with all the accoutrements of their culture out of context, stimulated the popular imagination and kindled belief in races of tailed people, dwarfs, giants, and even people with double heads (Clair 1968) that paralleled creatures of ancient mythology (Thompson 1968). The interest thus spawned was an opportunity, a platform, and a backdrop for showmen's creations. Promoters quickly began to exhibit what they claimed were examples of previously undiscovered types of humans: not only non-Western people but also, fraudulently, as a promotional strategy, Americans with physical anomalies.

The second major category of exhibit consisted of "monsters," the medical term for people born with a demonstrable difference. Lusus naturae, or "freaks of nature," were of interest to physicians for whom the field of teratology, the study of these so-called monsters, had become a fad. To the joy (and often at the instigation) of showmen, debates raged among scientists and laypersons alike as to whether a par-

6

ticular exhibit actually represented a new species or was simply a lusus naturae.

In the last quarter of the nineteenth century the blurred distinction between species and freaks of nature became moot; all human exhibits, including tribal people of normal stature and body configuration, as well as people who performed unusual feats such as swallowing swords, fell under the generic term *freak*.

Those twentieth-century authors who have written about the sideshow, mainly popular historians and humanities scholars, address the question "What were the various kinds of human freaks?" by concentrating on the physical characteristics of exhibits with anomalies (Drimmer 1973; Durant and Durant 1957; Fiedler 1978; Howard 1977). Their books and articles are organized like medical or special education textbooks, with headings covering such topics as little people (dwarfs and midgets), giants, hairy people, human skeletons, armless and legless wonders, wild men, fat people, albinos, Siamese twins, people with extra limbs, half men/half women, people with skin disorders, and anatomical wonders. They are eager to provide readers a quick course in genetics, endocrinology, and embryology. One of the most widely read, Drimmer's *Very Special People*, romanticizes exhibits by casting them as courageous warriors battling the disadvantage they received at birth. These writings, however, ignore exhibits *without* blatant physical anomalies, not to mention the social constuction of freaks.

The humanities scholar Leslie Fiedler, in his popular book *Freaks* (1978), still concentrates on exhibits with physical anomalies, but he breaks the mold of writers who focus on "freak" as a physiological condition. Rather, his mythological, psychoanalytic approach posits that human beings have a deep, psychic fear of people with specific abnormalities. Dwarfs, for example, confront us with our phobia that we will never grow up. Yet although Fiedler's study of "human curiosities" shifts the focus from "them" to "us," it also reifies "freak" by taking "it" as a constant and inevitable outpouring of basic human nature. Moreover, in his writing he slips back to treating the person exhibited as the subject of the study. His typology of human oddities does not stray from the traditional view of "freak" as a physiological condition, and it excludes exhibits with no physical anomalies. Thus, rather than penetrating the socially constructed dimension of the freak show, he merely mystifies it.

In answer to the question "What were the various kinds of freaks?" people who have been inside the exhibiting business use the physiological categories as well, but they also use the distinctions *born freaks, made freaks*, and *novelty acts* (Gresham 1948; Kelly 1950). According to this classification, "born freaks" are people with real physical anomalies who came by their condition naturally. While this category includes people who developed their uniqueness later in life, central are people who had an abnormality at birth: Siamese twins and armless and legless people are examples. "Made freaks" do something to themselves that make them unusual enough for exhibit, such as getting adorned with tattoos or growing their beards or hair exceptionally long. The "novelty act" (or "working act") does not rely on any physical characteristic but rather boasts an unusual performance or ability such as sword swallowing (the more contemporary versions used neon tubes) or snake charming.

In addition to these three main "types," sideshow people refer to "gaffed freaks": the fakes, the phonies—the armless wonder whose arms are tucked under a tight fitting shirt, the four-legged woman whose extra legs really belong to a person hidden from the audience,[10] or the Siamese twins who were in fact two (Fig. 2). When in public freak show personnel showed disdain for the gaff; their competitors might try to get away with it, but they would not. The "born freak" was publicly acknowledged as having esteem.

This is the standard typology as those in the business present it, and it has not changed over the last hundred and twenty years. More inclusive than other schemes, it is a good starting point for approaching the subject of freaks. Yet even though the "insiders'" way of categorizing differentiates freak show exhibits in the abstract, even they had difficulty applying the distinctions. Non-Western people, for example, were exhibited in freak shows on the basis of their cultural differences. Although showmen called them "freaks" and displayed them on the same platform as people with physiological and mental disabilities, their place in the commonsense typology is unclear. The categories did not, moreover, acknowledge the pervasive hype, fraud, and deception that was characteristic of the whole freak show enterprise. If taken at face value, the insiders' typology veils more than it reveals. It interests us not because it clarifies the freak show or the exhibits, but because it enlarges the subject and grounds us in the commonsense notions of the amusement world.

Exhibiting people, although often treated as an educational and

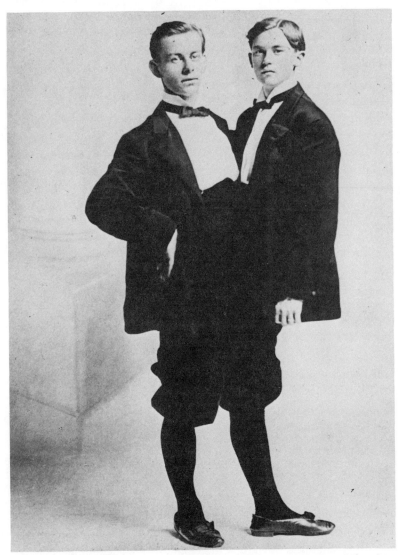

Fig. 2. Phony Siamese twins. Adolph-Rudolph were gaffs: joined twins are always identical. Note the dissimilar facial features. Photo by Frank Wendt, c. 1899. (Becker Coll., Syracuse University.)

scientific pursuit, was always first and foremost a for-profit activity. Presentors learned from the medicine shows that packaging of the product was as important as what was inside. Thus, using information from science, exploration, medicine, and current events, and appealing to popular images and symbols, promoters created a public conception of the exhibit that would have the widest appeal, attract the most people, and collect the most dimes. Every exhibit was, in the strict use of the word, a fraud. This is not to say that many freaks did not have profound physical, mental, and behavioral differences, for as we will see, many did; but, with very few exceptions, every person exhibited was misrepresented to the public. The gaff was only the extreme of this misrepresentation.

The major lesson to be learned from a study of the exhibition of people as freaks is not about the cruelty of the exhibitors or the naïveté of the audience. How we view people who are different has less to do with what they are physiologically than with who we are culturally (Sarason and Doris 1979). As with the tall Jack Earle, having a disability or another difference did not make the people discussed in this book freaks. "Freak" is a way of thinking, of presenting, a set of practices, an institution—not a characteristic of an individual. Freak shows can teach us not to confuse the role a person plays with who that person really is.

Why 1840?

By "freak show" I mean the formally organized exhibition of people with alleged and real physical, mental, or behavioral anomalies for amusement and profit. The "formally organized" part of the definition is important, for it distinguishes freak shows from early exhibitions of single attractions that were not attached to organizations such as circuses and carnivals.[11]

In the nineteenth century the United States was moving from an agrarian, family- and community-based society to one in which formal organizations like schools, factories, businesses, hospitals, and government agencies would dominate. During this time the organizations that would eventually house freak shows developed. It would be a distortion to state that in 1840 human exhibits changed all at once from unattached attractions to freak shows, for the process was slow and had been under way for half a century. But 1840 is significant because by that time the transition had progressed significantly and because, close to that date, P. T. Barnum became the proprietor of an organization in New York City, the American Museum, that looms large in the history of the American freak show. It was this establishment that brought the freak show to prominence as a central part of what would soon constitute the popular amusement industry.

Significantly, once human exhibits became attached to organizations, distinct patterns of constructing and presenting freaks could be institutionalized, conventions that endure to this day. The freak show thus joined the burgeoning popular amusement industry, and the organizations that made up that industry, housing as they did an occupation with a special approach to the world, developed a particular way of life. That culture is crucial to an understanding of the manufacture of freaks.

In Search of Freaks!

How does one go about studying freak shows? What types of material are available? Although many of the standard historical sources are useful (Flint 1972),[12] certain unusual sources deserve attention here because they help to introduce the concoction of freaks and the place of freak shows in American life.

One kind of information is found in abundance: the materials that were used to publicize the exhibits—handbills, newspaper advertisements, canvas bannerline posters, and the promotional photographs and advertising booklets that exhibited people sold as a way of supplementing their incomes.[13] At first glance these materials appear useless. They are so contrived, so obviously produced merely to win customers' attention that they can be easily dismissed as lies. But fraud is central to the freak show, and lies make good data—that is, if one knows that they are lies and if deception is the subject of investigation. After all, misrepresentation is integral to the manufacture of freaks.

FREAK PORTRAIT PHOTOGRAPHS

If you visited a proper American household of the 1860s to early 1900s, you would wind up sitting in an ornately decorated parlor (Seale 1981). There, often supported by their own stands, would be thick, elaborately crafted and lavishly decorated photograph albums containing formally posed, studio portraits (M. Mitchell 1979; Taft 1938). Pictures of family members filled most albums, but Victorian and post-Victorian Americans collected pictures of other people as well: statesmen, generals, performers, and, interestingly, freaks.

Nineteenth-century Americans suffered from "cartomania" (Bassham 1978, 3; Darrah 1981; McCullock 1981)—a compulsion to collect photographs. They bought pictures to fill their albums, which they spent hours looking over and showing to friends. The photo album was the television of Victorian homes: what Victorians viewed, what they collected, reflected their interests and tastes. Judging by the number of freak images produced, it is safe to say that human oddities were not only fascinating but quite acceptable as Victorian houseguests—as long as they stayed in their albums.

Prior to 1850, technology limited imagery production to two basic processes: one resulted in an image similar to the daguerreotype, the other rendered the calotype. Because glass negatives were not employed (daguerreotypes used no negative and calotypes employed paper), the production of high-quality multiple copies, and thus widespread marketing of photographs, was impossible. In 1851, however, the development of the collodion process, or "set-plate" technique, enabled photographers for the first time to make many prints from one exposure, and by the early 1860s the carte de visite (hence the word *cartomania*) was all the rage (Darrah 1981), with annual sales of 400 million in the peak years of their production (Mitchell 1979, 15).

Drawings and prints provide the earliest visual record of human oddities. Some daguerreotype images of freaks have survived the years—including Tom Thumb and the "Aztec children" (Harvard Coll.)—but it was not until the mass-produced carte de visite that a comprehensive record of human exhibits could be assembled. Popular freak show attractions of the 1860s posed for photographers and sold their carte de visite likenesses to Victorian Americans. Mathew Brady (Meredity 1970), premier early photographer, famous for his Lincoln portraits and his striking visual chronicle of the Civil War, made cartes de visite of Barnum's American Museum freak attractions (Kunhardt and Kunhardt 1977).[14] In his studio on Broadway, across from Barnum's landmark, he took pictures of popular authors, statesmen, dignitaries, and such freak show notables as Henry Johnson (What Is It? or Zip); Captain Bates and his wife Anna Swan, the married giants; Major Newell, the midget; Charles Tripp, the armless wonder; Admiral Dot; General Tom Thumb and his wife; Lavinia Warren; Chang and Eng, the original Siamese twins; Annie Jones, the bearded lady; the Lucasie albino family; and the Fiji cannibals. The Barnum freaks that Brady captured on film went on to be the prototypes of later freak exhibits.

By the late 1860s larger and clearer cabinet photographs were being produced, which reignited the collecting craze. Although the cabinet photo eventually replaced the carte de visite, enough of the smaller images remained in circulation in the 1880s to warrant at least a few pages for them in contemporary photograph albums.

In the last three decades of the nineteenth century, freak shows and photographers flourished (M. Mitchell 1979). Particular photographers took up freak portraits as a specialty. Human oddities would regularly climb the stairs to their top-floor studios (lighting was provided by skylights), carefully pose, and then they or their manager would pick the images to be duplicated.[15] In some cases thousands of reproductions would be ordered at one time.

They posed in front of one of various painted backdrops depicting scenes that ranged from jungle terrain to Victorian parlors. Props were selected, costumes worn, and the pose struck—all to reflect the image that the manager and the subject wanted to promote. Some exhibits were presented in an exotic mode, others in a way that aggrandized their status. Dwarfs were photographed in oversized chairs to appear smaller than life, and giants were shot in scaled-down chairs to appear larger. Fat people's garments were stuffed with rags to add to their size. In addition, negatives were doctored, with, for example, additional hair added to exhibits whose abundance of hair was their oddity (Figs. 3 and 4).[16]

Exhibits and managers would carefully review the proofs and give printing instructions that would enhance the image, perhaps to emphasize the oddity or to promote a particular presentation. On photographs in the Harvard Theater Collection, some of the cabinet pictures still bear the photographers' notes. On one photo of an albino woman, the instructions read: "Make half length and have the hair show as white as possible." On the back of an 1880s picture of R. J. James, "The Ohio Fat Boy," the instructions call for a retake with looser clothing to make him look larger.

In some photos, the freaks' managers posed with their exhibits. In others, the exhibit's family was included. Exhibited children often sat with their parents, and older exhibits appeared with spouse and children. In the 1880s and 1890s major cities had photography studios that catered to freak show clienteles. Because studios branded their photocards with their logo, it is relatively easy to compile a list of studios—from Lonma in Eastport, Maine, to Rulofon in San Francisco.[17]

In post–Civil War America, New York City was the freak show capital of the country, and the Bowery was its center. Photographers had to work hard to keep up with the demand for freak portraits. With thousands being sold, more New York photographers entered into the freak portrait business.[18] Yet one person stands out, in both the quality and the extent of his effort (Roth and Cromie 1980, 79; M. Mitchell

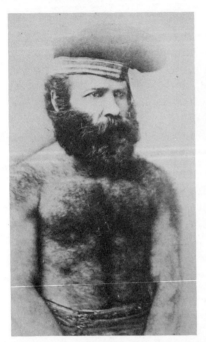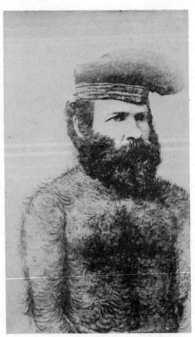

FIGS. 3 AND 4. Two versions of a hairy man. In producing the photo on the right extra hair was added to the exhibit. Photos by Charles Eisenmann, c. 1884. (Becker Coll., Syracuse University.

1979): Charles Eisenmann, whose photographic legacy is truly amazing.[19] Every major freak show attraction sat for his Bowery studio camera during the 1880s and 1890s, and many made repeated appearances. More photos by Eisenmann are available for study than by any other photographer, and major circus and theater libraries are rich with his images.

Showmen and exhibits cashed in on America's photo-collecting craze. Freaks placed photocards on the platform in front of them for sale, which, if a patron requested, could be signed, dated, and even inscribed with a personal message. The "armless wonder's" "footwritten" messages were in high demand. Ann Leak Thompson, the "armless lady," was famous for her catchy phrases: "I write poetry and prose holding my pen between my toes" (Harvard Coll.), or "Hands deprived, toes derived" (Becker Coll.).

Freaks sold thousands of these pictures, and because the markup was good, profits were high. The income was usually split between the

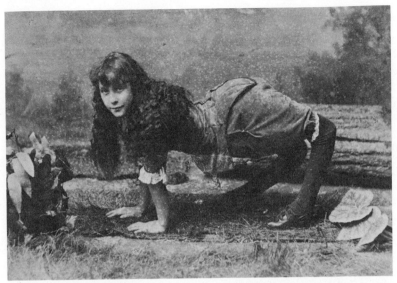

Fig. 5. Ella Harper, "the Camel Girl." Photo by Charles Eisenmann, 1886. (Becker Coll., Syracuse University.)

show's management and the attraction, although the most popular exhibits negotiated to keep a higher percentage of the cash. The photos provided benefits to the show besides the direct flow of cash, however. Not only were they good publicity, but selling them also provided the attractions with a diversion from the tedious routine of sitting on the stage. Photograph sales were also a tangible measure of the exhibits' popularity relative to others on the platform.

The great bulk of sales of freak portraits occurred at the exhibition proper. In the nineteenth century, however, pictures of particularly popular exhibits, such as Tom Thumb, could also be bought from the photographers and their agents (Kunhardt and Kunhardt 1977). Lavinia Warren, Tom Thumb's wife, was referred to as the most photographed woman in the world. She ordered fifty thousand pictures of herself at a time (Desmond 1954, 222) and these were widely available from photography vendors.

In some cases these freak portraits with their occasional handwritten messages are all that remains, the only communication left. The only evidence of Ella Harper, for example, is an Eisenmann cabinet portrait of a pretty thirteen-year-old with severe orthopedic problems, on all fours (Fig. 5). On the back of the picture is written: "I am called the camel girl because my knees turn backward. I can walk best on my hands and feet as you see me in the picture. I have traveled considerably in the show business for the past four years and now, this is 1886, I now intend to quit the show business and go to school and fit myself for another occupation" (Becker Coll.).

During the nineteenth century and into the twentieth, freak show patrons took their treasured photo souvenirs home and placed them in their albums. Often they wrote information on the back—the name of the attraction, his or her age or birthdate, where and when the exhibit was seen—as a reminder. While the reliability of this information is never certain, notated pictures can be helpful in tracing exhibits' stories. This misspelled note for example, was written on the back of a cabinet photo showing a young family consisting of mother, father, a five-year-old, and infant Siamese twins (Fig. 6): "The Jones twins. Born in Russianville, Ind June 25, 1889. Joined at buttock, had there own normal lags, they had but one rectum. They died while on tour with a carnival show when about 15 months old" (Becker Coll.). By means of the photo and notation, the twins could be identified as those described in an 1880s medical journal (Huff 1889).

Eisenmann and the other Victorian photographers left a rich collection of clear and elegant images that help us to understand freak shows and their place in nineteenth-century America. After the turn of the century, although the collecting craze declined, a market for freak photos persisted. The Barnum and Bailey Circus sideshow attractions, for instance, continued to sell cabinet-style photocards until at least 1916. With the invention of cheap, lower-quality processes to reprint pictures in a postcard format, however, and with the decline of the studio photographer, freak portraits began to figure less importantly in sideshow life. Nonetheless, well into the 1940s freak postcard portraits were regularly sold to promote the show and to supplement income—and Otis Jordan, "The Frog Man," was selling portraits at the New York State Fair in the 1980s.

Of course, most of the millions of freak portraits that were created have been destroyed (some probably by appalled spring cleaners), but they occasionally turn up still in attics and old trunks. They can be purchased at antique shops, estate sales, and through antique photographic dealers. For the student of freak shows these are an important resource, our most complete record of the one hundred years of freak show popularity.

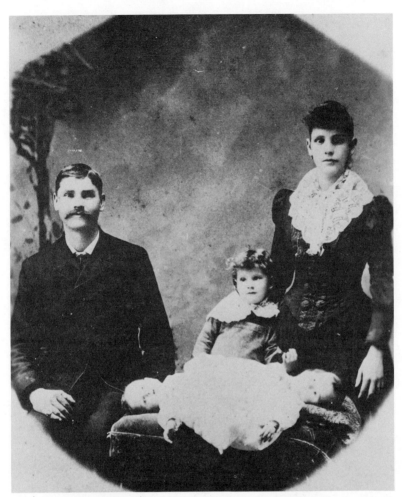

Fig. 6. The Jones Siamese twins. Family portrait, with the twins in the foreground. Photographer unknown, 1889. (Becker Coll., Syracuse University.)

"True Life" Pamphlets

Although freak portraits capture the visual dimension of presentation, they cannot convey the details of the stories constructed to explain the exhibits to the audience. Luckily, in addition to photos, exhibits sold biographical pamphlets from their platforms (Fig. 7). These pamphlets are not, however, as plentiful as the portraits, for two reasons. First, they were not as popular; while virtually every exhibit sold pic-

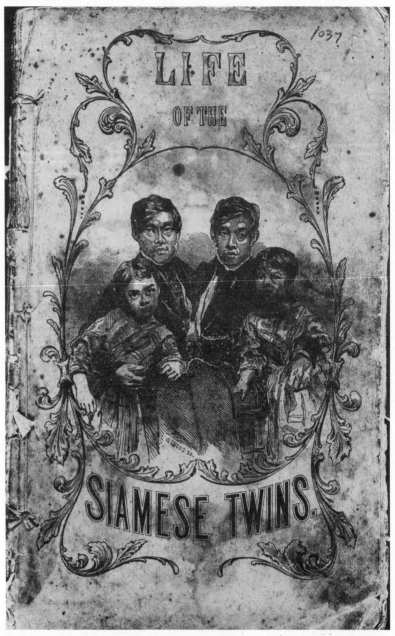

FIG. 7. Cover of Siamese twins' "true life" pamphlet. C. 1855. (Becker Coll., Syracuse University.)

tures, the sale of pamphlets was less pervasive. Second, unlike the photos, which were printed and mounted on enduring materials, the booklets were printed on inexpensive paper that disintegrated over the years. Nonetheless, extensive collections of these booklets exist, covering the period of our concern.[20]

The titles of these pamphlets reveal their content: "Biography, Medical Description and Songs of Miss Millie/Christine, the Two Headed Nightingale" (1883); "Sketch of the Life of General Decker, the Smallest Man in the World" 1874); "Life and History of Alfonso, the Human Ostrich" (c. 1903); "Life and Adventures of the Burdett Twins" (1881); "Interesting Facts and Illustrations of the Royal Padaung Giraffe-Neck Women" (1933); "Sketch of the Life, Personal Appearance, Character and Manners of Tom Thumb" (1854); "History and Description of Abomah, the African Amazon Giantess" (c. 1900); "Personal Facts Regarding Percilla the Monkey Girl" (c. 1940); and "What We Know About Waino and Plutano, the Wild Men of Borneo" (c. 1878).

With minor variations, by 1860 a pattern in contents had been established. First, a short biography of the subjects was presented: where they were born, what their early life was like, how they were discovered, and what the condition of other family members was. This part concluded with a description of the exhibit's recent history—where they had been shown, who had seen them, and how patrons had reacted to them. Second, a description of physical condition was given, commonly written by or quoted from a medical doctor or a person affiliated with the natural sciences. Third, the pamphlets contained endorsements from people—elected officials, newspaper editors, royalty, and clergy—who had seen the exhibit and vouched for its authenticity, interest, and propriety for public viewing. Medical personnel and scientists commented on the authenticity and scientific relevance of the curiosity. Fourth, if the exhibit was said to come from some exotic land, a brief history of its exploration and a short description of the geography, plants, animals, and native people would be included. In addition, most pamphlets contained drawings or photographs and, occasionally, songs or poems, either written by the freak or in celebration of the exhibit.

These "true life" pamphlets were filled with exaggeration, fabrication, and out-and-out lies. Their purpose was to promote the exhibit, to present the details of the story that had been created to draw potential patrons in. Like the freak photos, the stories were part and parcel of the freak image which the managers, promoters, and freaks themselves wanted to promulgate. Some pamphlets were forty and more pages long, going on in elaborate, fraudulent detail about the trek through the jungle that resulted in finding the lost tribe of which the exhibit was a member—when in fact the person was born and raised in New Jersey.

The "true life" pamphlets, like the freak portraits, changed over the years. Their length, the detail, the endorsements were greatest and grandest in the nineteenth and early twentieth centuries. After 1920 they went the way of the photograph, and the quality and elaborate detail of the prose was curtailed. Pamphlets that would once have been several dozen pages were reduced to sometimes only one folded page. In some cases the portrait and the "true life" pamphlet merged into a postcard format, with a picture of the freak on one side and a few paragraphs of biography and description on the other. The decline in the quality and detail of both photo and booklets parallels the decline of the freak show itself.

I have drawn extensively on the freak portraits and "true life" stories in the pages that follow. When juxtaposed with candid memoirs, interviews, letters, newspaper reports, and medical and scientific articles, the modes of presentation discussed in this book emerge.

The rest of the book is divided into two parts. Part One looks at the freak show as an institution, presenting a historical overview of its development as well as a discussion of the standard modes of presenting attractions.

Chapter 2 chronicles the development of the exhibition of human oddities from single, haphazard traveling exhibits to highly organized multi-attraction shows attached to such organizations as dime museums, circuses, world fairs, amusement parks, and carnivals—which together formed the popular amusement industry. Chapter 3 deals with the culture of that industry: the development of the amusement world, the perspective of its members, and their relationship to the social construction of freaks.

Chapter 4, which concludes Part One, is crucial to the rest of the book. There, in detail, the specific techniques and methods that showmen evolved to manufacture freaks are discussed. Central to their ploys were two major modes of presentation, the *exotic* and *aggrandized*. These are the focus of the chapter and provide the organizing framework for Part Two.

In Part Two are presented profiles of freak presentation, with three chapters devoted to presentations in the exotic mode and two in the aggrandized mode. While these chapters are mainly descriptive, each is loosely tied to an issue of more general interest. In Chapter 9, for example, "Self-Made Freaks," we see how competition affected the shape the exhibits took.

The five chapters of case studies are not meant to be an all-inclusive biographical encyclopedia of past exhibits. Rather, they are intended to illustrate and discuss the conventions of presentation that, put together, became the freak show. Because of this focus and the limitations of space, whole genres of freaks as well as particular exhibits have been left out. In addition, with exhibits that are discussed, only the barest details of the nonpresentation side of their lives are given.

Chapter 10, the conclusion, reviews major issues, for the most part by means of stories of exhibits and who were engaged in struggles, both real and fabricated, about their presentations.

I Freak Show: The Institution

2

From Tavern to Madison Square Garden
A Chronicle of the Freak Show in America

IN THE 1920s when Clyde Ingalls asked Jack Earle, the tall Texan, whether he wanted to be a giant, he was inviting him to join a well-established institution. Jack needed the freak show to become a giant. Not only did it supply the platform and the audience, but it provided the idea of "freak" and the patterns to construct an exhibit as well. While each freak had to be made separately, and each had a unique stamp, the freak show had developed the flexible mold, the instructions, and the perspective by which the exhibit could be constructed.

The Early Years

How, when, and why did freak shows start in the United States? Their closest antecedents were found at English fairs (Clair 1968; Frost 1971) where, already by the early Renaissance (Thompson 1968), almost all forms of human variation that would later adorn our sideshow platforms could be seen for a fee.[1] The seeds of the stylized presentations that became institutionalized in the nineteenth-century American freak show were found there too. Human oddities were shown as single attractions (as opposed to being part of a troupe) and traveled from fair to fair. In seasons when no fairs were held, rented rooms in taverns and other busy commercial establishments were their showcases.

In 1738 a notice appeared in colonial American newspapers in the Carolinas telling of an exhibit who "was taken in a wood at Guinea; tis a female about four feet high, in every part like a woman excepting her head which nearly resembles the ape."[2]

Decades before the revolution, then, human exhibits who were later to be called "freaks" were being presented (Vail 1956).

Eighteenth-century displays of "human curiosities" followed the English model. Although often they were one-person dis-

25

plays, they did not work alone. Managers or showmen who did the promoting, made the business arrangements, and collected the admission charge, accompanied them on their rounds. Some of these relationships were partnerships in which both the manager and the exhibit profited; others were more one-sided, with the manager exploiting his companion as a meal ticket. Some managers made a career of it, taking on one curiosity after another and aggressively recruiting for their business. Others were tied to one exhibit—their child perhaps, or another relative. Together they endured the hardships of the lonely treks from town to town seeking an audience. Occasionally they would meet other touring shows at fairlike gatherings, but for the most part there was little contact between different touring exhibits; there were none of the close-knit organizations that would shelter them later in the nineteenth century.

At the same time that showmen were on the road beginning to exhibit unusual humans, other roving entrepreneurs were traveling from town to town showing "animal curiosities." The beasts were representatives of unfamiliar species from far-off countries and the interior of what was to become the United States. The first lion was exhibited in 1716,[3] and the first elephant in 1796 (Vail 1938). Americans had to wait until 1837 to see the first giraffes, or cameleopards as they were called (Polacsek 1973; Pfening III 1973), and even by 1850 the evasive gorilla was yet to arrive.

Announcements for human and animal exhibits in the eighteenth century and through at least the first half of the nineteenth used the phrase "To the Curious" to grab patrons' attention. Animal and human oddities were referred to jointly as "living curiosities." In our present state of worldliness it is difficult to imagine a time when giraffes, for example, were an improbable marvel, but that is how citizens of those centuries greeted such living curiosities. Elephants, giraffes, orangutans, and many of the human oddities that were exhibited were simply out of the realm of eighteenth- and early-nineteenth-century Americans' experience.

It is not surprising that ordinary people did not know what to make of these strange beings, since the scientists of the day, most of whom were amateurs ("scientist" had not yet emerged in America as a full-time occupation [Daniels 1968, 7; Bates 1965, 30]),[4] did not know what to make of them either. Many of the exhibits had yet to be classified by taxonomists. Such fields as endocrinology, genetics, and anthropology were in their infancy. Some exhibits were referred to as "what is its" or "nondescripts," revealing both the showmen's promotional strategy and the state of descriptive science at the time.[5] Debates concerning whether a particular exhibit was a new species or a lusus naturae raged.[6]

People who viewed exhibits were vulnerable to any tale a showman might tell about the origin of the strange creatures they paid to gawk at. Having never seen a giraffe or a very small person with a distorted head, one might very well believe that they were from the moon, or from the dark crevices of one of the mysterious landmasses not yet penetrated by Westerners.

Nineteenth-century Americans, especially during the Victorian period, were enamored of "human curiosities." By the late eighteenth century the belief that lusus naturae were evil omens, or the workings of witchcraft, or a punishment for a parental transgression, was fading and being replaced with the idea that they were a part of God's great order of creatures and subject to scientific study and classification, as were all creatures. The developing science of teratology, the study of monsters, was bent on establishing a "scientific" classification of lusus naturae. But nineteenth-century discussion of cause remained primitive. Classification and nomenclature dominated scientific writing, with the question of what caused monsters to be born only a secondary issue.[7]

The fact that reputable scientists were interested in such things legitimized the public's interest in curiosities. When physicians and natural scientists visited freaks, as they often did, their comments served to fan widespread interest and debates as to the nature and origin of these creatures. Scientists, for their part, who did not then have the status they do today, gained visibility and authority by serving as "experts" in curiosity controversies.

Toward the end of the eighteenth century and into the nineteenth, the number and diversity of the humans displayed increased. Descriptions in newspapers and in diaries provide a fairly detailed picture of the kinds and nature of exhibits. Henry Moss, a black man from Virginia whose body was marked by white patches, exhibited himself in Philadelphia in 1796 and left a rather full record of the nature of the public's interest (Stanton 1960). Although Moss did not become the object of a debate concerning the distinction between "species" and "lusus naturae," he did quite a business showing himself for a price at Leech's tavern, at the sign of the Black Horse. People from all levels of society flocked to see him. Some of the most eager visitors were Benjamin Rush, Dr. Charles Caldwell, Dr. Samuel Stanhope Smith, and other members of the Philadelphia-based American Philosophical Society, one of the first and most prestigious scientific organizations in the United States. They saw Moss as providing evidence that might help to answer some of the pressing scientific questions of the day.

One raging controversy divided those who believed that all humans came from the same source, Adam and Eve, and those who posited a separate creation for each race. On the monogenesis side, one theory held that all people were created simultaneously but, as they spread out, became changed in appearance through differences in climate and living conditions. Those living in tropical countries presumably gained their color from the sun and outdoor living. Moss was regarded as proof of this theory, for if blacks had become dark as a result of the sun, when they lived in temperate climates they would begin to turn pale once more. The polygenesist Dr. Benjamin Rush, however, at a special meeting of the American Philosophical Society, declared that Moss offered no such proof. According to Rush's interpretation, the skin color of "Negroes" was the result of leprosy. Rush, then, believed that Moss was undergoing a spontaneous cure of the disease (Stanton 1960).

Our knowledge of Moss is limited to his appearance in a particular place at a particular time. We can trace Martha Ann Honeywell for a longer period. In 1798, at the age of seven, she appeared at the Museum of Gardner Baker in New York City, where she was described as "without any limbs. . . . Although she is thus conditioned, she can help herself with the greatest ease and facility to food of all kinds, can take a glass and convey it to her mouth and help herself to drink, can work various kinds of needlework and any kind of plain sewing to the astonishment of all who see her" (Vail 1956, 59). There are records of her being exhibited, accompanied by her mother, in Salem, Massachusetts, in 1809. In August 1828 she began a long run at the Peale Museum in New York, lasting into 1830. During the 1830s she was exhibited in "all the principal cities of the Union" ("Historical Rings" 1871).

Honeywell's case is interesting because it illustrates a significant change that occurred in the first decades of the ninteenth century. Her career is spotted with appearances at organizations called "museums." Other curiosities followed a similar pattern, and by the mid–nineteenth century, in urban centers, museums dominated as the place to view human curiosities.[8]

Early Museums

In the last decades of the eighteenth century and the first decades of the nineteenth, a few industrious dilettante scientists began to open museums in major American cities. Originally started as edifying educational and scientific institutions these establishments typically contained a hodgepodge of exhibits including paintings, stuffed animals, live animals, wax figures, mechanical devices, light shows, and artifacts brought back by sailors and explorers. For the most part they were owned and managed by serious amateur scientists, who were at least as interested in the advancement of knowledge as in profit. Nevertheless, these museums depended on admission receipts for their operating budgets and, in some cases, for the maintenance of the curator's family. Yet the public interest that existed for these "cabinets of curiosities" (Bell 1967) was not always sufficient to keep them solvent.

Human curiosities had been included as museum displays from the start. As with Henry Moss, they were of scientific interest because they represented specimens, data to be examined in quest of answers to the pressing scientific questions of the day. Moss, native Americans, and non-Western peoples were relevant to debates concerning the classification of human races and the place of various humans in the great chain of being (Stanton 1960; S. Gould 1981; Gossett 1963). Other exhibits such as Siamese twins or people born with missing limbs and other congenital abnormalities were of interest as part of the science of teratology.

Although human oddities—albinos, dwarfs, people born with missing limbs or extra limbs, joined twins, people with excess hair, people with tattoos, Native Americans, non-Western people—were displayed at these early museums, they were not the featured attractions. Peale, for example, who started a museum in 1786 in Philadelphia (Sellers 1980, 22), exhibited albinos and other "human curiosities" but believed that they attracted too much frivolous attention. He thought that the proper subject of science should be regularly occurring specimens, not the unusual (Sellers 1980, 42). The public seemed not to share Peale's and other serious scientists' taste, however. Human oddities, concerts, and novelty acts drew more paying customers than did dull cases of stuffed birds and dusty artifacts (Allen 1980).

Throughout the first half of the nineteenth century, Christian convention frowned on theater and other forms of pure recreation. Lauded instead was attending lectures, studying science, and engaging in edificatory activities. In some cities theaters were actually prohibited. But the public craved entertainment, and the museum provided a cover of "rational amusement" (enjoyment while learning) that legitimized people's having fun (Sellers 1980). Drama and musical productions, freaks, and other more entertainment-oriented features gradually took over the program.

Early museums had lecture rooms in which scientists would speak to the visitors, and sometimes the exhibits would be displayed and discussed. Gradually, however, the lecture platform became a stage where music and plays were performed (Odell 1927, vols. 2 and 3; Allen 1980), and by the mid 1800s museum lecture halls, accommodating thousands at a sitting, featured dramatic productions and entertainment alone. The cabinets of curiosities and the human curiosity exhibits were maintained merely as a museum front (Ryan 1915; Skinner 1924).

Some human oddities, even at midcentury, remained independent enough of museums to exhibit themselves in rented rooms and halls, but eventually this became unusual as they became almost completely absorbed by museums.[9] This change is significant. Prior to their absorption by museums, human curiosities floated precariously, without roots. They existed hand to mouth, lacking the permanence that an organizational base could provide. Moreover, as long as each exhibit remained independent and had only limited contact with other freaks, no community or culture of showpeople could develop. By becoming attached to museums, however, and later to circuses, showmen and exhibits were incorporated into a burgeoning industry, the popular amusement industry. They thus joined a segment of society that was in the process of developing a way of life apart from the mainstream. Connections were no longer confined to the simple partnership between exhibit and manager. A "freak show" was emerging as a larger collectivity. As the museum brought together people who had a stake in maintaining the enterprise, the "freak show" took on a life of its own, becoming institutionalized as part of an increasingly complex urbanizing America. The patterns that developed at this time would endure throughout the history of the freak show.

The museum newspaper ads and handbills that appeared with increased frequency during the first half of the nineteenth century reveal a diversity in the physiological, mental, and cultural characteristics of the exhibits. Attractions included Calvin Phillips, "famous American Dwarf Child"; Sally Rogers, "deprived of the use of hands and feet"; Jeremiah Daly, an "albino from Ireland"; Patrick Magee, "remarkable for his extraordinary height"; Chang and Eng, "Siamese Double Boys"; Calvin Edson, five feet two inches tall, weighing sixty pounds; Joice Heth, "of 161 years" and the former "nurse of Gen. George Washington"; O'Connell, the tattooed man; two "Cannibals of the island in the South Pacific"; "Young Indian Chiefs of the Onondaga Tribe"; Sena Sama, sword swallower; Casper Hauser, "half man, half monkey"; Master Barber, "the whiskered child"; two "Snow White Negroes from Brazil"; Mr. and Mrs. Randall, "The largest giant and giantess in the world"; and Mlle. Fanny, "the connecting link between man and brute creation."[10]

About some we know nothing more than their name, a description of their novelty, and the place they were exhibited. But about others we know more, and from what we know it is clear that, like their predecessors and heirs, the exhibits were not always what they purported to be. Joice Heath, for example, the first human oddity that Barnum ever exhibited, was not the 161-year-old nurse of George Washington; more accurately she was an 80-year-old fraud. Mlle. Fanny, who was exhibited dressed in Sunday finery complete with a parasol, was less of a mystery than her exhibitors suggest: she was actually an ape.

By the mid-1800s museums and showmen, now appearing in ever greater numbers, had begun to compete for customers. Indeed, the state of science and the Jacksonian frame of mind which so relished trickery (Harris 1973) provided an excellent opportunity for emerging showmen to embellish their exhibits with presentations that were in some cases half-truths and in others out-and-out lies. Although such fraudulence was present far back in the days of Renaissance English fairs, mid-nineteenth-century America provided the ideal venue for humbug to be institutionalized as a fine art and as a basic and lasting part of the freak show. No one was more systematic and successful at it than Phineas Taylor Barnum.

P. T. Barnum's American Museum

In 1840 many cities in the United States had museums. And many were struggling to survive. Those that were solvent had made the transition from science and education to entertainment and amusement while still maintaining the trappings of the museum's respectability. But even owners and managers who had made the transition had not been bold in embracing and publicizing this new form of museum. Some museum managers simply lacked the calling and skill of showmen to make the successful transition. Barnum, however, seized on the idea of the museum as an amusement center and launched his American Museum into the national spotlight (Fig. 8). Thus were the stodgy "cabinets of curosities" transformed into the new "dime museum."[11] Barnum's skills as a promoter and public relations man even earned him the title of "father of modern day advertising" (Presbrey 1929).

Barnum went into the museum business in 1841 when he purchased the failing Scudder's American Museum,[12] on the corner of Broadway and Ann streets in the heart of bustling New York City. Opposite the museum was the most prestigious hotel in New York, the Astor House, headquarters for many visiting dignitaries, statesmen, and prosperous business leaders. Four blocks north was Delmonico's Restaurant, the city's best. In between was City Hall. The offices of the *Tribune* and the *Herald* were nearby, as would be the photography studio of Mathew B. Brady and the lithography studio of Currier and Ives. Brady photographed the human curiosities that Barnum displayed in his museum. Currier and Ives, using the familiar style and technique of their popular lithographs, made advertising posters of freaks. Barnum's American Museum, then, in which freaks were the major attraction, was a central part of mainstream America at mid-century, and the fame of its celebrity owner was second to none. The American Museum was not a sleazy operation on the fringe of Victorian America; it was, rather, quite fashionable and most legitimate.

Almost overnight Barnum transformed the museum into an entertainment center where families would come with picnic lunches to spend the day. He accomplished this feat by introducing more and more diverse human oddities and entertainment (Fig. 9). Gypsies, albinos, fat boys, giants, dwarfs, and native Americans were soon on the payroll. Barnum advertised aggressively and made up outlandish stories about his exhibits; he decorated the facade of the museum with

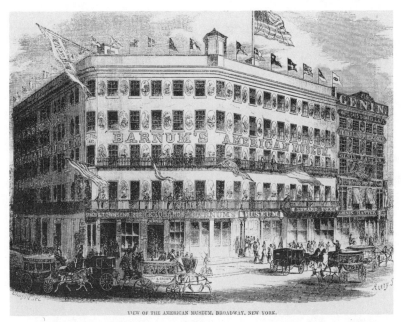

VIEW OF THE AMERICAN MUSEUM, BROADWAY, NEW YORK.

FIG. 8. Barnum's American Museum. This engraving of the Broadway establishment was published in *Gleason's Pictorial*, 1853.

bright banners depicting the attractions and had a band play out-side—all practices that became a standard part of the freak show.

The American Museum thrived. By 1850 it was the premier attrac-tion of New York City—and it looked the part. A splendid chan-deliered lecture hall had been built, accommodating three thousand. There the patrons could be educated and amused by "scientific dem-onstrations," skits, magic shows, lectures, ballets, and such edifying drama productions as *Uncle Tom's Cabin* and *The Drunkard* (Saxon 1983, xiv). The 1860 catalogue and guidebook lists thirteen "human curiosities" among the exhibits (*Barnum's American Museum* 1860, 106–112), including an albino family (the Lucasies), "The Living Aztecs" (Maximo and Bartola, brother and sister with microcephaly), three dwarfs, a black mother with two albino children, "The Swiss Bearded Lady," "The Highland Fat Boys," and "What Is It?" (or, more properly, Henry Johnson, a mentally retarded black man whose career we will trace in Chapter 5).

Fires were common during the period, and the American Museum was plagued by them. In 1868, when the museum burnt to the ground, Barnum retired from the museum business. Although the circus auto-

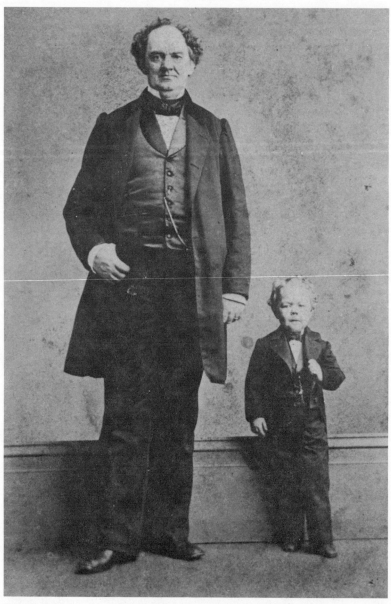

FIG. 9. P. T. Barnum and Commodore Nutt. Nutt was a dwarf and a popular "curiosity" at the American Museum. Photo by Gurney, c. 1863. (Becker Coll., Syracuse University.)

FREAK SHOW: THE INSTITUTION

matically comes to mind at the mention of the name Barnum, the museum was his primary calling. His association with the circus is only secondary, and often his name was more involved than his person. The American Museum was his first love and his major claim to fame: he had transformed it from a failing antique into a major new form of amusement, hosting an estimated forty-one million customers. The enterprise was more than a success. It was a national force.

Barnum charged twenty-five cents admission, not the ten cents of latter-day dime museums. Except for this minor discrepancy, however, Barnum's edifice contained all the elements that dime museums would capitalize on in the forty or so years of their great popularity, starting in the 1870s and continuing through the turn of the century. The American Museum—the biggest, best, and best known of all curiosity museums—became the dime museum's prototype (Wilmeth 1982).

Dime Museums

The upheaval caused by the Civil War led to major social and economic changes. By the late 1860s European immigrants were pouring into the country, and most settled in the cities: between 1860 and the close of the century, the number of urban-dwellers had burgeoned from five million to twenty-five million (M. Mitchell 1979; Weber 1965). This immigration, along with industrialization, created the modern American metropolis.

Starting in the 1870s dime museums proliferated, reaching their peak in the 1880s and 1890s. They operated from coast to coast, and any decent-sized city had one. New York City was the dime museum capital, however (Fig. 10), and the Bowery, an entertainment district replete with German beer gardens, theaters, vendors, photography studios, and various other amusement establishments, had more dime museums than any place in the world (M. Mitchell 1979).[13] One observer estimated that scattered about New York City "were half a hundred dime museums" (Isman 1924, 25).[14] Some became semipermanent establishments located in their own buildings, changing owners and names occasionally; others, located in rented stores, were more short lived. Their changing titles and transient nature make compiling an accurate list impossible.[15] Many, particularly those in the Bowery, played to immigrant laborers who were packed into nearby tenements. But dime museums were not just for the poorly educated and non–English speaking (Allen 1980). G. B. Bunnell's Museum on Broadway and 9th, for example, which one observer referred to as the

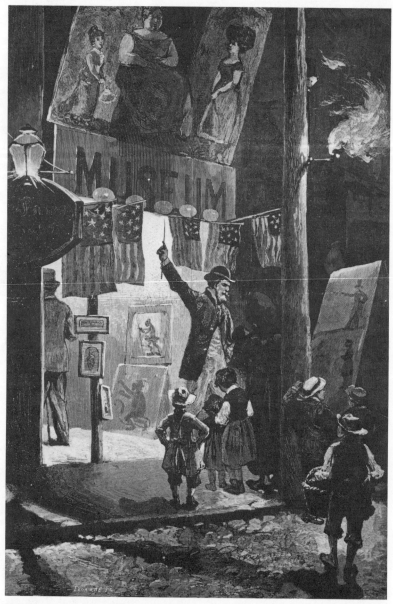

Fig. 10. Bowery dime museum. This view of the showman and his establishment appeared in *Harper's Weekly*, February 26, 1881.

FREAK SHOW: THE INSTITUTION

aristocrat of the genre, served a more sophisticated patron (Isman 1924). (Bunnell also had museums in Brooklyn and Jersey City.) While the lower-rung museums would book whomever they could, Bunnell—who cultivated his resemblance to P. T. Barnum assiduously—was very selective when it came to hiring his variety performers and freaks (Isman 1924, 75).

Although New York had the most dime museums, other cities such as Boston (Allen 1980), Philadelphia, and Chicago had a good number as well.[16] There were even national chains and booking agents to facilitate the movement of human curiosities, variety acts, and acting troupes from establishment to establishment. George Middleton and C. E. Kohl ran museums in New York, Chicago, Milwaukee, Cincinnati, Louisville, St. Paul, Minneapolis, and Cleveland (Middleton 1913). Other well-known museums include the Miracle Museum in Pittsburgh, Drew's in Providence, Keith and Batchelder's in Boston, and Bradenburgh's in Philadelphia (Looney 1976). There were dime museums coast to coast.

The best attractions played New York; other museum managers followed New York's lead by imitating new attractions and promotion strategies. Through New York booking agents and trade journals help-wanted ads, attractions were distributed throughout the country (Metcalfe 1906, 9).

The freak show was the main attraction of most dime museums of the period 1870–1900, and the human oddity was the king of museum entertainment (Hartt 1909, 108; McNamara 1974; Wilmeth 1982). Museum managers, under increased competition not only from other museums but also from circus side shows and other amusement organizations, often promoted the shabbiest of human oddities and gaffed freaks as scientific sensations and singular attractions. Following the lead of earlier freak promoters, most notably P. T. Barnum, they raised fraud, misrepresentation, and exaggeration—the hard sell—to new heights.

The genuine freak show greats drew large salaries and pulled in the crowds. In the 1880s, Jo-Jo, "The Dog-Faced Boy," a person with a great excess of hair on all parts of his face and body, commanded so much interest that a New York museum manager crowded twenty-three shows into each day (Isman 1924, 45). But there simply were not enough Jo-Jos to go around. Despite the fact that "freak hunting" ("Freak Hunting through India" 1894) was now a full-time occupation, sending managers and their agents searching the world for people with anomalies strange enough to make them a premier attraction, there was a freak shortage (Allen 1980; "Are You a Freak?" 1907). As we shall see, this shortage had important implications for those who climbed onto the freak show platform and the way they were presented. Novelty acts, non-Western exotics, self-made freaks, and gaffs filled in the ranks, and bizarre hyperbole dominated.

Urban areas like the Bowery became dens of gambling, deception, prostitution, and other sleazy goings-on much attacked by progressive reformers. The dime museums were in the thick of such activity, running various confidence games and even some semipornographic displays (McNamara 1974). Soon their embellished displays and wild claims about their attractions got out of hand. The reading public was increasingly bombarded with accounts of the fraud and duplicity behind the banners (Alden 1896; Harlow 1931), and eventually "respectable" citizens began to desert the dime museums, leaving them to the immigrants and country bumpkins.

As the nineteenth century yielded to the twentieth, the urban dime museum began its downward turn. Urban audiences now had a wide variety of popular amusements to choose from. The forms of entertainment that before had used the museums as a facade no longer needed such protection. Popular song and dance acts, variety entertainment, and popular drama now competed on their own against the establishments that had nurtured them. As circuses, street fairs, world's fairs, carnivals, and urban amusement parks, all of which exhibited freaks, began to collect the dimes to which museum proprietors had once enjoyed almost exclusive claim, museums evolved—some into vaudeville houses, others into theaters (Allen 1980).

Dime museums did remain popular, if in a state of decline, through at least 1910. Those that remained after World War I were operating in diminished quarters in storefronts. By the thirties they were, with few exceptions (such as Huber's Museum at Times Square, New York, the Newark Dime Museum, and Philadelphia's Eighth Street and South Street museums), strictly vagabond shows. Freak attractions dominated. The roving dime museum would rent vacant stores in small cities, stay for a few weeks or sometimes months, and then move on when business slacked off (Fig. 11). Their names—The Odditorium, Austin and Kuntz's Palace of Wonders, Lauther's Oddities on Parade, and Gross's Cavalcade of Wonders—often disguised their dime museum origins, but even into the forties there were probably a dozen traveling freak shows with the word *museum* in their titles.

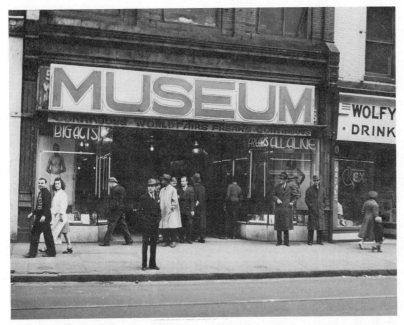

Fig. 11. Dime museum. A 1941 dime museum in temporary storefront quarters in Norfolk, Virginia. The photographer, John Vachon, worked for the Farm Security Administration. (Library of Congress.)

In the late 1930s, *Billboard*, the major weekly amusement world magazine, still devoted a special column—entitled "Museums"—to reporting the activities of these nomad shows. The January 16, 1937, issue, for example, reported that F. W. Miller's World's Fair Museum was playing at Fort Smith, Arkansas, and that the manager had procured a "honey" of a building in the heart of the business section. Opening-day business was the best of the season, the article claimed. Featured were Susie, the "elephant girl"; Alfred, the "green alligator boy"; Bet, the "frog boy"; Babe Lee, the "fat girl"; Bobo and Kiki, the "monkey children." Lady Vivian was swallowing swords, and Prince Le Roi was lifting weights with his "iron-eye lids." Andrew Marro's Traveling Museum was in Lynn, Massachusetts, with Kanga, half man–half monkey, and Nocturn, the human ostrich. Carl Lauther's Museum was in Florence, South Carolina. Exuding showmen's hype, the article told readers that "they were breaking all records." The truth of the matter was that they were the dying remnants of a breed that, although it had given birth to the freak show, had lived and prospered in another age.

The Circus

As a sideshow, the freak show was an integral part of the circus. The large sideshow that was attached to the best known and most prestigious circus, Ringling Brothers, Barnum and Bailey—known in the business as the "big one"—symbolizes the pinnacle of the practice and its visibility and acceptance in American life.

When the "big one" started its season at Madison Square Garden in New York City, it symbolized the coming of spring. Indeed, to appear in "the Garden" at this premier event in the amusement world was the ultimate sign of distinction in the freak show business (C. Fox and Parkinson 1969, 57).

The circus as we know it is a conglomeration of many elements— roving jugglers, aerial artists, clowns, trained animals, menageries, museums—that existed independently in the eighteenth and early nineteenth centuries. Whereas in 1820 there were only a few circus-like shows touring the United States, by the turn of the century there were close to a hundred. Until the 1850s all circuses had only one ring. W. C. Coup is credited with introducing the second ring and thus moving the American circus along the path of "the bigger, the better," which ultimately led to the three-ring extravaganza.[17] Coup also was the first to transport his circus by railroad, an innovation that led to mammoth troupes of performers and animals crisscrossing America. The five Ringling brothers opened their first show in 1884, thus founding an enterprise that was to grow until it had consumed much of the competition. The Ringling outfit, which included the "big one" and other top circuses, dominated the industry for forty years.

For people in rural areas the circus's arrival in town and the county fair were the only amusement they had. From 1850 to 1900 the number, size, and scope of circuses exploded, its tents swelling to accommodate, in the big top of the larger shows, twelve thousand people (C. Fox and Parkinson 1969, 25). During its golden era, from roughly 1870 to 1920 (Wilmeth 1982, 52), the circus was the major organization of popular amusement for rural Americans (Sweet and Habenstein 1973).[18]

By the 1920s the circus was in a real decline as a major form of amusement. There was competition: the cities had amusement parks; even small towns had movie houses and vaudeville tours; and the radio was becoming a force. During the depression attendance dropped significantly. By the end of the 1930s economic hard times and union demands were making the circus less and less economically viable. Although the "big one" remained under canvas until 1956, it, along with other circuses, was significantly changed. The big parade had disappeared, and the Big Show was no longer the main attraction in the American amusement world.

Single human oddities started hooking up with traveling circuses in the early 1800s, but it was only toward midcentury that they were organized into anything like the sideshow as we know it. The first organized touring freak shows were simply traveling museums. The first circus to advertise as a menagerie, circus, and museum was Waring, Raymond and Co., in 1837 (Pfening, Jr., 1985). Soon museums began to travel with circuses as concessions. Colonel Wood, for example, who had operated dime museums in Philadelphia, appeared with the Spalding and Rogers Circus in 1858 under the title "Col. Wood's Museum." George Bunnell, the important New York City museum operator, had the sideshow with the Stone and Murray Circus in 1869. In 1875, Bunnell and his brother owned and operated the "Place of Wonders" sideshow with a circus that traveled under Barnum's name.[19]

W. C. Coup, who first worked in the traveling Barnum Caravan Museum show in 1852, had the sideshow privileges in a number of circuses. In 1861 he was with the E.F.J. Mable Circus, and in 1866 with the Yankee Robinson Circuses. In 1869 he joined with Dan Costello Circuses, and two years later Costello and Coup persuaded P. T. Barnum to to allow them to use his name for their circus, which became P. T. Barnum's Museum, Menagerie, and Circus. In this circus the museum was prominent, with twenty vans of waxworks, dioramas, mechanical figures, and such human oddities as Admiral Dot, a midget; Colonel Goshen, a giant; Ann Leak, an armless wonder; and Baby Esau, a bearded girl. The next season Coup took P. T. Barnum's Great Traveling Exposition on tour by rail. Here the museum was housed in a separate tent on the midway (Pfening, Jr., 1985).

As late as 1876 most of the museums and sideshows that traveled with the major circuses were independently owned ("Number of Colossal Organizations" 1876), but very soon the museum part of the traveling circus changed. Fewer were operated by concessionaires. By 1880 the animals were in their own tent and the inanimate curiosities had been dropped. Human oddities now combined with variety entertainment acts to form the sideshow, the main attraction of the midway.

Tent size and the number of sideshow attractions began to increase

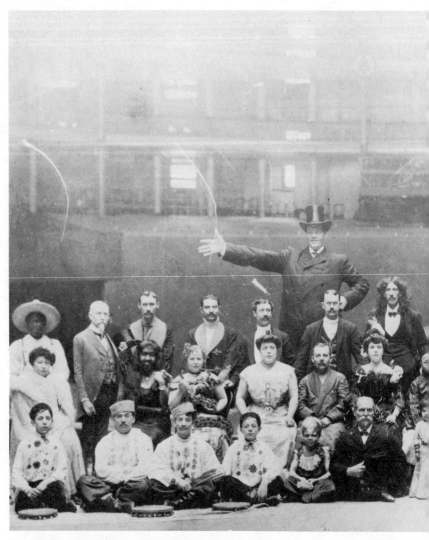

FIG. 12. Barnum and Bailey Circus sideshow group, 1903. The troupe consisted of forty-seven attractions including the Hovarth Midgets; Eli Bowen, "The Legless Wonder"; Charles Tripp, "The Armless Photographer"; Krao, "The Missing Link"; Henry Johnson, "What Is It?"; and the Korean Siamese twins. Photographer unknown. (Circus World Museum, Baraboo, Wisconsin.)

FREAK SHOW: THE INSTITUTION

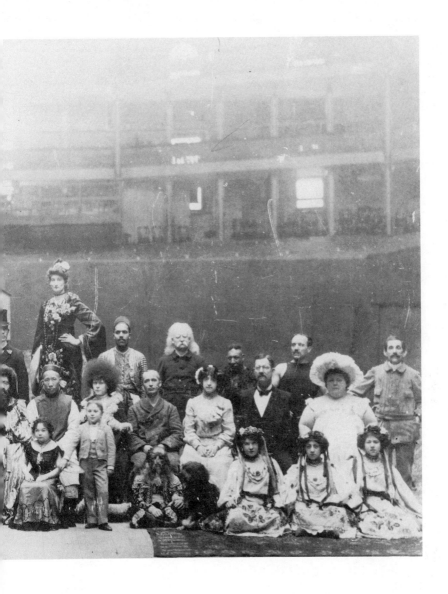

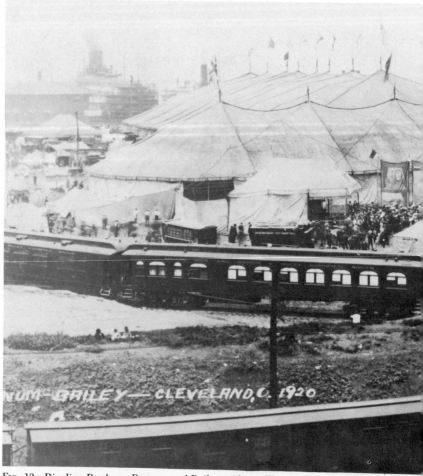

Fig. 13. Ringling Brothers, Barnum and Bailey midway. The sideshow (on the right) dominated the area outside the entrance to the big tent (far left). Note the word *museum* on the bannerline. Photographer unknown, 1920. (Circus World Museum, Baraboo, Wisconsin.)

around 1890, with most sideshows in large circuses now comprising twelve to fifteen exhibits plus a band (Fig. 12). Bands with black musicians, blackface minstrel bands, and troupes of dancers dressed as Hawaiians were used to attract crowds and provide a festive atmosphere inside the freak show tent. Even though the word *sideshow* gradually replaced *museum* in circus lingo, some circuses continued to use *museum* on their freak show banners through the 1930s.

FREAK SHOW: THE INSTITUTION

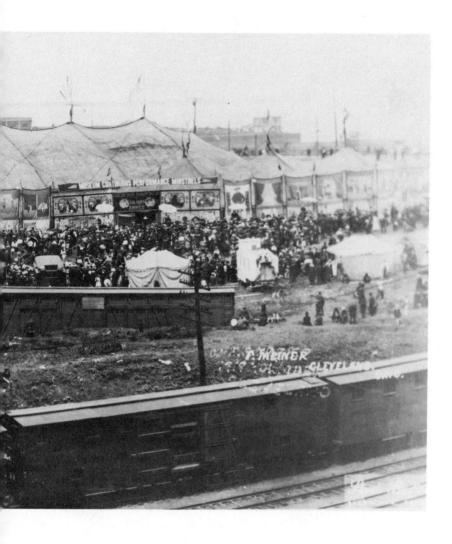

(In the vocabulary of the circus world, the sideshow is also referred to as the "kid show" and the "ten in one." The origin of the term *kid show* is unclear. The term *ten in one* derives from the fact that in the sideshow a number of attractions—often more than ten—can be seen for one price. In addition to "ten in one" shows, circuses had "pit-shows," in which one human oddity would be displayed for the price of admission. Many of these had an audience walkway around a cen-

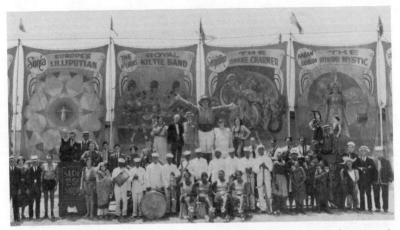

FIG. 14. Hagenbeck-Wallace Circus sideshow, 1933. The picture of the troupe in front of the bannerline and showing the ticket sellers' stands was taken in the Bronx, New York. Photographer unknown. (Hertzberg Coll., San Antonio Public Library.)

ter pit where the exhibit performed. When sideshows were in their prime, some circuses had both a large "ten in one" and various pitshows. The expression *String show,* another name for a multiple-exhibit freak show, is used mainly in carnivals.)[20]

By the 1870s most circuses had a freak show, and eventually the circus became a major venue for the exhibition of human oddities. The pattern for the type and nature of sideshow exhibitions had been set by the earlier dime museums, which preceded the circus and had so dominated the early freak show market. In this sense sideshows were just what the name implies: something on the side, an addition to the circus's main show.[21] Indeed, of all the many thousands of circus posters that are left as memorabilia of the circus's golden era, fewer than a dozen feature the sideshow.[22] Yet this is not to say that the sideshow was not large and an important source of revenue.

Prior to the big-top performance, before the gates for the main show even opened, the freak show tent was doing business with the early arrivals (Fig. 13). This tent was long and oval (large ones were 80 by 120 feet and took ten people to erect), and one of the long sides edged the path that led to the entrance of the big top, the tent where the main show was held. At the turn of the century this path came to be called the "midway.")

The sideshow continued as a standard circus fixture into the 1950s (Fig. 14). Ringling Brothers, Barnum and Bailey Circus had one that

FREAK SHOW: THE INSTITUTION

traveled with the show until 1956, but then the "big one" folded its tents and played only indoor engagements. After 1956 they had a sideshow only at their opening at Madison Square Garden.

The Great World's Fairs

International expositions, or world's fairs—mammoth displays of the commerce, industry, art, history, and culture of participating countries held in major cities of the world on grounds especially constructed for these great co-operative ventures—began in the second half of the nineteenth century. Sponsored by governments and entrepreneurs, these displays of human industry and progress caught the imagination of people all over the world.

Historians point to the beginnings of the world's fair as the large display of commerce and industry held in London in 1851 (Rydell 1984; Benedict 1893). Most agree that the magnificent Centennial Exposition, held in Philadelphia in 1876, was the first major world's fair hosted by the United States (Rydell 1984). There was, however, a minor exhibition held in New York City in 1853, and interestingly, P. T. Barnum, back from a successful European tour with Tom Thumb, was persuaded briefly to take over the financially troubled "Association for the Exhibition of the Industry of All Nations" as president. Although later exposition directors, namely those of the elegant 1876 fair, purposely shunned the incorporation of entertainment and amusement, Barnum, foreshadowing later expositions, wanted to include not only musical and dramatic artists but also freaks. Barnum's efforts to revive the troubled fair failed, however. As he put it, "It was a corpse long before I touched it" (Barnum 1872, 382). He resigned in 1854 and the concern soon went into liquidation.

America entered the world's fair business properly in the spring of 1876 with the official opening of the Centennial Exhibition in Philadelphia. On the first day 186,672 visitors came to the fairgrounds, and by its conclusion six months later, ten million—or one-fifth the population of the United States—had seen the exhibition (Rydell 1984, 10).

The main fairgrounds, with massive, ornate architecture and acres of agricultural, industrial, and cultural exhibits, are important to the history of the freak show in two ways. The first is very direct. Included in the exhibition were native Americans and other "exotic" people from around the world. Although they were not displayed as a paid sideshow, as they had been in dime museums and the circus, the line between "scientific" ethnological displays of the world's people and sensational exploitation of the exotic for profit was blurred at Philadelphia (Rydell 1984). The organizers did not intend that visitors should be attracted to the fair merely to gawk at these people, but gawk they did, and all under government sponsorship. The inclusion of exotic people at the Centennial Exposition, then, laid the groundwork for native people's becoming sideshow exhibits at later fairs and helped to legitimize the practice for showmen.

The second aspect of the fair that is important to the history of the freak show does not relate directly to the official exhibits. The throngs of people that were expected to visit the exposition attracted hordes of enterprising businessmen and, most notably for us, showmen. Never before had so many itinerant showmen been gathered in one place for so long. Fair organizers fought to keep the main exhibition grounds free from the influence of what they considered to be the darker side of American culture—the independent showmen, vendors, and various entrepreneurs of the entertainment and amusement world. But outside the fairgounds, especially on Elm Avenue, just across from the exposition's main building, small businesses proliferated. On this street for almost a mile were ramshackle restaurants, small hotels, saloons, amusement booths, food vendors, and dime museums with freak shows. Although most knew this midwaylike area as "Centennial City," some referred to it disparagingly as "Shantyville" and "Dinkeytown" (Hilton 1975, 195).

As world's fair patrons went to and fro, showmen called out, hawking their wares. Many of the freak show greats were actually present on Elm Avenue. Visitors reported seeing such classic attractions as "The Wild Men of Borneo," "The Wild Australian Children," and "The Man-Eating Feejees," as well as a 602-pound fat lady whose name has escaped history (McCabe 1876). Fair-goers who tired of the splendor of the educational and uplifting main attraction simply strolled down to Shantyville, where food was cheaper and attractions less stodgy.

In September, Shantyville was leveled by a fire. Nevertheless, future fair organizers learned a lesson from the freewheeling amusement street. People wanted more at their international exhibitions than enlightenment, and they would pay for it. Perhaps there was a place for a midway at world's fairs too.

The next world's fair hosted by the United States, the great Columbian Exposition of 1893 in Chicago, attracted a large contingent of showmen to its periphery, but it also had its own amusement area on the fairgrounds proper. World's fairs had to turn a profit. Thus, despite some opposition, organizers of the Chicago fair included amusement concessions as a financial necessity.

The official amusement area was the Midway Plaisance, a broad thoroughfare extending seven-eighths of a mile to the east of the great White City (the present site of the University of Chicago). As opposed to the substantial buildings of the rest of the fair, the midway concessions were mere temporary structures, some no more than shacks. Payment of one fifty-cent admission charge (a hefty amount in those days) got a visitor into the fairgrounds, and for all but a few of the nonmidway exhibits there was no additional charge. The midway concessions, in contrast, were all pay as you go, with showmen sitting on high stools spieling to the passing crowds. "Hagenbeck's Arena and World's Museum" featured trained pigs and lions that rode horses (*Official Souvenir Programme* c. 1893); there was an ostrich farm and an international beauty show ("40 Ladies from 40 Nations").[23] One concession offered hot-air balloon rides. Yet with all this novelty, none was to generate more interest than George W. Ferris's engineering marvel, the giant Ferris wheel. The first of its kind, at a height of 264 feet and a capacity of over two thousand people it dominated the center of the midway.

The most numerous exhibits on the midway were the so-called foreign-villages. In these one could, for the price of admission, see foreign nationals dressed in their native attire and in surroundings that were supposed to replicate their home environs. There were, of course, the Irish, German, and Viennese villages, but these did not have the sideshow flavor of the exhibits of non-Western people. These "natives" were displayed with an emphasis on the bizarre and primitive. The "Dahomey Village," with "mud-daubed huts, on which are scraped queer animals and bird figures" (Starr 1893, 619), housed sixty-nine "native warriors"—the same tribal people who had fought so valiantly when the French made a move to colonize West African land just prior to the fair's planning (Schneider 1982, 97). Featured on a central platform inside this "village" was a war dance. The advertising banner for the exhibit pictured the Dahomans in ferocious poses wearing grass skirts and carrying menacing spears.

The Dahomey warriors were not to be outdone in their savagery, for up the midway were the "cannibalistic Samoans in all their primitiveness" (Doenecke 1973, 542). These tropical specimens of "un-

civilized and semi-barbarous humanity" had for company representatives of colder climates, for a "Lap and Esquimaux village" were
featured. Robert Rydell, who has extensively studied the portrayal of
non-Western people at international expositions, states that the "native villages" at the Columbian fair provided "a quasi-scientific basis
for the American image of the nonwhite world as barbaric and child-
like" (Rydell 1984, 67).

Before the opening, vendors and showmen flocked to Chicago and
the area around the fair. There they prospered, serving the thousands
of construction workers and the curious citizens who were allowed to
visit while the exposition was under construction. Additional amusement shows opened for the fair season, including dime museums with
their freak shows (Middleton 1913);[24] and just outside the grounds,
on a fourteen-acre site, Buffalo Bill's Wild West Show performed to
large audiences (Appelbaum 1980, 103; Sayers 1981, 53). While very
little information exists about the showmen who worked the area
around the fair, it is known that they congregated around the Buffalo
Bill operation.

The Midway Plaisance had the aura of the amusement world, together with its hype and humbug. The women in the World Congress
of Beauty were not from "40 nations" (Appelbaum 1980). Many of the
Egyptian "hoochy-koochy" dancers were likely locals (Doenecke
1973, 537), and one, the famed Fatima, is alleged to have been a female impersonator (McKennon 1972, 34). The Ostrich Farm featured
ostrich-egg omelettes made from chicken eggs, supplied each day just
before daylight by a local poultry farmer (McKennon 1972, 39). As
one New York Times reporter put it, "The late P. T. Barnum should
have lived to see this day" (Rydell 1984, 61).

The Columbian Exposition contributed to the growth and popularization of the freak show in many ways.[25] Although the variety of
human oddities on the Midway Plaisance was less extensive than on
circus and dime museum platforms, many "exotic" peoples, mainly
from the non-Western world, were on display. The great fair thus set an
important precedent, and soon similar exhibits were prominent features of dime museums and circuses. Most notable was the incorporation in the Barnum and Bailey Circus of 1894 of a "Great Ethnological
Congress of Savage and Barbarous Tribes," a display of "primitive"
people rivaling that in Chicago.[26] The people who were part of this
"Congress" were exhibited in the menagerie tent (the freak show tent
being too small to accommodate them all) before and after the big-top

FREAK SHOW: THE INSTITUTION

shows ("Strange Sights at the Circus" 1894). Such displays of exotic people remained a part of circus and other freak shows through the 1930s.[27]

The native village displays at the Chicago fair also included such attractions as sword swallowers, snake charmers, and fire eaters, novelty acts that were already part of circus and dime museum "freak shows" and would remain so through the period of our concern.

By including popular amusement rides, sideshows, and other concessions as part of the exposition proper, the fair legitimized this type of amusement. In addition, the introduction of such innovations as the huge Ferris wheel gave a boost to the popular amusement industry in general. And the unofficial amusement zone that developed around the Buffalo Bill Wild West show provided showmen with an opportunity to work together and forge alliances that would lead to a new wave of popular amusement development in the twentieth century.

The Midway Plaisance meant the difference between profit and loss for the Columbian Exposition (Appelbaum 1980). The concessions far outdid prefair estimates, providing $4 million of the total revenue. The midway's success earned it a crucial place in future world expositions. Moreover, it launched a new form of popular amusement in which the freak show would loom prominently.

A succession of international exhibitions followed the Chicago fair: Atlanta in 1895; Nashville in 1897; Omaha in 1898; Buffalo in 1901; St. Louis in 1904; and on and on until the 1933–1934 Century of Progress International Exposition in Chicago and the 1939–1940 New York World's Fair. With each fair the amusement sections got larger and fell more under the control of the showmen. "Native villages" remained a part of the amusement section, although at the turn of the century interest in Dahomey savages waned, only to be replaced by interest in native Americans who fought the last battles of the West and indigenous Filipinos, who were exhibited as dog-eating missing links (Fig. 15) (Everett 1904; Benedict 1983). These "native villages" became even less authentic; often American-born blacks were employed to pose as "savages" (Dufour 1977; Holtman 1968), and, as we shall see in Chapter 7, the exploitation of tales of "savagery" quickly grew to almost unbelievable lengths.

Increasingly the showmen, who at one time had been limited to the fairs' periphery, were on the midway bringing other "human curiosities" to center stage. Although it is unclear which American world's fair officially incorporated the first circuslike freak show, dwarfs and

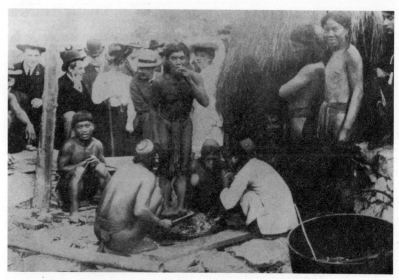

FIG. 15. Dog-eating natives. The fairgoers at the 1904 St. Louis Exposition gawk at Igorots from the Philippines eating dog meat. Photographer unknown. (Author's collection.)

hairy people were on display at the 1901 Pan American Exposition in Buffalo (Barry 1901), and the midway of the 1915 Panama Pacific International Exposition in San Francisco included a "Midget Village" and a dime museum "freak show" (Dufour 1977, 11).

Throughout the 1920s and 1930s, freak shows were a main feature of world's fair midways. The 1933–1934 Chicago Exposition had a pitshow that featured a "Live Two-Headed Baby"—in reality, a Siamese twin infant in formaldehyde (Dufour 1977, 62). The same exhibition boasted a "Believe It or Not Odditorium" featuring twenty-five human oddities, which, drawing on the publicity generated by the Robert Ripley syndicated newspaper feature, grossed over $900,000 (Fig. 16) (Dufour 1973, 85).[28]

After the Century of Progress, traveling dime museums and sideshows adopted names to cash in on the fame of the Chicago world's fair of 1933–1934 (Pfening 1983). Although some managers actually worked freak shows in conjunction with the fair and many of the exhibits that went on the road had appeared at the exposition, most merely used the title as showmen's hype. These names include Miller's World's Fair Museum, White and Bryan Odditorium, World's Museum, Peter Korte's World's Fair Museum, and Ray Marsh Brydon's World's Fair in Miniature (Fig. 17).[29]

FREAK SHOW: THE INSTITUTION

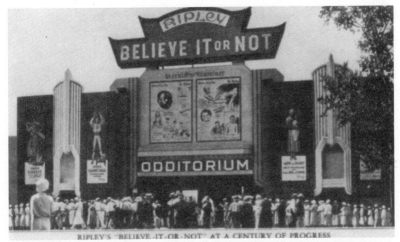

RIPLEY'S "BELIEVE-IT-OR-NOT" AT A CENTURY OF PROGRESS

FIG. 16. Odditorium. This photo is from a postcard sold in 1933 at the Chicago Century of Progress World's Fair. The "Ripley" show featured "human oddities." Photographer unknown. (Goldman Coll., Baltimore, Maryland.)

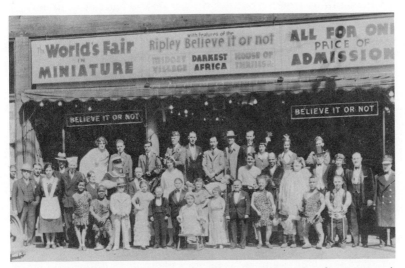

FIG. 17. "World's Fair in Miniature." Ray Marsh Brydon's touring dime museum in the fall of 1934 in a downtown storefront location. The use of Ripley's name was unauthorized. Photographer unknown. (Circus World Museum, Baraboo, Wisconsin.)

Lou Dufour and Joe Rogers, veterans of many international expositions, in which they managed various exotic village and freak show
exhibits, secured exclusive rights to the exhibition of freaks at the
1939–1940 New York World's Fair. They used the title "Strange as It
Seems" for their air-conditioned sideshow, which had 100 feet of midway frontage and was 150 feet deep. Inside were fourteen stages, each
containing two exhibits. Attractions included Marvello, the "finger-
less pianist"; George White, the "ossified man"; Frances Murphy, the
"bearded lady"; Betty Broadbent, the "tattooed woman"; "Chief Amok
Headhunter"; the Williams Family, the "leopard-skinned wonders";
Forrest Layman, the "armless wonder"; Jank Haggar, "with the twelve-
inch monkey tail"; Lipo Sul, the "lion-faced Chinaman"; and Frieda
Pushnik, the "limbless half-girl" (Dufour 1977, 123–124). As with
the earliest world's fair attractions, all were not what they appeared to
be. Frances Murphy, the bearded lady, it was revealed after an encounter with the police, was really a man.

Amusement Parks

By the mid-nineteenth century, summer resorts had begun to develop
near major cities (Mangels 1952). At first merely bathhouses, clam
shacks, and family hotels connected to metropolitan areas by crude
roads and modest ferries, by the late 1800s some had become bustling
entertainment centers with boardwalks, midways, saloons, dance
halls, rides, variety halls, fun houses, and freak shows. Early resort
business was dominated by individual vendors and showmen who
would present their offerings on the promenades and side streets.
Later though, large, corporately owned and managed amusement
parks dominated.

The model for the amusement park was cast by the Midway Plaisance at the 1893 Columbian Exposition in Chicago. Various aspects
of the exposition were copied, and in some cases virtually trans-
planted, to the burgeoning amusement resorts (Funnell 1975). The
forerunners of today's Disneyland and theme parks, these resorts
offered a lavish environment consisting of ornate buildings and decor,
along with a variety of rides, shows, and experiences, all within one
huge fenced area. A small payment gained a visitor admission, with
individual attractions available for an additional charge.

Urban centers were ready to supply the humanity to fill the amusement parks, promenades, and streets, and to provide the "freak

shows" on the streets of these urban resorts and in the amusement parks with customers. By the end of the nineteenth century middle-class America had largely shed the belief that fun for fun's sake was wrong, and customers were thronging to these urban playgrounds. The many new immigrants, too, some of whom had money to spend on amusement, were eager to partake in diversions from working-class life (Peiss 1986). By 1910 most major cities had at least one amusement resort, providing leisure activity that was a mixture of a midway, city entertainment district, and resort recreation area. In 1919 there were an estimated 1,500 amusement parks (Wilmeth 1982, 30); these were a central part of the urban working class's world.

Amusement parks could be found in all major cities: at Boston's Paragon Park and Revere Beach, Philadelphia's Willow Grove and Atlantic City, Atlanta's Ponce de Leon Park, Cleveland's Euclid Beach, Chicago's Cheltenham Beach, St. Louis's Forest Park Highlands, Denver's Manhattan Beach, and San Francisco's The Chutes (Kasson 1978; Mangels 1952). Yet although many of these parks could boast of their size and splendor, none could compare on any dimension to the famed New York City mecca, Coney Island.

Coney Island became a bustling resort in the 1870s when its connection by railroad to New York City finally allowed New Yorkers to visit for the day (Yriazi 1976). As crowds kept coming, entrepreneurial showmen expanded their activities. The beginnings of Coney Island's amusement ambience can be traced to the Bowery of Manhattan. In keeping with that beginning, one of Coney's busiest streets went by the same name—"Bowery," a street with bars, variety theatres, vendors, and freak shows (Peiss 1986).

The elaborate, mammoth, self-contained amusement park was one feature of Coney Island that made it stand out (Mangel 1952). In the resort's heyday it had three such parks: one was the Steeplechase, which opened in 1897; the second, Luna Park,[30] opened in 1903 (or, more accurately, reopened, since it replaced the smaller and earlier Sea Lion Park) and was followed quickly in 1904 by the third—and the park of greatest interest to us—Dreamland. It is difficult to capture the size and grandeur of these establishments and the spirit and size of the crowds that patronized them—the rides, extravagant shows, ornate buildings, millions of electric lights, huge dance floors, and thousands of people. Dreamland alone had a thousand electric lights, a 25,000-square-foot ballroom, and a 375-foot tower that furnished a fifty-mile view. Luna Park in its first year of operation had four million paying visitors (Pilat and Ranson 1941, 149).

Coney Island saw its first freak show in 1880 (McCullough 1957, 252; "Our Summer Resorts" 1881). A circus man who had brought his unemployed troupe to the beach for a holiday was struck by the business potential. Setting up banners, he began a practice that would prosper at Coney Island for at least sixty years. From these small beginnings, Coney Island became a center for freak shows. During the period 1910–1940 no single place in the world had more human oddities on exhibit. For older exhibits, for those who did not want to endure the hardships of the traveling shows, it became a place to settle down. Such renowned freaks as Lavinia Warren, the famous wife of General Tom Thumb, and Henry Johnson (Zip or Barnum's original "What Is It?") were last seen on the platforms of what became a honky-tonk extravaganza.

Although minor Bowery-type museums featuring human oddities were at Coney Island before the turn of the century, it was the big amusement park that launched them as a major aspect of the Coney Island scene. When Dreamland opened, one of its most popular attractions was "Lilliputia," a complete village scaled to the size of the three hundred dwarfs that worked there. Everything was in miniature, from a firehouse to the lifeguard stand to the toilets in the private homes. The midget city was a big draw, and it launched Samuel W. Gumpertz's career as the most important freak show promoter of the nineteenth century.

In a style similar to the displays at world's fairs, Gumpertz brought people from the non-Western world to be exhibited in Dreamland. In addition, he combed the world for people with physical anomalies to display. He made thirty-one trips abroad in search of freaks and imported 3,800 sideshow attractions; these he displayed at Coney Island as well as leased to circuses, museums, and carnivals here and abroad (Johnston 1933). He also set up "Dreamland's Big Circus Side Show" within the park (Kasson 1978).

When Dreamland amusement park burned down in 1911, Gumpertz immediately went into his own freak show business, building his Dreamland Sideshow as an independent enterprise on a section of the fifteen-acre charcoal lot that had once contained the park (Fig. 18). Gumpertz's show was a big success—in 1920 as many as thirty thousand patrons a day took the ten-cent, twenty-minute tour through the Dreamland Sideshow (McCullough 1957, 267). He added attraction

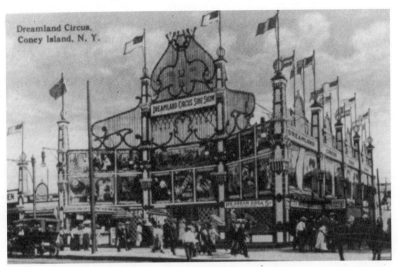

FIG. 18. Gumpertz's Dreamland Sideshow. A 1914 postcard view of this popular Coney Island attraction. (Raymond Coll., Baltimore, Maryland.)

after attraction, and soon the show had more exhibits than any in the history of the business. Other freak shows quickly opened up and down two of the main business streets in Coney Island, Bowery and Surf (Kyriazi 1976, 75).

In 1922 "Professor" Sam Wagner opened the World's Circus Freak Show, which proved so successful that Wagner soon succeeded Gumpertz as godfather of the Coney Island freak show. Gumpertz, however, had met John T. Ringling at the 1893 world's fair in Chicago, and in the 1930s he became the boss of the Ringling circus empire. The twenties, moreover, saw a decline in the bustling Coney Island and other amusement centers as movies and other mass entertainment diversions competed for the crowds. Coney Island continued as a throbbing resort, but physical deterioration was setting in and the subway brought a crowd with less money and more honky-tonk taste. The heyday of the self-contained amusement park had passed. Whereas in 1915 it was common for twenty thousand spectators to visit a Coney Island freak show on a warm Sunday, by 1930 an operator would be lucky to get eight thousand. Showmen dropped prices to attract more customers, but that only added to the deterioration (Traube 1936, 40).

In the late 1930s, New York Park Commissioner Robert Moses tried, as he saw it, to clean up the park. One of his moves was to ban ballyhoo and outside lecturers. The year 1938 saw three major sideshow operators brought to trial for violation of the ordinance: Wagner, who was still operating the World's Circus Freak Show; Dave Rosen, manager of the Coney Side Show; and Fred Sindell, owner of the Place of Wonders Freak Show (Uno 1938). Although it rebounded in the forties, Coney Island never returned to what it had been.

Carnivals

The history of the carnival is intimately interwoven with other amusement organizations. Because of the splendor and prominence of some of the other branches of the industry, and the carnival's own reputation of being cheap and sleazy (Dadswell 1946, 27; Easto and Truzzi 1974)—hardly the stuff for serious historians—the carnival has taken a backseat in the chronicle of popular amusement (McKennon 1972).

Carnivals developed during the last decade of the nineteenth century and the first part of the twentieth. Not every town was large enough to support an amusement park like Coney Island. The carnival provided for small-town America what the large amusement park provided for the urban masses.

The word *carnival* originally referred to street festivals and celebrations like Mardi Gras. While this sense embodies the freewheeling, involving, and participatory atmosphere that promoters hoped to create, we are concerned here with a carnival consisting of a traveling group of sideshows, games of chance, shooting galleries, and mechanical rides organized, but not entirely owned, by one person. Although aspects of the carnival existed in circuses, world's fairs, local and state fairs, and other amusement organizations prior to the carnival's official birth in the early 1890s, it was the organized amusement-company version that went on to be such a remarkably successful twentieth-century industry.

In the 1800s, before formally organized carnivals were developed, showmen traveled independently, turning up at fairs and other celebrations. Medicine shows, variety acts, wax museums, games of skill and chance, and even crude riding devices, the forerunners of the spectacular Ferris wheel and lavishly crafted merry-go-round, operated as independent traveling attractions that went from town to town by wagon. With the coming of the railroad in the 1870s, these showmen left the muddy roads and began booking on a regular route that included local fairs, festivals, and celebrations (McKennon 1972, 23). And with the railroad came the promoter, a person who would work with local businessmen and town officials to produce festivals and fairs, engaging the independent showman to play particular towns. Promoters, along with more organized agricultural and other fairs, began bringing independent amusement operators together regularly.

The Columbian Exposition of 1893 brought independent showmen, who had flocked to the fair site to get a crack at the crowds, into a cooperative work effort for the long six-month season. The showmen working the Midway Plaisance, too, not only shared the same grounds and experiences but even met to discuss common problems. It was at this exposition of 1893, in the area around Buffalo Bill's Wild West Show, that the idea for a collective amusement company was first discussed and the carnival as we know it was born (McKennon 1972).

Otto Schmidt is credited with first organizing independent showmen from the Chicago fair into a traveling unit. His season opened in Toledo, Ohio, but because of financial difficulties he never made the planned closing date in New Orleans. Schmidt returned to Chicago, got refinanced, and started off again, this time with a much-improved show. He called his carnival the Chicago Midway Plaisance Amusement Company. Included were thirteen attractions, some direct from the Midway Plaisance, with at least one freak show (McKennon 1972, 47).

This entourage played fairs in New York and New England, but because of poor organization and management it closed, bankrupt. Although this first carnival was not a success, it provided the model for other carnivals, and a number of showmen affiliated with it went on to become well-known carnival operators. Following Schmidt's lead, but more successful in organization and business acumen, others formed carnivals and took to the road, playing on streets and at agricultural fairs.

Agricultural fairs in the United States had begun back in the early nineteenth century, and gradually most states and counties had developed their own fairs. The formally organized carnival, however, provided an efficient method for earning revenue. The carnival owner either provided the fair sponsor with a percentage of total income or paid a flat fee for concession privileges. This partnership proved an enormous boon to both parties, and into the twentieth century major carnivals formed the financial base of state and county fairs.

In the 1902 season seventeen organized carnivals were on tour; by 1905 there were forty-six (Dadswell 1946, 25); and by 1937 an estimated three hundred carnival units roamed the United States (Hewitt 1937). The trend was almost the reverse of the circus: as the number of circuses declined, the number of carnivals soared.

Human oddities were exhibited at early carnivals, but they were always pitshows. At first, carnivals did not attract the prime freak exhibits; instead, second-rate wildmen, geeks (see Chapter 7), and other minor freaks dominated. The carnival, not yet well established, could not lure the exhibits from the more popular circuses, amusement parks, and other turn-of-the-century popular amusement enterprises. Around 1904, as carnivals became larger and more lucrative, "string shows" or "ten-in-one freak shows" became common. The carnival sideshow was a copy of the circus sideshow. One price bought admission to a number of attractions, all arranged on platforms inside a large tent with a bally in front. Also like the circus, the carnival freak show employed the elaborate bannerline as a come-on—and many added the word *circus* to this advertisement to distinguish these shows from the less interesting and earlier pitshow.

As the carnival developed, the largest show on the carnival midway was almost always the freak show (Easto and Truzzi 1973), which was considered central to the financial well-being of the operation. In their heyday in the 1920s and 1930s, these shows were financed by the carnival office itself to ensure that there was a good show (Fig. 19). State fair freak shows reached huge proportions, especially in large, jam-packed state fairs like those in Minnesota, Wisconsin, and Ohio.

Dime museums, circuses, fairs, amusement parks, and carnivals were the best places to see a freak show from 1840 to 1940, but there were other places to see them as well. Circuslike "wild west" shows, for one, had sideshows with human oddities. And toward the end of the nineteenth century vaudeville began to compete with popular amusement organizations for their audiences. While vaudeville houses never included full-scale freak shows, human oddities were sometimes included on their programs, especially novelty acts (mind readers, knife throwers, sword swallowers, and the like), which fit nicely into the vaudeville format. Exhibits whose primary interest lay in their physical abnormality, however, did not fare as well. As we shall see, the Hilton Sisters, the attractive and musical twentieth-century Siamese twins, made it in the vaudeville circuit in the 1920s and 1930s, but they were the exception.

Human oddities were not able to break into the lucrative and rap-

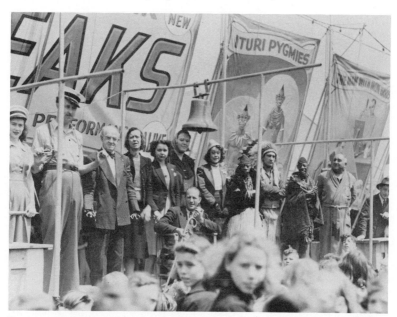

Fig. 19. Carnival freak show. Photographer unknown, 1930s. (Circus World Museum, Baraboo, Wisconsin.)

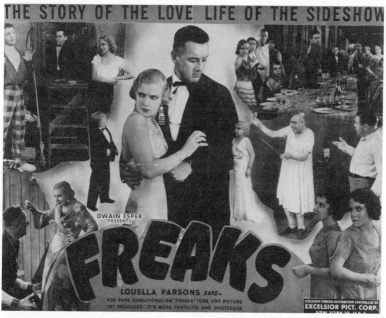

Fig. 20. Poster ad for the film *Freaks*, c. 1932. (Becker Coll., Syracuse University.)

idly developing movie industry either. A few mass-audience films featuring freaks were released in the 1920s and 1930s, including Tod Browning's *Freaks* (Fig. 20) (also *The Barker, Unholy Three,* and *Sinners Holiday*), but they failed at the box office. In the early 1940s a serious, semiautobiographical love story starring the Hilton Sisters, *Chained for Life,* bombed.

The Decline and Demise of the Freak Show

Throughout the nineteenth century and into the twentieth, showmen were not taken to task for their impropriety in exhibiting humans in the freak show. On the whole, the practice was quite acceptable to a broad range of the citizenry, including the upper crust. The pious avoided such displays, of course, but not because they had anything in particular against freak shows—they just frowned on any sort of frivolous amusement. To the showmen's great delight, physicians and other scientists were particularly interested in human anomalies, and their commentary provided good advertising copy. But all this was to change. During the first decade of the twentieth century were heard early rumblings of discontent with the practice of exhibiting people with physical and mental differences for profit and amusement. These changes can be understood only within a larger social context than that of the amusement world.

The turn of the century saw the rediscovery and application of Mendel's laws of genetics to human traits. Hair color and texture, it was discovered, as well as such unusual characteristics as excess toes and fingers, were inherited in a way that paralleled the pattern Mendel had discovered in peas. This new perspective was accompanied by the rise of the eugenics movement, a vicious use of social Darwinism which cautioned the nation that because modern societies protected their weak, the principle of survival of the fittest was not working (Ludmerer 1972; Haller 1963). The weak, the imperfect, the social, mental, and physical misfits, they warned, would, if left unchecked, breed at such a rate as to outnumber the better breeding stock. People who were physically and mentally imperfect would hand down their inferiority to the next generation. One of the solutions the eugenicists advocated was "negative eugenics," that is, keeping the bad gene carriers from breeding, through counseling, sterilization, and incarceration. The eugenics movement promulgated the idea that physically and mentally inferior people were far from being benign and interesting; rather, they were a danger. Many were segregated in large state-financed and physician-run custodial asylums that grew and multi-plied during the first quarter of the twentieth century (Scheerenberger 1983; Wolfensberger 1975).

Some human anomalies were linked to genes. In addition, early in the century a number of scientific and medical discoveries suggested other causes of physical and mental differences. The endocrine sys-tem, the ductless glands that secrete hormones to regulate growth, secondary sex characteristics, and certain body functions, was one particularly important discovery. Another was the X-ray, which helped probe the physiology of deformity. These discoveries began to de-mystify the human anomalies. At the same time, continuing explora-tion of the continents increased Americans' knowledge of the world and its people, thus undermining the myths and legends of lost tribes of giants and pygmies and natives with tails. The knowledge acquired in these decades provided an approach to the question of the cause of human variation that challenged earlier notions embedded in the idea of the "human curiosity" and the "lusus naturae."

A parallel series of events was equally significant in changing ideas about human variation. Like the freak show, physicians had become organized (Starr 1982) and by 1900 were well on their way to pro-fessionalizing. At the same time, they were beginning to lay claim to authority over a wide range of human processes and conditions, in-cluding many forms of human differences (Conrad and Schneider 1980; Szasz 1961). Human differences became medicalized as patho-logical—as "disease."

The eugenics movement and the medicalization of human differ-ences had major implications for the freak shows. Although the reper-cussions were not felt immediately, as the freak show moved through the twentieth century these larger social, political, and medical events became significant factors in its decline.

The first hints that the freak show platform might be affected by the changing social milieu was in 1908. Tody Hamilton, the flamboyant chief press agent for Barnum and Bailey Circus, in conjunction with its Madison Square Garden opening, sent out a press release an-nouncing: "SAD NEWS FOR OLD CIRCUS FREAKS—No more Curio Hall or Alluring Barkers for Barnum and Bailey's Show this Year." Papers across the country carried the story of how the Greatest Show on Earth was eliminating the freak department. The key reason Hamilton gave for the closing was "the large number of letters received by the circus criticizing exhibition of 'human abnormalities' as part of the big show and expressing the wish that something more elevating might be substituted" ("Sad News" 1908). Deceitfully, knowing that his proposal would not be well received, Hamilton suggested a substitution: for the freak show, a tropical garden exhibit with cages containing rare birds.

A few days later, and with equal fanfare, Hamilton announced that they had reversed their decision—when the circus opened it would have its freaks after all ("Circus Freaks Get Rehearing" 1908). Why the about-face? The management told the public that it had been bombarded with sympathetic letters from irate sideshow fans demanding that the show remain open. But the truth was, the freak show had never really been canceled—the whole episode was merely Hamilton's way of publicizing the show's opening.

Although the fabricated closing was merely a publicity stunt, it was precipitated by a real attack, not from the general public but from the scientific community. An article, "Circus and Museum Freaks, Curiosities of Pathology," had appeared in the widely circulated *Scientific America Supplement* (1908). It was very different from earlier scientific writings on freaks. Previously, scientists had limited their commentary to specific exhibits, describing them and reflecting on their scientific importance. This article, in contrast, not only commented, it criticized: "Most of these humble and unfortunate individuals, whose sole means of livelihood is the exhibition of their physical infirmities to a gaping and unsympathetic crowd, are pathological rarities. . . . A more refined and a more humane popular taste now frown upon such exhibitions" (p. 222). Although there is no evidence that the sentiment expressed was widespread, the article signals the first wave of the medical profession's attack on the freak show. The assault redefined exhibits as "humble and unfortunate" "pathological rarities," a far cry from the interesting "curiosities" or "lusus naturae" they had been in the past. The author declared that the exhibits were "sick" and to be pitied, that human oddities were not benign curiosities, they were pathological—diseased. The implication was that freaks' proper roles were not as public exhibits, but as patients of physicians, to be viewed on hospital rounds and in private offices, by appointment only.

The *Scientific America Supplement* article had a pretentious tone of authority. The message was clear: exhibits were no longer open to public speculation. The scientific community, the physicians, knew what the exhibits "had." While the public might question how much they actually did know, they had a scientific-sounding vocabulary which asserted that they were in charge. Bass, the "ossified man," had, according to the article, "polyarthritis deformans"; the "elastic skin man," "generalized dermatolysis"; the "dog-faced man," "hypertrichosis"; Chang, the "Chinese giant," "acromegaly"; "and the 'wild men of Borneo' and Barnum's 'what is it' we now recognize in the maturer years of professional experience, as cases of microcephalous idiocy."[31]

Hamilton got the publicity he was seeking with his announcement. One might say that he turned the criticism into an opportunity, but there were repercussions. A columnist for *The Nation* took the announced closing seriously and jumped on the anti—freak show bandwagon, reiterating to a larger public the idea that freakishness "was generally a disease." As people would do in years to come, the columnist suggested that the passing of the freak show was not a tragedy but rather a healthy tendency in the move to rid us "of the morbid and unwholesome in our life" ("Amusements at the Abnormal" 1908). Hamilton may have turned the criticism around, but the seed had been planted.

In April 1914, an encounter unlike any previously recorded took place between a group of doctors and several freak show promoters. The Barnum and Bailey show was opening in New York. A circus official had invited representatives of New York's College of Physicians and Surgeons for what the doctors thought was to be a private viewing of the freak show attractions. But when the fifteen students and Drs. Theodore Janeway, Walter James, and R. A. Lamberg arrived at ten o'clock on the appointed morning, they discovered that they were not alone: the publicity department had invited the press to cover their visit and to listen to the physicians' comments. In fact, the whole affair had been concocted as a media event. When the physicians discovered this, they walked out. They declined to be used in the showmen's promotional schemes.

Some reporters salvaged a story by treating the physicians' walkout humorously. The "living skeleton" was quoted in the *New York Herald* of April 17, 1914, as saying, "Of course there is little that they could teach me about my condition. I find it very remunerative and I feel perfectly comfortable and it costs but a little for my food. Sometimes I am amply satisfied with an olive for dinner" ("Physicians Quit Lecture" 1914). But the event could not be shrugged off so easily. Physicians had always been willing participants in such events, and although they would continue to participate at a reduced level through the 1930s, the respectable scientific community was asserting its control and dissociating itself from the public exhibition of people.

By 1922 the general public could read articles in the popular press that explained the "sickness" behind human exhibits. In an *Illustrated World* article entitled "Side-Show Freaks as Seen by Science" (Gilliams 1922), a lengthy explanation of the pituitary and thyroid glands' functions in producing freaks is discussed.[32] By the early thirties the medicalized view of human differences had become so pervasive that Browning's 1932 film *Freaks*, which starred many sideshow attractions, started with the statement that freaks' abnormalities were gradually being eliminated by medical science. A 1932 *New York Times* film critique remarked: "The difficulty is in telling whether it should be shown at the Rialto—where it opened yesterday—or in, say, the Medical Centre."

By the late 1930s the transformation of those with physical and mental anomalies from curiosities to diseased people was complete (Johnston 1934b, c). From a 1937 article in *Colliers*, "Side Show Diagnosis" (Lees 1937), readers could confirm that "practically all side show freaks . . . can be found fitted snugly between the pages of some medical textbook. Curiosities they may be, but what they more certainly are is sick" (p. 22).

The shifting meaning of abnormality fanned by scientific discovery and the accent of medical authority is basic to understanding the decline of the freak show. Competition from other forms of amusement contributed to its decline as well. Others have offered simpler explanations, the most popular being that showmen just ran out of exhibits (Lentz 1964)—that is, medical intervention had become so effective that there were no longer enough exhibits to supply the enterprise with its raw material. Although there may be some truth to this theory, the incarceration of human oddities in asylums and a declining interest in freak show careers on the part of potential exhibits probably had more to do with the scarcity than did any cures.

The question arises whether medical intervention actually resulted in reduced numbers of people with physical and mental anomalies. Certainly, the prevalence of certain conditions declined, but, as in the case of thalidomide, others were created. In addition, medical technology made it possible for people who otherwise would not have survived to live to adulthood. Thus, while the medical profession may take some credit for the decline of the freak show, it was actually accomplished more by social and political means than by medical ones.

By 1940 the freak show was "on the ropes." The organized public exhibition of people with physical, mental, and behavioral anomalies had become less profitable and, for some, not amusing. The dime museum, which had nurtured the practice of displaying freaks in its infancy and remained its guardian through young adulthood, was dead. The circus, amusement park, and carnival still existed, but their prominence had been undermined by the Great Depression, their own amusement world practices, and competition from other forms of popular entertainment. Sideshows declined precipitously compared to their host organizations. Whereas in its prime the freak show had been the main attraction of the midway, by 1940 it was losing its audience. In fact, respectable people were turning their backs on the show. Once the freak show, packaged as rational entertainment, had legitimized and provided a cover for theatrical undertakings; by the forties it had become morally bankrupt.

Our brief chronology of the freak show is a mere sketch of the institution's development. Exhibits of human curiosities changed from single traveling attractions to freak shows as they joined the emerging amusement organizations of the nineteenth century. Their popularity helped launch dime museums and circuses, and later, amusement parks and carnivals. These organizations in turn provided a stable home for the freak show, allowing the development of standard exhibits, methods, and modes of presenting human anomalies.

The early association of human curiosities with museums and science gave the mature freak show its pseudoscientific aura, complete with inside and outside lecturers and attractions who posed as natural-scientific and teratological exhibits. The exploration of the globe that was occurring concurrently with the development of the freak show, moreover, resulted in Third World exhibits being incorporated into the freak show as both exhibits with anomalies and cultural oddities. Yet whereas nineteenth-century science supported and legitimized the growth of the freak show, twentieth-century science began to undermine it by medicalizing human variation and stripping exhibits of their mystery.

As the various freak shows prospered, competition escalated. Exhibits therefore became more innovative, relying increasingly not only
on variety acts, but also on exaggeration, misrepresentation, and
gaffs—aspects of the freak show that were present in its earliest days.

With this barebones history of the freak show behind us, the next
chapter fills in some details as we look at the growth of amusement
world culture. Why and how did it develop? What were the characteristics of the showmen's approach to the world? How did their culture
shape the construction of freak exhibits?

3

"Step Right Up"
The World of Popular Amusement

GIL ROBINSON, son of the famous circus owner and manager John Robinson, tells this tale of 1860s circus life with his father's company. One morning a "remarkable-looking specimen" of a young man came to the circus grounds asking for a job. "His hair was at least a foot and a half long, and his whiskers looked like a haystack after a cyclone." The man's potential as a wild man exhibit having been noted, he was immediately hired, given a dollar to bind the bargain, and instructed to report for work that afternoon. About one o'clock he returned, but Gil could hardly recognize him. His wild man attributes, his whiskers and long hair, were missing. When asked what had happened, the naive man proudly announced that he had spent his dollar at the barber to get cleaned up for the show (Robinson 1925, 77).

Embodied in this simple tale, and hundreds of others that make up the folklore of the amusement world, is a basic theme: the world can be divided into two groups of people—those who are "with it," and those who are not. Those who are know the working of the show and are ready to exploit a situation's money-making potential for all it is worth. Those who are not are naive, dumb to the ways of showmen.

Freak shows were attached to larger organizations—circuses, carnivals, dime museums, and amusement parks—that together formed the bulk of the popular amusement industry. While there were important differences among these organizations (Easto and Truzzi 1973), people who worked in the industry shared a way of life, developing a culture, a world view, an argot, and a set of practices that set them apart and provided a justification for the way they treated customers. This chapter explores their special perspective on life and how it relates to the social construction of freaks.

When I refer to the "amusement world," I mean the people who worked in the popular amusement industry, their way of life, and their worldview. The people who shared that world are the "showmen." Although this term is sometimes used more narrowly to refer only to the flamboyant promoters, managers, and owners, I prefer to use it in a more general sense. The slick operators may personify the showmen, but they share the title with other members of the amusement world. By using the terms *amusement world* and *showmen* in this broadened sense, I do not mean to say that everyone who worked for amusement organizations shared exactly the same perspective or way of life. But freak show personnel were "showmen" incarnate, and their approach to life exemplified the amusement world perspective. Most freak exhibits actively participated in the fraudulence of their presentations. Some even exclusively managed and promoted their own careers.[1] The great majority of freaks were in fact themselves showmen.[2]

I refer to show*men* because that was the term people in the industry used. Naturally, however, women were part of the business. While they seldom filled leadership positions,[3] women were well represented in other roles; particularly as performers and freak show exhibits. As the use of the generic word *showmen* for both men and women suggests, then, the amusement world was strongly male-dominated.

The Making of the Amusement World

Individual exhibits of human oddities became part of the emerging circus and dime museum in the first half of the nineteenth century. The last quarter of that century saw the development of the amusement park and carnival, which completed the roster of popular amusement enterprises housing freak shows. The popular amusement industry quickly became a world unto itself.[4]

During the 1800s the *New York Clipper*, a weekly magazine, functioned as the industry's unifier. By the end of the century, however, it had been replaced by the weekly *Billboard*. Both were bulletin boards for posting coming events, help-wanted ads, and for-sale offers. Photography studios advertised specials on bulk-ordered freak portrait cards, and shows in need of human oddities placed freak-wanted ads. *Billboard* printed route lists of the traveling shows, with details of who was playing where and how they were drawing. It contained regular columns devoted to dime museums, amusement parks, circuses, and carnivals. While *Billboard*—or "the bible," in amusement world vernacular (McKennon 1980, 15)—stands as a tangible symbol of the

FREAK SHOW: THE INSTITUTION

mutual interest that members of these businesses shared, the basis of their unity was much deeper and more profound.

INTERLOCKING ORGANIZATIONS

Academics and showmen alike have come up with definitions that present the illusion of a clear separation between the circuses, carnivals, amusement parks, and dime museums.[5] As the last chapter documented, although these organizations did function as semidistinct entities with unique aspects, from the beginning and through the 1930s there was significant overlap. Established dime museums, for example, often went on the road with circuses as sideshows or, alternatively, had circus acts as part of their entertainment. Large carnivals sometimes included a small circus as one of the shows on the midway. Amusements parks had many of the rides and games of chance one would find on the traveling carnival. Although historians write separate volumes on the origins of the circus and the carnival, for example, the differences in these chronicles often have more to do with definitions and perspective than with what is covered.

In addition to the tremendous structural overlap, from the beginning of the evolution of the popular amusement industry showmen hopscotched from one type of organization to another.[6] A person might work one year in a circus, the next in a dime museum, only to move to the midway of a world's fair for a year, and then back to the circus. Some showmen had, at any given time, multiple affiliations.

From the people who owned and managed to their hired hands, the boundaries between organizations remained permeable. The biggest entrepreneurs of the amusement industry were affiliated with a range of organizations. P. T. Barnum, the father and patron saint of the amusement industry, traveled with a small circus prior to launching his dime museum career (Fig. 21). Later he worked with world's fairs, and still later became associated with the circus. Another famous amusement world executive, George Middleton, had a similar career. In 1880, after traveling with Adam Forepaugh's circus, he went to New York City where he started a successful dime museum. He had worked there for two years "when the circus fever came over me again and I wanted to travel, so I sold the dime museum . . . and went out on the road again with a circus" (Middleton 1913, 72). After two years of that he teamed up with C. E. Kohl and established dime museums across the country. During the 1893 world's fair they opened a dime museum in Chicago in conjunction with the great Columbian Exhibition. The

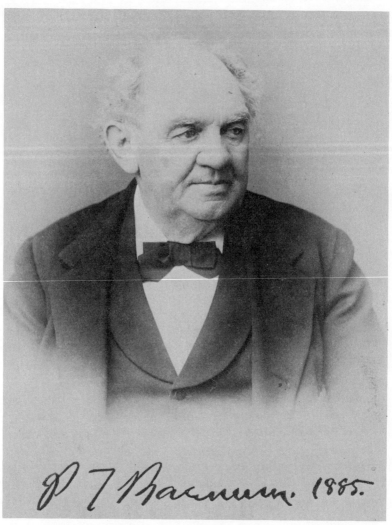

FIG. 21. P. T. Barnum. Photo by Charles Eisenmann, 1885. (Author's collection.)

roster of famous manager/owner/promoter showmen who switched organizations is long—Sam Gumpertz (M. Smith 1935), W. C. Coup
(1901), Ray Brydon (Pfening, Jr., 1983), William Tobey (J. Jordan
1925), and Joe McKennon (1980) are on it[7]—and far exceeds the list
of those who remained exclusively "circus," for example, or exclusively "carnival."[8]

Lower-level personnel too—performers, freak show exhibits, talkers, and ticket sellers—frequently switched organizations, encour-

FREAK SHOW: THE INSTITUTION

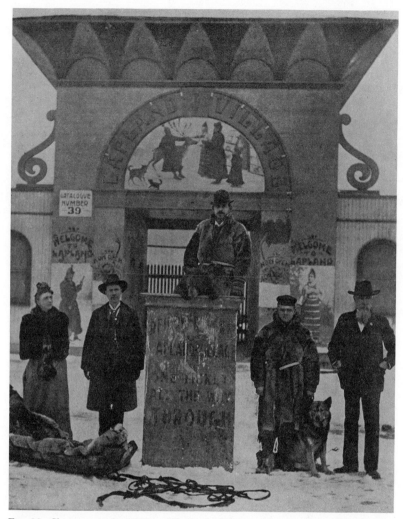

Fig. 22. Showmen at the 1893 world's fair in Chicago. Photographer unknown. (Author's collection.)

aged by the seasonal schedule of traveling companies. Many enterprises provided employees with room and board during the season, but the showmen's prospects for the winter months were bleak. Some, of course, turned a handsome profit in the regular season and could enjoy the winter vacation;[9] most, however, wanted or needed to work. Stationary dime museums, amusement parks near cities, and world's fairs often remained open during the off-season and could absorb some laid-off workers (Fig. 22).

The various types of amusement industry organizations had their golden years as well as their periods of decline. As dime museums were fading, amusement parks and carnivals were hitting their stride; in the twentieth century, the circus experienced serious declines while the carnival expanded. Showmen's careers were affected by these changes. Many who left the dime museums and circuses became attached to amusement parks and carnivals.[10]

Circus historians treat the circus as a separate and autonomous organization, not as part of the amusement industry. Certain segments of the circus, especially after the turn of the century, did remain exclusively "circus" and looked down on carnival and other amusement folk as "low life" (Dadswell 1946, 35; McKennon 1972). In this century, several upper executives of the more prestigious circuses as well as their star performers, many of whom were European, developed airs of superiority (Bradna and Hartzell 1952), even shunning others from their own company who were not part of the elite.

The freak show showmen were never part of the elite. They identified much more with the industry as a whole than with a particular organization. Most amusement industry workers, like their freak show counterparts, were not committed exclusively to any specific type of show—they were simply in the amusement business, waiting for each week's *Billboard* to check out employment prospects and see where their itinerant friends were working. Despite minor differences in vocabulary among the various segments of the industry, the amusement world as a whole had its own extensive vernacular (Maurer 1931; Bradna and Hartzell 1952; Dadswell 1946; McKennon 1980). The words and phrases embodied participants' approaches to the world and helped solidify membership.

ON THE ROAD

Many of the organizations that employed amusement workers were traveling establishments that moved from town to town with their troupes of showmen. An amusement industry circuit developed early on to route human oddities and novelty acts through dime museums and amusement parks around the country, and freak show attractions and others were soon shuffling from establishment to establishment along well-defined routes. Toward the end of the nineteenth century, and becoming more of an influence in the twentieth, booking agents entered the scene to facilitate these moves.

Amusement personnel lived close together, sharing meals and

FREAK SHOW: THE INSTITUTION

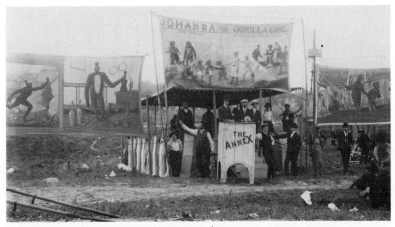

Fig. 23. Barnum and Bailey showmen. Pitshow front, with crew. Photo by Fred Glasier, c. 1905. (Ringling Museum of the Circus, Sarasota, Florida.)

lodging (Fig. 23). Cookhouses (actually tents) and on-site accommodations provided by the management became a regular feature of circuses in the late 1860s (Robinson 1925, 125, 126), and after the 1870s, when circuses began moving by rail, these became extensive and elaborate. Owner-provided, on-site room and board later became a feature of other traveling shows.

From the 1860s through the 1930s, many mobile shows practiced what was called the "boil up" (McKennon 1980, 19), a ritual that vividly illustrates how close the nomad-showmen lived. "Boil up" occurred on Sundays, when amusement businesses were forced to close under blue laws. The troupers stripped and boiled all their clothes in large buckets while they bathed in a waterhole or a makeshift bathhouse. The purpose was to get rid of body lice. On days off, fires with boiling pots over them marked the show's camps.

Traveling shows that did not have cook tents and company-owned sleeping arrangements were put up in boardinghouses and hotels. Typically, the show's manager would rent whole facilities and the troupers would room together. In the case of permanent amusement businesses, it was common for showmen to live together in nearby boardinghouses or on the premises. Many dime museums had facilities for itinerant staff. In 1868, when a nighttime fire destroyed Barnum's American Museum, twenty people, mainly exhibits and performers, had to be evacuated from their sleeping quarters ("Barnum's Museum Fire" 1868). Two young dime museum performers, Weber and Fields, left this description of the room and board arrangements of the Keith Batchelder Dime Museum in Boston in the early 1880s. It suggests the close proximity of the performers and their close relationship with the museum owner's family:

> Freaks and performers slept, ate and dressed in the attic, and paid six dollars a week to Mom Keith, who oversaw that floor and waited on table, assisted by a chubby, eight year old boy—their son Paul. Eight by ten partitions in which actors both dressed and slept lined the walls and opened upon the dining-room table, occupying the center of the attic floor. (Isman 1924, 81)

Even circuses that had their own mobile sleeping facilities rented whole boardinghouses or parts of hotels for the troupers when they were in a city for a long stop, or even as a once-a-week treat ("The 'Wild Boy' Tamed" 1903). A number of boardinghouses in new York City at the turn of the century catered to amusement world clientele ("Freaks Touch Elbows" 1888).

Traveling carnival performers either were provided with food and accommodations by the owner or manager of the unit with which they were associated (the "ten-in-one," say) or lived in mobile units on the fair or carnival lot. People who worked amusement parks were accommodated on the premises or in nearby homes and hotels that catered to that clientele.

To return to a point made earlier, not all those who worked the amusement industry mixed and were part of one big undifferentiated family. As the industry moved into the twentieth century and circuses consolidated and became extravaganzas, the more prestigious operations developed a social structure in which the preeminent acts remained aloof from the other showmen. With the Ringling Brothers, Barnum and Bailey Circus operation, for example, the cookhouse and sleeping arrangements were officially segregated so that people were kept with their own kind ("Circus Side Show Brought up to Date" 1931). Elite performers and management ate and slept separately; likewise, members of the freak show had a table of their own, as did the roustabouts and the clowns.[11] These arrangements not only made people's places clear but also served to keep those who were "with it" from those who did not want to identify with the amusement world.

The interlocking of amusement organizations and the close personal contact showmen had with one another provided the conditions

FREAK SHOW: THE INSTITUTION

for the development of the amusement world—an occupational culture with a particular worldview and a distinct set of practices. As these amusement organizations became self-contained enclaves, showmen grew isolated from the rest of society and more dependent on themselves for direction and values. But these were not the only factors that helped forge the amusement world. Adding to the solidarity and isolation, and giving a special, mischievous edge to their approach to life, was the rejection and out-and-out hostility showmen encountered from outsiders.

Showmen's Relations with Outsiders

Showmen were never fully accepted or trusted in the communities in which they made a living. While early circuses and dime museums were more acceptable to puritanical Americans than theaters, many people nevertheless perceived them as "against the laws of God," as decadent dens of moral corruption. Museums snuck in through the back door to enter the amusement business disguised as edifying, morally uplifting institutions. They became more entertainment-oriented only as puritanical influence and public tastes changed. Although this blurred identity combining education and amusement kept them from most of the direct attacks that circuses often suffered (Thayer 1976), they did not entirely escape moral crusaders' accusations of being immoral and dangerous.

NEWSPAPERS

In the first half of the nineteenth century, opposition to traveling amusements was so pervasive that newspapers freely editorialized against them. In February 1826 the *Connecticut Observer* stated, "It may be admitted that in some respects the circus is free from the evils connected with the theater; while perhaps, it has new evils of its own. Still, there are, in our view, objections equally applicable to both" (Thayer 1976, 19).

On into the century the press rode herd of traveling shows by seeking out and reporting various forms of skulduggery that were endemic to the operation. During the 1893 world's fair, in a crusade against what it termed "highway robbery," the *Chicago Tribune* regularly attacked the independent, itinerant showmen who had set up outside the gates (McKennon 1972, 42).

CHURCHES

Some churches waged vehement anticircus campaigns. Opposition from the pulpit was common and, indeed, extended far back in amusement world history. Barnum recalled one Sunday in 1836 when, while traveling with the Aaron Turner Circus, he attended a church in Lenox, Massachusetts. The preacher roundly denounced circuses, saying that "all men connected with them were destitute of morality" (Barnum 1855, 179).

Church groups published booklets containing anti–amusement world propaganda. *The Circus*, a publication of the American Sunday School Union, Philadelphia, written about 1840 to teach children the evils of the traveling life, reveals the details of antishowman sentiment. The booklet tells the story of two young children, brother and sister, who meet a man passing out circus handbills. They go home and show the fliers to their father, hoping he will take them to the show. The father sits them down and explains why he will not:

> The men who belong to [the circus] are generally idle and worthless people, who move about from place to place, and get their living by taking money of many persons who cannot afford to spend it so foolishly. Then there is a great deal of drinking and gambling about the circus. . . . I always think it is a very sad thing for a village when a circus comes into it. Besides all this, it makes all the boys who see it, want to do just as the men do; and some of them get so fond of seeing such shows that as soon as they get a chance, they join themselves to the circus, and then there is no hope of making them useful men. (American Sunday School Union c. 1840)

Clerical opposition to the traveling shows, although on the decline, continued through to the end of the century (Robinson 1925, 59). Into the 1900s, clergy denounced from their pulpits particular practices of carnival midways (George 1938, 56).

LEGISLATION

Disapproval of the circus and traveling shows soon made its way into legislation. State laws, originally designed to control the theater, were often applied to other traveling shows (Sweet and Habenstein 1973), and a few states passed legislation specifically directed at circuses as well. Until 1860, Connecticut had expressly banned them (Thayer

1981). In states with restrictive legislation, traveling shows played on the sly, moving about with little publicity of their route, almost like outlaws. Vermont's ban lasted until 1865, and even then licensing and fee requirements stifled business, making showmen feel unwanted and exploited. Not until 1933 were all anticircus laws, except those regarding towns' rights to license circuses, repealed in that state (Thayer 1981). Town ordinances, including taxes and prohibitive restrictions, existed throughout the history of the amusement industry. Corrupt town officials and law officers often used these ordinances to extort payoffs and special favors; they also overlooked illegal and fraudulent amusement world practices in exchange for bribes. The corrupt relationship between the law and the showmen did little to engender respect in the amusement world for the supposedly morally superior "towner."

HEY, RUBE!

Antagonism toward traveling showmen was not confined to the press, the clergy, and moral reformers, nor was it limited to verbal assault. W. C. Coup, a veteran nineteenth-century showman, recalled traveling about the country:

> It was no infrequent occurrence to be set upon by a party of roughs, who were determined to show their prowess and skill as marksmen with fists and clubs if required. As a consequence showmen went armed, prepared to hold their own against any odds. Not once a month, or even once a week, but almost daily, would these fights occur, and so desperately were they entered into that they resembled pitched battles more than anything else. (Coup 1901, 7)

From the origins of the amusement world in the early nineteenth century well into the twentieth, showmen were frequently attacked by belligerent town hooligans. Although some attacks were precipitated by a patron who discovered that he or she had been cheated, no specific event was needed to provoke abuse. Town folk felt a general hostility toward showmen, who were considered footloose outsiders with no home and questionable morals. In addition, sectional feelings were a constant menace. In the South, for example, showmen were universally regarded as "Yankees" (Coup 1901, 12).

Coup soon had ingrained in him the showman's "prevailing sentiment that we were constantly in the 'land of the Philistines,' that the hand of every man was against us, and that our only safety was in perpetual alertness and ready determination to stand together and fight for our rights on the slightest signal of disturbance" (Coup 1901, 9). Showmen's memoirs are filled with accounts of battles with the "towners" (Saxon 1979; Sweet and Habenstein 1973, 586). In the most hard-fought encounters, clubs and guns were used, and death was the result.[12]

The phrase "Hey, rube!" became part of the amusement world lexicon before the Civil War (Robinson 1925, 126), and it remained a frequent cry into the twentieth century (Tully 1927). "Rube" is the derogatory expression people in the amusement world use for those who are not "with it." Thus "Hey, rube!" was the showman's battle cry when it came time to fight the towners.[13] While the brawls (or "clems") eventually waned, traveling showmen continued to be regarded with suspicion through the 1940s. Lewis (1970) reports that even in the 1960s carnival people felt rejected by towners, with hotels and motels accepting showmen reluctantly.[14]

As the country became more urbanized and immigrants flocked to its shores, people grew more tolerant of the amusement world. The vehement attacks died down, but even in the twentieth century progressives viewed popular amusement as a "social problem" that needed careful watching. In 1913, the amusement industry was subjected to one of the progressives' famous surveys. The resulting report gave the circus this faint endorsement:

> Its familiar traveling zoo, its clowns, trained animals, acrobats, and aerial performers have important educational and amusement value, and the fact that the circus is attended by so many parents with children acts as a moral disinfectant. The further fact that a high degree of skill and steadiness are required by many of the performers, tends to check some of the excesses which other traveling amusement troops often indulge in. (Edwards 1915, 122)

The criticism never completely stopped; controversy and exposé remained a part of the public's relationship with the amusement world (see George 1938).

Showmen knew they were not trusted. They were well aware of their dubious status in the communities they worked. What they had to

FREAK SHOW: THE INSTITUTION

offer—the excitement, the entertainment, the fun, the bribes—was enough to compensate the hosts. But although the showmen were allowed to practice their trade, they were never accepted—they were merely tolerated.[15]

It is important to note that the hostility directed toward showmen had nothing to do with the practice of exhibiting people with physical, mental, or behavioral abnormalities for amusement and profit. The deception and stealing that freak show personnel engaged in were what provoked attack; the propriety of human exhibits per se did not become an issue until well into the twentieth century.[16]

Forging Solidarity

The litany of abuse that showmen endured was pervasive. But this narrative of their troubles is not intended to evoke sympathy for their plight. As we shall see shortly, it could easily be argued that they got what they deserved, that what was said about them was true. But to understand the showmen's approach to patrons and their view of the world, the circumstances of their existence must be taken into account. The blurring lines between the various types of organizations and the showmen's career patterns led to an occupational identity that transcended organizational bounds. The largely itinerant nature of the industry, combined with the close living conditions of the traveling troupers, provided the conditions for the forging of an occupational culture—an amusement world. External hostility—the attacks by the press, the clergy, government officials, respectable people, and hooligans alike—was another element in welding showmen into a unity, a particular spirit of "us" against "them."

Showmen's Worldview and Practices

"Towner," "rube," "yokel," "mark," "sucker"[17]—showmen used these words to refer to individuals outside the amusement world. These are not words of admiration, or even neutral words; they are words of contempt (Maurer 1931, 328). Showmen did not like the marks and seldom associated with them. To "take" a mark whenever and wherever possible was the showman's way of life (Taylor 1958a, b). "Trouper" and "with it" were the words showmen used for themselves, words that connoted solidarity and community. Although troupers working with different companies were in competition and sometimes used ruthless tactics, like ripping down posters and under-

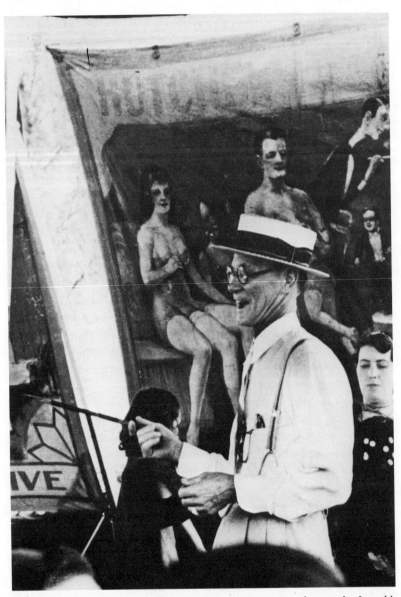

FIG. 24. Sideshow talker. This Farm Security Administration photograph of an old-timer showman was taken by Russell Lee at the Louisiana State Fair in 1938. (Library of Congress.)

FREAK SHOW: THE INSTITUTION

mining stellar attractions with phony imitations, ultimately showmen split humanity into two parts: those who were "with it," and those who were not.

Showmen were shrewd, worldly, clever, and too adventurous to be confined to a single location, regular work hours, or the rest of the trappings of conventional life (Fig. 24). They used expressions like "circus fever" and "sawdust in my blood" to indicate that being in the amusement world was more than an occupation, it was an addiction, something only those who were "with it" could understand. As one showman put it, "Circusing is sort of a disease. Few men, once victims, are every permanently cured" ("Grifting Isn't So Good" 1924). Rubes, in contrast, were naive and dull; they lived humdrum lives and knew little of the world outside their little town. They had not experienced the amusement world and the ways of the showmen.

Showmen worked long, hard hours and followed a grueling schedule of moves. But what they did was not necessarily considered hard work in the amusement world—and hard work was not thought to be the crucial element of success. *It Was Better Than Work*, the title of a circus press agent's autobiography, expresses that idea (Kelly 1982). Being clever, knowing the tricks of the trade, being skilled in the techniques employed to dupe the rubes—that was key to success.

What was success? It was, very simply, making money. Nate Eagle, freak show entrepreneur extraordinaire, tells the story of his negotiations with John Ringling North over salaries for himself and a troupe of midgets he managed. He captures the spirit of the showmen's humor and motivation both when he tells North, "I must confess, or acknowledge, that I'm just one of those terrible heels you may have heard about—I like money" (Taylor 1958b, 39). Making money was playing to a larger crowd today than yesterday, making towners give up more cash here than they had in another town.

But many showmen had sufficient entrepreneurial skills to have made a handsome, even better, living in the conventional world. Making money wasn't everything. Success meant prospering *as part* of the amusement world. Much of the pleasure came from being clever as only showmen were clever—wheeling and dealing, grifting and gaffing, keeping the suckers from penetrating the secrets of the amusement scene. It was a showman-get-sucker world. Being "with it" meant knowing the angles, having an advantage. The thrill was beating them at your own game (Fig. 25).

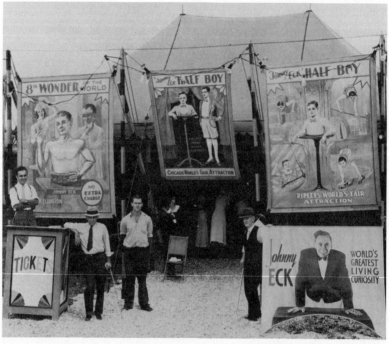

Fig. 25. Showmen with the Johnny Eck exhibit. Photographer unknown, c. 1932. (Mark Feldman Collection, Baltimore, Maryland; courtesy of Warren Raymond.)

PRACTICES

In 1917 the well-regarded and popular Sells-Floto Circus featured in its sideshow a two-headed man (Fig. 26) (Lifson 1983; Rusid 1975). He had a second, smaller head growing from the top front of what might be termed his normal head. The upper one, although not fully developed and lacking animation, had a face with eyes, nose, and mouth. The audience was told that the man had been able to see, talk, and hear with his upper head until he reached the age of twenty when, for no apparent reason, the upper head had atrophied.

This freak was a tremendous draw, and the talker's spiel made him even more appealing to the crowds. He was proclaimed to be a refugee who had followed General Pershing out of Mexico after Pancho Villa's raiders forced him and his family of seven from their little ranch. For three years, until he was struck with a serious illness, this attraction pleased crowds and brought in a fortune.

The two-headed Mexican was a fake. His name was Pasqual Pinon, and prior to being recruited as a freak he was a poor Texas laborer.

FREAK SHOW: THE INSTITUTION

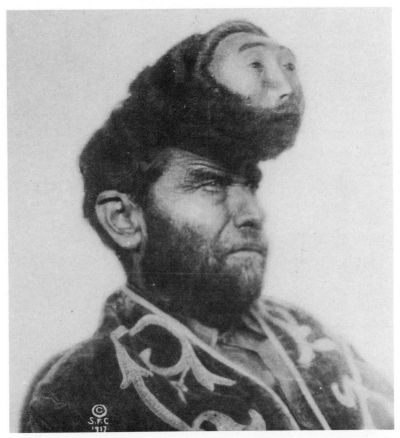

FIG. 26. Pasqual Pinon, "the two-headed Mexican." This picture was sold when he was on exhibit in the Sells-Floto Sideshow in 1917. Photographer unknown. (Becker Coll., Syracuse University.)

One account of this fraud asserts that Pasqual's second head was really a tumor that was outfitted with facial features (Braden 1922, 674). Another states that he was merely rigged with a well-made false head (Lifson 1983). Whatever the case, the showmen got the rubes.

The two-headed Mexican story illustrates one form of blatant deception in which showmen engaged. As we shall see in Part Two, showmen working the freak shows systematically and pervasively misrepresented their exhibits to the public. But this form of deception was minor compared to other of their activities, some of which were outright criminal. These practices are discussed here in brief to provide a sense of how the misrepresentation of freaks fit into the larger pattern of the amusement world. These practices were carried out in various areas and departments of amusement industry organizations and occurred from the ticket window to the big show, inside the main tent, and at the many concessions and sideshows on the midways. Although freak shows were often the center of the action, none of the practices were exclusive to the freak show.

"Grift" is a word that showmen used to refer to all the forms of illegal and fraudulent money-making activities in the amusement world, including rigged games of chance, pickpocketing, and short-changing (Inciardi and Petersen 1973; McKennon 1980). Interestingly, grift does not include misrepresenting freak exhibits to the public in order to entice customers into the tent, nor does it include promoting acts that did not exist. "Fibs" like these were standard in the amusement world, so standard that there was no special word for them. Illustrating showmen's humor and morality in regard to fraudulent presentations, Nate Eagle, in a discussion in which he dissociated himself from any grift, proclaimed, "I would much rather talk a man inside a tent to see nothing than shortchange him" (Taylor 1958a).

Grift was so pervasive in the amusement world that a pejorative phrase existed to refer specifically to organizations that had no grift: the "Sunday school show" (Dembroski 1973). One nineteenth-century con artist estimated that prior to 1900 some traveling amusement organizations derived 80 percent of their profits from grift. An "anonymous circus grifter" whom the sociologist Edwin Sutherland interviewed in the 1930s stated that in the early twentieth century all circuses except Ringling and Barnum and Bailey had grifting (Inciardi and Petersen 1973), and another circus old-timer estimated that from the turn of the century to World War II, not necessarily a period with the highest grift, about half the circuses had owners or managers who practiced grift (Sharpe 1970, 35). In other segments of the industry—especially the carnival, where grifting flourished during the 20th century—the figure may be higher. In addition, many of the owners and managers who did not encourage grift were not especially rigorous in their attempts to control it but instead turned their backs on the dealings of concession owners who were part of the show. Finally, a great deal of grift went on in spite of the owners' and managers' attempts to eliminate it.

The most widespread form of grift was systematic shortchanging by

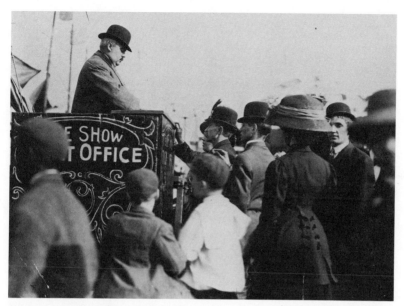

FIG. 27. Lew Graham selling freak show tickets. The top of the ticket stand is above patrons' eye level. Graham managed major circus freak shows from the early 1890s through the early 1920s. His employers included the Barnum and Bailey Circus, Ringling Brothers' Circus, and Ringling Brothers and Barnum and Bailey Combined Show. Photographer unknown, c. 1905. (Pfening Coll., Columbus, Ohio.)

ticket sellers. I say "systematic," because this form of grift—and indeed, most others—was not a matter of an individual stealing: it was a normative and calculated part of the show's economy (Irwin 1909, 51). In many freak shows, for example, ticket sellers were paid no salary and in fact were required to give the manager money for the privilege of shortchanging the customer. Owners depended on the grift operation to keep salaries down and provide cash (Inciardi and Petersen 1973; Sharpe 1970).

A variety of approaches were used in shortchanging. The most common, and the one requiring the least direct deception, was the "walk-away." Unbeknownst to them, customers were actively encouraged to leave ticket sellers' counters without their change. To promote "walk-aways," ticket sellers—and freak show ticket sellers most characteristically—operated on stools behind high counters (Fig. 27). They could thus deliver change in a place that was hard to reach and impossible to see—and easy for the patron to forget.

Giving customers less change than they had coming was facilitated by placing the coins above eye level. Other techniques involved methods of counting back change that confused customers (Tully 1927). If the mark was buying more than one ticket, for example, the addition could be handled so as to hike the price. Shortchanging was also accomplished by handing back folded bills and substituting tokens for coins. All these practices were easier owing to the crowd atmosphere surrounding the vendors and the eagerness of ticket buyers to move on. Showmen also employed "shills" to work the crowds by pushing and generally heightening agitation in the queues. Ticket seller–shortchangers were skilled at their profession. Not only did they master quickness of the hand, but they knew how to confront people who complained, cool the mark, and generally turn the tables on the rube.

Shortchanging wasn't the only illegal practice that went on. In fact, it was probably the most innocuous. Amusement organizations also had pickpockets buzzing about the grounds. Although some were not affiliated with the organization and its management, others operated with its blessing, paying for the "dip" privileges. Throughout the second half of the nineteenth century it was common for local newspapers to report a tally of the number of victims and the amount of cash lifted. [18]

Another form of grift was the rigged game. The wheel of chance was controlled by a foot pedal; the pea that was supposed to be under the shell might in fact be under the table; the bottles to be knocked over had lead bases. This kind of grift was part of the carnival from its inception. Frequent advertisements in *Billboard* at the turn of the century read, "Everything goes!"—invitations for crooked-game operators. In addition to the games of chance on the midway, more serious gambling often occurred at special, out-of-the-way locations. Loaded dice, marked cards, crooked dealing, and other forms of hustling were all employed in pursuit of the mark.

The examples of grift are endless. There were elaborate con schemes—one involved phony diamonds which the rubes were led to believe were real. Rubes were forced to pay for services they thought were free, or to pay extra to see special attractions that did not exist. Showmen even stole directly from town merchants.

Other aspects of amusement organizations' operations and the lifestyle of showmen were offensive or illegal as well. After the turn of the century the kooch show or girlie show, some of which were clan-

FREAK SHOW: THE INSTITUTION

destine, became a standard part of the traveling amusement industry. The constant travel also made carnivals and circuses excellent hideouts for criminals (Dadswell 1946). And some amusement organizations sold bootleg liquor and had prostitutes traveling with them.

Although it has been claimed that amusement organizations had largely cleaned up their operations by the 1930s (Gresham 1948, 103; "The Grifting Isn't So Good" 1924), nevertheless, drinking, gambling, kooch shows, gaffs, and grift remained pervasive, albeit sometimes behind the scenes—and sometimes unbeknownst to owners.[19] Sam Gumpertz was supposedly running the epitome of a clean show when he was manager of the Ringling Brothers, Barnum and Bailey Circus in the mid 1930s. But two people who worked as ticket sellers for that circus's freak show contend that shortchanging of customers was a regular practice (W. Wood 1980, 18; Holtman 1968). Wood reports that Clyde Ingalls, the manager of the freak show (Fig. 28), shortchanged customers, taking slugs from a whiskey bottle he kept hidden in the ticket box. No one ever claimed that the fraud and misrepresentation in the presentation of freaks was ever cleaned up—and it never was.

JUSTIFICATIONS

Hearing of the showmen's illegal and deceptive practices, one might ask, "How could they be so unscrupulous?" Our discussion of the amusement world, how it was forged and the perspective that was embodied in it, provides a partial answer. For amusement world people it was "us" versus "them," and anything was permissible. Their practices of deception flowed from this belief that "anything goes." In addition, as with other semi-isolated subcultures (youth gangs, convicts, drug addicts) whose practices are at variance with those of the mainstream, a defense of their ways became articulated and served to insulate showmen from outsiders' attacks. These standardized "accounts"[20] were then used to justify what others might consider to be reprehensible practices.

The justification that flowed most directly from the showmen's perspective was that their patrons "got what they deserved." As illustrated in this chapter, showmen felt deeply the hostility they encountered from towners. At times they were ridiculed, chastised, even beaten—and in addition they were forced to pay bribes and protection to the so-called law enforcement authorities. In the showmen's

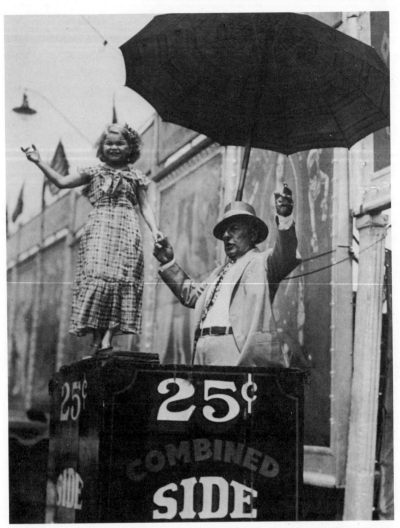

Fig. 28. Clyde Ingalls on ticket stand. Ingalls took over from Lew Graham as manager of the Ringling Brothers and Barnum and Bailey Combined Side Show. Standing with Ingalls is one of the Doll Family. Photographer unknown, c. 1930. (Pfening Coll., Columbus, Ohio.)

eyes, therefore, the rubes' hostility earned them what they got. Furthermore, twisting the story some, the showmen believed that the rubes would do the same thing to them if they could. Hoke Hammond, an old-time grifter, put it this way in a 1922 interview: "I never yet

FREAK SHOW: THE INSTITUTION

saw a rube who wasn't trying to do me, to take advantage of me at every turn, and to play the meanest kind of tricks and frauds on me. That's why it is hard to make grifters believe it's wrong to trim thousands when they are out to trim him" (E. Smith 1922, 12).

The "they deserved what they got" theme was also used in a different, and contrasting, context from the way Hoke used it. Here, grifting, rather than being a form of self-defense, was regarded as a normal reaction to the mark's stupidity. As showmen put it, anyone who could be fooled and cheated so easily was so dumb that he deserved to be taken. The logic here derives from the famous adage "A sucker is born every minute." If so many of them were born, they must have been born for some purpose. Clearly, that purpose was to be preyed upon.

In addition to the "they deserved what they got" line, showmen justified their fraudulence by saying that their practices did not really harm anyone. Taking this belief one step further, showmen even discussed their activities as actually benefiting locals. That is, rubes enjoyed being taken—it was a thrill for them, a break from their ordinary, humdrum existence. Showmen provided some spice in their lives, an opportunity to take risks and be touched by the amusement world. Following this line of thinking, people who ran freak shows justified their misrepresentation of exhibits by reasoning that if they did not lie, people would not enter the show. People had to be coaxed into spending a dime; but once they did, they received much more entertainment than they had paid for (Gorham 1951, 5; Circus Side Show Brought Up to Date 1931). Nate Eagle went so far as to tell an interviewer that even if he offered "an authentic two-headed baby" that turned out to be rubber, the audience had its money's worth in the incomparable thrill of anticipation (Taylor 1958b). In misrepresenting exhibits, showmen were doing rubes a favor.

In support of the account denying any harm was the doctrine that showmen were basically honest men. They even had an honor code of sorts. Part of the code involved selectivity in choosing victims, or at least so showmen claimed. A rigged-game operator remembered: "I never let a very old man or a younster or a girl or a woman play my game" (E. Smith 1922). Eddie Martin, shortchange artist for Yankee Robinson Circus, told his fellow worker Adrian Sharpe that in all his life he had never shorthanded a woman, a cripple, or a fool. Turning the explanation back into a "they deserved what they got" account, he finished his remarks by saying: "A fool had sense enough to count his change. The only person you can short is a man too smart to count his change" (Sharpe 1970, 32).

Not all justifications were directed at the customers. Showmen took the position that they did nothing that was very much different from what other businessmen did. As one carnival press agent put it; "Carnivals do not differ greatly from some of our own local stores when it comes to making suckers of the public. One of my friends in the merchandising business, puts regular two dollar dresses 'on sale' with blasting newspaper advertisements at twice the price customarily charged" (Dadswell 1946, 39).

Showmen did not define themselves as evil. Groups that defy societal norms seldom do. Their worldview and the justifications that grew from it helped make good work out of corrupt deeds. Some observers have even suggested that "the born showman is so earnest in manner and gesticulation, so leathern of lung, and so profuse—not to say incoherent—in opulent adjectives before potential patrons, that he at length believes implicitly in every statement he himself makes" (FitzGerald 1897a, 320).

Not all showmen participated as fully, not all organizations were as systematically involved, but to some extent everyone in the amusement world joined in tricking the public one way or the other. The exaggerated advertising, the humbug, the misrepresentation of freak exhibits constituted the mildest form of chicanery. The serious grifters went in for systemic stealing, cheating, and other illegalities—and all with management's blessing and cooperation.

The showmen's whole approach to their audiences can be summed up in one word: deception. They exaggerated, they appealed to curiosity and to status, and they used principles of persuasion and group dynamics to get customers to perform for them. One might be tempted to agree with showmen that some of their antics did not differ much from those of businessmen in other lines of work. To a certain extent this is true. Even modern high-power, hard-sell sales practices parallel those of the earlier showman. But the difference lay in the extent of their deception and the repertoire of their skulduggery. These systematic and accomplished liars, these Machiavellian small-time capitalists, had their own style of deception. They worked the crowds and took their patrons with turns of phrase and techniques of trickery developed and refined over the years. They loved it, and they took great

FREAK SHOW: THE INSTITUTION

pride in the power they had over those they duped. They were also light-hearted and delighted in dipping into their large repertoire of "Did you hear the one about the rube who . . ." jokes.

As the popular amusement industry developed during the nineteenth and early twentieth centuries, although the various segments of the business remained somewhat distinct, there was a blurring of forms. Showmen moved freely between organizations, and few felt committed to only one type of show. They lived together and traveled together, sharing a close community with strong barriers and antagonisms against outsiders. The culture they formed emphasized the distinction between those who were a part of this world and those who were not. Their worldview stressed hostility toward the customers, and justified and promoted illegal and fraudulent practices directed at the patrons. This chapter has described the nature and conditions that accompanied the development of that worldview, as well as various forms of grift and fraudulence that were an accepted part of the showman's way of life. Siamese twins attached by a corset (Johnson 1934c) and other forms of freak show deception were just part and parcel of the amusement world, an extension of the showman's approach to life. In the next chapter we will look in detail at freak show practices, at the fraudulent ways in which showmen constructed freak show exhibits.

4

Exotic and Aggrandized
Modes of Presenting Freaks

AT THE HEIGHT of the freak show's popularity, people strolling in urban entertainment districts or down midways were sure
to hear the strong voice of a freak show lecturer spieling to the
crowd:

> All for the insignificant sum of one dime, two nick-
> els, ten coppers, one-tenth of a dollar—the price of
> a shave or a hair ribbon. . . . The greatest, most
> astounding aggregation of marvels and monstrocities
> gathered together in one edifice.
>   Looted from the ends of the earth. From the wilds
> of darkest Africa, the miasmic jungles of Brazil, the
> mystic headwaters of the Yan-tse Kiang, the can-
> nibal isle of the Antipodes, the frosty slopes of the
> Himalayas, and the barren steppes of the Caucasus!
>   Sparing no expense, every town, every village,
> every hamlet, every nook and cranny of the globe
> has been searched with a fine-tooth comb to provide
> this feast for the eye and mind. A refined exhibition
> for cultured ladies and gentlemen. No waiting, no
> delays. Step up, ladies and gentlemen, and avoid
> the rush! Tickets now selling in the doorway. (Isman
> 1924, 79)

The best of these "talkers"—or "outside lectures" or "blowers"
(Bradna and Hartzell 1952, 236)—were orators who had mas-
tered the art of persuasion (Taylor 1958a,b,c; Wiley 1931). Their
job was to attract the crowd, to grab attention with their modu-
lating voices and slick talk. Using exaggeration and misrepresentation, they told passersby of the wonders that awaited them
for the price of one thin dime.
  The outside talkers were important advertisers for the freak

show. But they were only a small part of an elaborate system of promoting and presenting—constructing—freak exhibits that became standardized during the second half of the nineteenth century (Pfening 1977). This chapter explores the methods employed—the patterns and practices that became the freak show in the nineteenth century and defined it in the twentieth, vestiges of which can still be found in the few wilted shows of today. The physical aspects of the freak show—the bannerline, the inside of the tent—will be described, but the chapter's focus is on the content of the presentation, what the patrons were told about the exhibits, the messages embodied in the poses and exhibits took, and the routines they employed.

Clyde Ingalls, manager of the Ringling Brothers, Barnum and Bailey Sideshow in the 1930s, once said, "Aside from such unusual attractions as the famous three-legged man, and the Siamese twin combinations, freaks are what you make them. Take any peculiar looking person, whose familiarity to those around him makes for acceptance, play up that peculiarity and add a good spiel and you have a great attraction" (Beal 1938, 242). Ingalls points out that showmen produced freaks, but by using the three-legged man and the Siamese twins as exceptions he overlooked one thing: even with exhibits with blatant physical anomalies, freaks were what you made them. How they were packaged, how they were dressed, how they acted, and what the audience was told about them—their presentation was the crucial element in determining their success, in making a freak.

By using imagery and symbols they knew the public would respond to, showmen created for the person being exhibited a public identity, a presentation, a front, that would have the widest appeal, attract the most people, collect the most dimes. To accomplish this feat they took people—some of whom had abnormalities, but others who had only the desire to live the life of a trouper—and make freaks out of them.

Showmen fabricated freaks' backgrounds, the nature of their conditions, the circumstances of their current lives, and other personal characteristics. The actual life and circumstances of those being exhibited were replaced by purposeful distortions designed to market the exhibit, to produce a more appealing freak. In some cases mere fibs were told, with only a minor detail of the person's true identity altered—the albino from Australia was really from Brooklyn; the European midget prince actually came from an American family with modest means. In other cases half-truths were the rule. For example, Pirmal, a man from India who appeared in American freak shows at

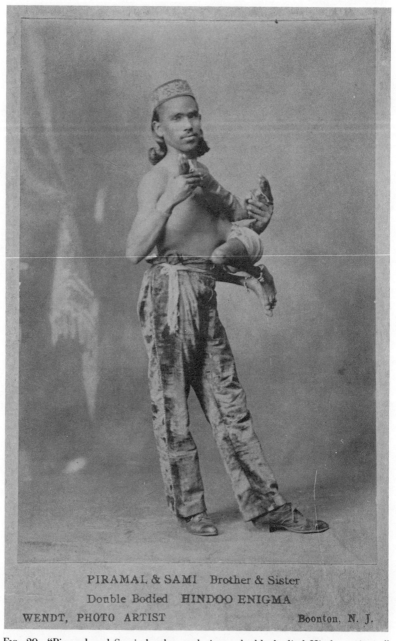

PIRAMAL & SAMI   Brother & Sister
Double Bodied   HINDOO ENIGMA
WENDT, PHOTO ARTIST   Boonton, N. J.

FIG. 29. "Piramal and Sami, brother and sister, double bodied Hindoo enigma."
Photo by Frank Wendt, c. 1902. (Becker Coll., Syracuse University.)

the turn of the century, actually had an underformed, atrophic, parasitic twin growing from his chest. But the twin's sex was, as always with Siamese twins, the same as the host's, not female as the audience was told. Misrepresenting the sex was just a ploy to heighten interest in "Pirmal and His Sister Sami, the Double-Bodied Hindo Enigma" (Fig. 29). William Durks, a 1930s carnival attraction (Lewis 1970, 73) took advantage of his severe cleft palate by painting a third eye in the crevice of his flaw and promoting a successful career as "the man with three eyes" (Mannix 1976, 154).

In other cases the deception was merely exaggeration—in publicizing size, inches were added to the height of giants (a twelve-inch inflation was common) or subtracted from that of dwarfs (McWhirter and McWhirter 1969, 10–12). In a similiar vein, young children who were presented as dwarfs were said to be older than they actually were, and young people presented as giants had years subtracted from their actual age. Thus dwarfs were made shorter for their age and giants taller. It was also common for giants to wear lifts and tall hats to make them appear taller. These tricks of deception were standardized, just the run-of-the-mill conventions of the business. The gaffed freaks, such as the Siamese twins who, in protest, walked off the stage on opposite sides, was only the extreme of fakery.[1] In the end, whether only a few white lies were used or distortion was all-pervasive, the presentation dominated showmen's approach to an exhibit.

This chapter concentrates on the two major patterns by which exhibits were presented to the public: the *exotic*, which cast the exhibit as a strange creature from a little-known part of the world; and the *aggrandized*, which endowed the freak with status-enhancing characteristics. Just as these modes were central to the freak show, so are they central to this book. The five chapters that follow (Part Two) contain graphic illustrations of presentations in the two modes. In Chapter 5, for example, we meet the Davis Brothers, who were exhibited in the exotic mode. Both were short and mentally retarded, but one was born in New York, the other in England. From 1852 until 1905 they were exhibited in dime museums and circus sideshows as the "Wild Men of Borneo" (Randall 1937). In Chapter 6 we meet the five-year-old, Connecticut-born Sherwood Stratton who, displayed in the aggrandized mode, became the eleven-year-old, English-born General Tom Thumb.

Promoting the Show

Before I discuss these two modes of presentation more explicitly, additional background on the freak show's physical arrangements, organization, and forms of promotion is necessary.

Since electronic advertising was either unavailable or impractical, it was necessary to use written publicity to promote the exhibits. Most shows had publicity men who hung posters, placed advertisements in merchants' windows, distributed handbills and couriers, placed ads in local papers, and staged publicity events. With traveling shows, this promotion was done by advance men—publicity men who arrived in town to promote the show a few days before the rest of the troupe arrived.

Not many posters featured freak shows, but printed handouts regularly introduced freak attractions to the public. Dime museums used handbills (one-page handouts distributed in the streets to publicize their attractions) extensively. Traveling shows frequently used advance couriers (publicity announcements in newspaper format distributed in advance of the show's arrival); in addition to advertising the big-top attractions, circus couriers—those distributed by Barnum affiliates, for example—often contained short, pithy, stylized descriptions of the featured freak attractions.

During the 1881 circus season, townspeople across New England were handed a courier featuring "The Unquestionable Goliath of the Century, CHANG, THE CHINESE GIANT, Undoubtedly the Tallest, Largest and Finest Proportioned Giant the Age Has Produced, Standing Nearly 9 Feet High in His Stocking Feet" (Fig. 30).

In a courier from about 1885 (Ringling Coll.) was found the fabricated "true life" story of "Jo-Jo, the Dog-Faced Russian Boy." Jo-Jo's real name was Theodor (or Fedor) Jeftichew, and he was truly a sight to behold, for from every part of his face grew long thick dark hair (a hairiness that was inherited). But his presentation was pure show world hoopla. The first few paragraphs of the courier story provide some of the flavor of this type of handout:

> By special permit from the Czar of all the Russias, we exhibit for the first and only time in the New World.
> THE MOST PRODIGIOUS PARAGON OF ALL PRODIGIES SECURED BY P. T. BARNUM IN OVER 50 YEARS. THE HUMAN—SKYE TERRIER THE CROWNING MYSTERY OF NATURE'S CONTRADICTIONS. This Incarnate Paradox, be-

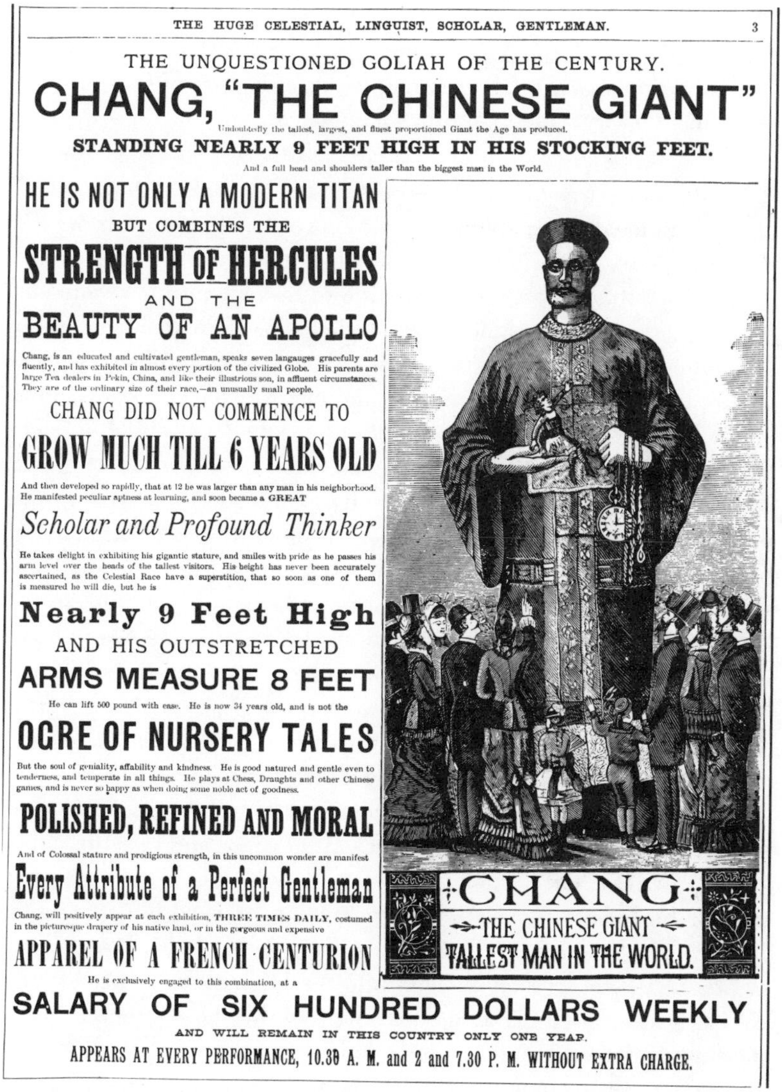

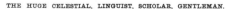

THE HUGE CELESTIAL, LINGUIST, SCHOLAR, GENTLEMAN. 3

THE UNQUESTIONED GOLIAH OF THE CENTURY.

CHANG, "THE CHINESE GIANT"

Undoubtedly the tallest, largest, and finest proportioned Giant the Age has produced.

STANDING NEARLY 9 FEET HIGH IN HIS STOCKING FEET.

And a full head and shoulders taller than the biggest man in the World.

HE IS NOT ONLY A MODERN TITAN

BUT COMBINES THE

STRENGTH OF HERCULES

AND THE

BEAUTY OF AN APOLLO

Chang, is an educated and cultivated gentleman, speaks seven languages gracefully and fluently, and has exhibited in almost every portion of the civilized Globe. His parents are large Tea dealers in Pekin, China, and like their illustrious son, in affluent circumstances. They are of the ordinary size of their race,—an unusually small people.

CHANG DID NOT COMMENCE TO

GROW MUCH TILL 6 YEARS OLD

And then developed so rapidly, that at 12 he was larger than any man in his neighborhood. He manifested peculiar aptness at learning, and soon became a GREAT

Scholar and Profound Thinker

He takes delight in exhibiting his gigantic stature, and smiles with pride as he passes his arm level over the heads of the tallest visitors. His height has never been accurately ascertained, as the Celestial Race have a superstition, that so soon as one of them is measured he will die, but he is

Nearly 9 Feet High

AND HIS OUTSTRETCHED

ARMS MEASURE 8 FEET

He can lift 500 pound with ease. He is now 34 years old, and is not the

OGRE OF NURSERY TALES

But the soul of geniality, affability and kindness. He is good natured and gentle even to tenderness, and temperate in all things. He plays at Chess, Draughts and other Chinese games, and is never so happy as when doing some noble act of goodness.

POLISHED, REFINED AND MORAL

And of Colossal stature and prodigious strength, in this uncommon wonder are manifest

Every Attribute of a Perfect Gentleman

Chang, will positively appear at each exhibition, THREE TIMES DAILY, costumed in the picturesque drapery of his native land, or in the gorgeous and expensive

APPAREL OF A FRENCH CENTURION

He is exclusively engaged to this combination, at a

CHANG
→ THE CHINESE GIANT ←
TALLEST MAN IN THE WORLD.

SALARY OF SIX HUNDRED DOLLARS WEEKLY

AND WILL REMAIN IN THIS COUNTRY ONLY ONE YEAR.

APPEARS AT EVERY PERFORMANCE, 10.30 A. M. and 2 and 7.30 P. M. WITHOUT EXTRA CHARGE.

FIG. 30. Chang the Chinese giant. Picture from an advance courier for P. T. Barnum's Greatest Show on Earth, 1881. (Becker Coll., Syracuse University.)

fore which Science stands confounded and blindly wonders, was found about thirteen years ago in company with his Dog-Faced Father, living in a remote cave in deep Kostroma Forests of Central Russia. They were first discovered by a hunter, and a party was formed who tracked

MODES OF PRESENTING FREAKS

99

them to their cave, and, after a desperate conflict, in which the savage father fought with all the fury of an enraged mastiff, their capture was effected. . . .

In addition to free printed handouts, various traveling shows placed paid ads in local newspapers. Large circuses had publicity crews who not only wrote and designed the paid ads but also wrote press releases about new attractions and human interest events, which were distributed to newspaper offices. The stories were often accompanied by a fistful of free tickets to serve as an inducement to publish.

Circus press agents like Tody Hamilton, Dexter Fellows (Fellows and Freeman 1936), Roland Butler (Plowden 1982) and Bev Kelly (Kelly 1982) were revered by showmen for their shrewd, trickster ways. They staged outrageous publicity stunts and then issued press releases to eager reporters, who often printed them verbatim. Freak birthday dinners, marriages between human oddities, medical and scientific examinations of curiosities, and, as we shall discuss in Chapter 10, a freak protest were all staged by these agents to spark interest and gain free publicity. Human-interest stories accompanied by photographs of freaks were a regular part of newspaper coverage well into the twentieth century. Circus press agents created stories, and local papers, hungry for copy, gobbled them up.

This written material was the first advertising assault. It was designed to heighten general awareness of the show and lure the public to the premises. The second line of assault was outside the freak show proper. Early on, attention-grabbing signs were used to decorate the facades of all freak show establishments (Pfening 1977; Weedon and Ward 1981). These soon evolved into the bannerline, a row of large canvas paintings strung along the length of the show's front and supposedly depicting the attractions inside (Fig. 31).

The bannerline paintings were wildly distorted representations. Exhibits with certain physical anomalies, for example, were often promoted as being part human and part beast: male exhibits with poorly formed arms were billed as the "The Seal Man"; with poorly formed legs, "The Frog Man"; with excesses of hair, "The Lion Man" or "Dog Boy"; and with a genetic anomaly that resulted in ectrodactylous hands (split down the middle with middle finger and metacarpal bone missing), "The Lobster Man." Banners advertising these exhibits showed the body of the animal with a human head.

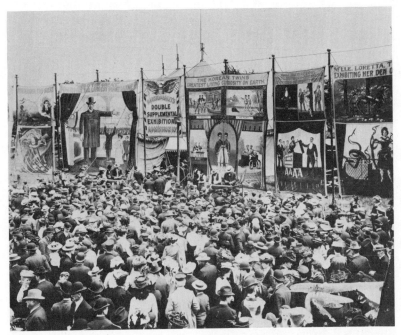

Fig. 31. Bannerline for Barnum and Bailey's Sideshow. Milling crowd begin to crowd the ticket sellers. Note the bannerline exaggeration. Photographer unknown, c. 1903. (Harvard Theater Collection, Cambridge, Massachusetts.)

Some banners gave the impression that an attraction was alive when in fact it was in a jar, preserved. Other banners depicted exhibits in thick jungle fighting wild animals or battling with their captors. Still others showed the exhibit dressed elegantly and being received by nobility. Bannerline paintings of midgets depicted exhibits as being so small that they could stand in the palm of a normal-sized person.

The outside advertisement for one carnival exhibit, "The Pig-Eyed Man," suggested that marks would actually see a person who was part swine. Inside was a man with his eyes bandaged. The lecturer, dressed in doctors' whites, explained to the rubes that the exhibit before them had just had the first pig to human cornea transplant.

When a British visitor to Boston was strolling past a dime museum in 1885, a banner advertising a "three-legged man" caught his eye. The exhibit was pictorially represented as possessing three symmetrical legs in a row, all three fashionably attired. The visitor entered to find that although the exhibit did in fact have three leg like appendages, the third was useless, shriveled and so small that it could easily be concealed (J. Wood 1885, 763).

One late-nineteenth-century observer summed up the effect of the dime museum facade thus: "The external promise is far in advance of the internal performance" (Campbell 1896, 466). As we shall see, the content of these and other promotional ploys grew out of the mode of presentation the showmen worked within in creating the exhibit.

The talker and his spiel introduced this chapter. (People who are "with it" and write about the amusement world are redundant in pointing out that "barker" is not a word that insiders use.) His call to the crowd was the next line of assault in promoting the freak show (C. Fox and Parkinson 1969). Be it in front of a dime museum, a circus sideshow, or a freak show that was part of an amusement park or carnival, the talker always employed a "bally" (also called a "ballyhoo"), one of the exhibits, who came out front to lure customers closer. A scantily clad woman with a python around her neck, a blatantly deformed person in colorful dress, or a flamboyant fire eater would serve the purpose. On a midway, the bally stood on the bally platform, a small stage four feet off the ground, which stood at the center of the bannerline and close to the entrance.

Attracting a crowd around the outside talker and his bally was necessary for getting patrons, but the crucial maneuver involved transforming the attentive observers into paying patrons, a manipulation they called "turning the tip." This feat required clever verbal transitions and deceptive ploys. The marks watching the bally were told, "If you think what you are seeing is good—wait until you get inside." Shills, show employees planted in the audience, then bought tickets in an attempt to get the real customers moving.

In the typical show, ticket sellers flanked the entrance. The talker directed the audience to the high, boxlike sellers' stands, where tickets were sold from large rolls the employees held in their quick hands. (The arrangements were slightly different for dime museums, where crowds were not as thick and the intensity not as great.)

Ticket purchasers would then be moved quickly inside, where the exhibits were lined up around the periphery on raised platforms (Fig. 32). (In the case of some dime museums, the audience might have to climb stairs to another floor to reach "the hall of curiosities.") An inside lecturer would greet the incoming crowd, drawing its attention to each exhibit in turn and telling fabricated tales about each attraction.

102   FREAK SHOW: THE INSTITUTION

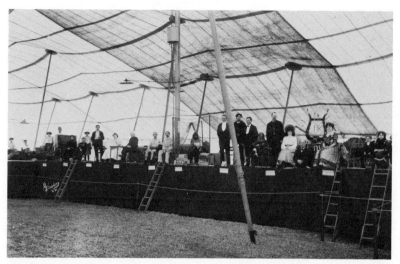

Fig. 32. Inside 1904 sideshow. When this photograph was taken, the Barnum and Bailey Sideshow exhibits were on the platform waiting for the first rubes of the day. Note the photographs on display and for sale in front of some of the exhibits. Photo by Fred Glasier. (Ringling Museum of the Circus, Sarasota, Florida.)

Although some freaks would just sit observing the observers, most actively performed. The wild man would look ferocious, pace up and down, and growl; the armless women would demonstrate her prowess with her feet. With some, the lecturer might break from his monologue to let the exhibit provide autobiographical comments. Certain exhibits played musical instruments, sang, danced, or performed novelty acts. But whatever they did, however they appeared, their act had to correspond to the fabricated image that was created for them, and it had to be short. The inside lecturer had to keep the crowd moving to make space for the next batch of customers.

The audience was not rushed so fast as to deprive them of the opportunity to buy souvenirs from the "curiosities." The carefully posed freak photographic portraits and fabricated "true life story and facts" booklets which were so central to the presentation of the exhibit (see Chapter 1) were readily available. In addition to these artifacts, exhibits sold other trinkets. In this century, for example, giants took to selling huge rings, allegedly the size of their finger, and some midgets sold miniature Bibles as momentos.

One last aspect of the freak show, which became standard at the end of the nineteenth century, was the "blowoff." Usually part of the finale, the blowoff consisted of yet another attraction patrons could view—if they paid the additional charge. The added exhibit was puffed up extravagantly to lure the mark into surrendering more change. In some cases showmen actually kept their best exhibits for the blowoff, but more often it was an optical illustration: the headless women was a favorite. In some minor shows the blowoff was promoted as "for adult males only," giving the impression that the customer was buying a peek at nudity—which in some instances he was. More often, however, it was just a trick to get the man to pay more.

The pitches that freak show promoters used in selling tickets contained the same general appeals other entrepreneurs employ in promoting other shows, cars, or even vacuum cleaners (Bogdan 1972).[2] Exhibits were presented as unique, or the best of their kind, or one of a category never seen before. Most giants were presented as the tallest in the world, and most dwarfs as the shortest. All exhibits were recommended by, or associated with, prestigious people and organizations—scientists, doctors, clergy, newspapers, and professional organizations. Additionally, people were told of the great popularity of the exhibits—of the need to act quickly so as not to miss the chance of a lifetime. Freak shows were heralded as more than frivolous amusement: they were morally uplifting, educational, and prudent. The price was right as well, too much of a bargain to pass by, particularly if one believed the talker's description of the great time and expense involved in getting the exhibits from far-off lands, not to mention the high salaries some of the human oddities allegedly received. These ploys, many of which have become the clichés of the sales industry, were liberally injected into the promotion of exhibits.

Some general tactics of promotion were unique to the freak show world. Believing that exhibits were better draws if kept from public view, some managers allowed their freaks to show themselves only when on stage. Prior to the invention of the automobile, this practice resulted in the expression "carriage freak" (Ford 1904), which referred to exhibits arriving and departing in covered horse-drawn carriages and never appearing in public.

Modes of Presentation

In addition to the appeals and strategies already discussed, showmen developed two highly stylized modes of presenting freaks: the exotic mode and the aggrandized mode.[3] By "mode of presentation" I mean a standardized set of techniques, strategies, and styles that showmen used to construct freaks. These two modes, then, provided the for-

FREAK SHOW: THE INSTITUTION

mulas for the fabrications that made up the "true life stories," the staged appearance, the freak portraits, the banners, and other aspects of the freak promotion.

THE EXOTIC PRESENTATION

In the exotic mode, showmen presented the exhibit so as to appeal to people's interest in the culturally strange, the primitive, the bestial, the exotic. Promoters told the audience that the exhibit came from a mysterious part of the world—darkest Africa, the wilds of Borneo, a Turkish harem, an ancient Aztec kingdom. In a few outrageous cases, the place of origin was claimed to be extraterrestial: in the 1920s and 1930s, Eko and Iko, brothers with albinism and dreadlocks, were presented as ambassadors from Mars discovered near the remains of their spaceship in the Mojave Desert (Mannix 1976, 130); and giants and dwarfs in one Coney Island exhibition were dressed in strange costumes and included in the "Trip to the Moon" display.

The geographic place of origin was most often in the non-Western world, but occasionally American venues such as native American villages or the wilds of the far western mountains were used. The lecturer and the "true life story" booklet would tell of the person's origins, giving specific and purposefully erroneous and distorted information about the life and customs of the freak's alleged homeland and his or her place in that society. Tales of albinos, for example, contained accounts of their having been either worshiped or, more usually, prepared for sacrifice (*The History and Life of Unzie* 1893). The sacrifices were cut short by an explorer who saved the albino's life by rescuing him or her from the tribe. Some stories were so elaborate they took forty pages to tell.

Dressed in a style that was compatible with the story, the exhibit would behave consistently with the front. "Wild men" or "savages" might grunt or pace the stage, snarling, growling, and letting off warrior screams. Dress might include a loincloth, a string of bones around the neck, and, in a few cases, chains—allegedly to protect the audience from the beast before them. In the case of people who were supposedly from the Middle East or the Orient, the presentation and the performance would be characteristically more sedate, with the freak acting out in exaggerated, stereotypic ways the presumed mannerisms and customs of the countries they represented. Here the dress consisted of flowing robes, turbans, and silks.

Freaks displayed in the exotic mode appeared in their photos in front of a painted backdrop depicting jungle scenes or exotic lands. Papier-mâché boulders, imitation tropical plants, and other touches of exotica often added a three-dimensional flair to the set.

The stories used in presenting exhibits were created to maximize interest. Because the period of concern was a time of intense world exploration and Western expansion, news events provided some of the scripts and descriptions for the presentation of freaks. Thus, when Stanley and Livingston were lost in the "dark continent" and the imperialist British were fighting those they were colonizing, the "savage African" was a popular motif (Lindfors 1984, 1983a, 1983b). Late in the nineteenth century and early in the twentieth, when the United States took the Philippines from Spain and was fighting the indigenous people, a Philippine backdrop was prominent.

An important source of stories to be used in the promotion of freaks was the scientific reports and travelogues of nineteenth- and early-twentieth-century natural scientists. Pre- and post-Darwinian discussions about the place of human beings in the great order of things and the relationship of the various kinds of humans to each other and to baboons, chimps, and gorillas were in the air (S. Gould 1981; W. Jordan 1968; Gossett 1963). Scientific writing on classification and anthropological reports about the "races of man" and "missing links" (Stanton 1960; Greene 1959) provided the ideas for show decorations and for details of the plots to be presented in the exotic mode.

While the different-species explanation was the most popular in presenting "exotic" exhibits, scientists provided a broader range of theories for showmen to choose from. Exotic-mode explanations of people who were blatantly different or who had obvious physical and mental disabilities were sometimes bolstered by the "hybridity" theory, for example (Warkany 1959). This theory posited that certain malformations were the result of crossbreeding man with beast. The comparisons showmen made between exhibits' malformations and certain animal structures ("the seal man," for instance) also implied a biological link. Another popular explanation which fit nicely with certain exotic presentations was the "atavistic" or "throwback" theory. The basic premise here was that humans could give birth to children who were reversions to more "primitive" forms of life, including less-developed species of humans (S. Gould 1981).

Natural scientists who examined freaks were often asked to authenticate subjects' origins and credibility; their commentaries then frequently appeared in newspapers and publicity pamphlets (Altick 1978, chap. 20). Some exhibits were presented to scientific societies for discussion and speculation (see Altick 1978, 284–287; Warren 1851; Bouvé 1880). The use of the word *museum* in the title of many freak shows attests to the association of this form of entertainment with natural science (Betts 1959), as does the practice of calling freak show lecturers "professor" or "doctor" (Pfening, Jr., 1983). The linking of freak exhibits with science made the attractions more interesting, less frivolous to puritanical antientertainment sentiments, and more believable.

In the most blatant distortion under the exotic mode, native-born Americans were misrepresented as foreigners—Ohio-raised dwarfs from Borneo; a tall, black, North Carolinian from Dahomey. But the exotic mode was not employed only for native-born Americans. Many of the exhibited freaks actually were from the non-Western lands, and some were even born in the countries the promoters claimed they were ("Freak Hunting through India" 1894; Johnston 1934c). Here the distortion and misrepresentation came in the exaggerated details of the culture and the person exhibited with the odd, bizarre, erotic, and savage being highlighted (Rydell 1984). Favorite themes included cannibalism, human sacrifices, head hunting, polygamy, unusual dress, and food preferences that were disgusting to Americans (eating dogs, rodents, insects, and dirt). If the culture of origin was sedate and the people's practices not shocking, the promoter's imagination could fix the situation by lies and extravagant, overstated claims.

Non-Western people with demonstrable physical differences—those who were very tall, very short, without arms and legs, Siamese twins, and so on—were exhibited within the exotic motif through emphasis of their anomalies as well as their "strange ways." But many freaks who were brought from abroad had nothing "wrong" with them physically. They were generally referred to as freaks and often shared the freak show platform with people we would describe as having disabilities, but all that made them freaks really was the promoters' racist presentations of them and their culture (Butler 1936).

In the exotic mode, promoters showed seemingly unlimited imagination. A wide variety of motifs were used with a multitude of variations on a theme, of which missing links, wild men, savages, lost tribes, animal people, harem refugees, and escapees from death or torture are but a few.

THE AGGRANDIZED PRESENTATION

In the exotic mode the emphasis was on how different and, in most cases, inferior the person on exhibit was. With the aggrandized mode the presentation emphasized how, with the exception of the particular physical, mental, or behavioral condition, the freak was an upstanding, high-status person with talents of a conventional and socially prestigious nature. Under this mode some exhibits were presented as prototypical Americans—the prim and proper girl next door, or the down-home, really tall Texan—and others as sophisticated ladies and gentlemen from abroad. One, some, or all of the following attributes were fabricated, elevated or exaggerated, and then flaunted: social position, achievements, talents, family, and physiology.

Freaks in the aggrandized mode were given high-status titles such as "Captain," "Major," "General," "Prince," "King," "Princess," or "Queen." Since Americans looked up to Europe and England as being culturally superior, changing common-sounding names to those suggestive of European or British birth was common. In some exhibits' aggrandized-mode presentations, the public was told that the freak was highly educated, spoke many languages, and had snobbish hobbies such as writing poetry or painting. In addition, the exhibits were linked with well-known and high-status people in Europe and the United States. Having had an audience with royalty or with the president was a commonly fabricated and flaunted accomplishment. Of course, similar claims were made for freaks cast in the exotic mode, but with the aggrandized the publicity suggested that the exhibit belonged in the same social circle as celebrities. These were no mere scientific specimens, but a loftier breed entirely.

The aggrandized-status mode meant dressing the part as well. For some exhibits this involved expensive jewelry and stylish clothes— top hats and tails, evening gowns, furs, and other accoutrements of fine taste lavishly displayed. For others it merely entailed being very clean, neat, and respectably dressed.

Another way of enhancing the exhibited person was to flaunt conventional, but status-significant, organizational affiliations and attainments. Membership and offices held in the Masons, Eastern Stars, the Daughters of the American Revolution, and churches were mentioned in lectures and pamphlets and listed on the backs of freak photographic portraits. An Eisenmann photograph of Anna Leak Thompson, "The Armless Lady" (M. Mitchell 1979), pictures her with insignia from her father's Masonic chapter as well as a "footmade" embroidered shawl decorated with religious symbols. Some of the "human curiosities" also wore pins and displayed other symbols of their affiliations while on the platform.

Performances in the aggrandized-status mode were of two types. The first involved doing tasks that one might assume could not be done by a person with that particular disability. A man without legs, for example, might walk and perform acrobatic feats using his arms. The emphasis was on how the person exhibited compensated for the disability. The second kind of performance was more standard show business and included such talents as singing, dancing, and playing a musical instrument (see Chapter 7). The emphasis in this type of performance was on the superior talents and accomplishments of the freak. As we shall see, troupes of singing, dancing, and acting midgets became quite common in freak shows in the twentieth century.

Status aggrandizement was also accomplished by emphasizing the normalcy of the freak's spouse, children, and family life. Many of the photographic portraits that exhibits sold show them with their families against a sitting-room backdrop with stuffed chairs and other symbols of middle-class status. "True life" booklets and the lecturers' descriptions sometimes dwelled on the exhibit's family role and on the accomplishments of the spouse and children. In the case of child freaks, the normalcy of the parents and siblings was portrayed. Sometimes the parents were displayed along with the freak.

People who were exhibited in the aggrandized mode tended to be presented as physically normal, or even superior, in all ways except the one anomaly that was their alleged reason for fame. Emphasis, especially in the presentation of midgets and giants, was placed on the fact that a person was—as the showmen would say—"physically attractive and perfectly formed in every way, and, in no way distasteful so as to offend the audience."

In discussing the aggrandized-status mode of promoting freaks, I do not mean to suggest that all the exhibits were actually devoid of the status-enhancing characteristics attributed to them. In fact, it was easier to succeed in using this mode if the person's characteristics were somewhat compatible with the front. If a woman was charming, a countess, had a wonderful voice, wrote poetry, dressed impeccably, was married to a king, and had five talented and handsome children—and was a midget—a promoter would not have to fabricate anything to enhance this person's status. Yet, while the freak show was not devoid of Europeans or attractive middle-class Americans, most of the recruits were people of lesser station (Bradna and Hartzell 1952, 241). And even those who were truly outstanding could benefit from some embellishing and uplifting.

With the exotic-mode presentation, stories were borrowed from imperialistic excursions and natural-scientific explorations. On occasion physicians were called on to examine the specimen, but for the most part the freak was presented as belonging in the domain of anthropologists or zoological and philosophical classifiers. In the aggrandized mode, in contrast, teratology provided the scientific underpinnings for the presentation (see G. Gould and Pyle 1896; Jones 1888). Medical testimonials and pronouncements were generally used as part of the status-enhanced presentation, and lengthy quotations by such experts sometimes appeared in the "true life" booklets as well. Emphasis was always on the fact that the anomaly was a specific condition and did not reflect on the integrity or morality of the exhibit or on his or her parents.

In the nineteenth century the question of what caused the condition if raised, was most frequently addressed with the theory of "maternal impression." Lecturers and "true life" booklets attributed traumatic or significant events experienced by a pregnant woman as an important teratogenic factor.[4] Two different, but closely related, explanations for deformities fell under the maternal impression theory. In one, the "photographic" theory (Warkany 1959), the form the child took was directly related to the kind of experience the mother had had. The explanation provided for one woman's giving birth to Siamese twins was that she had become upset during her pregnancy at seeing dogs unable to disconnect while copulating. Lionel, "The Lion-Faced Boy" (a man with thick hair all over his face who was exhibited during the first decade of the twentieth century), it was explained to the audience, was born that way because his mother, while pregnant, had observed Lionel's father being mauled to death by a lion. In the other maternal impression explanation, the specific circumstances of the fright or distress experienced by the expectant mother had no direct or necessary relationship to the morphology of the abnormality. Thus Charles Stratton blamed his small size on his mother's grief over the death of the family dog.

The theory of maternal impression was alive and well in late-nineteenth-century America, and not only in the freak show (Jessup 1888). In Keating's 1889 *Cyclopedia of the Diseases of Children* a whole chapter, "Maternal Impressions," is devoted to case descriptions (Warkany 1959).

Maternal impression and many other nineteenth-century teratological explanations of congenital abnormality may not have been more valid than earlier theories, but they were more humane and harmless, for they castigated neither the child nor the parent. They were also more scientific, in that the causal factor was less rooted in religion. A deformed child, according to these newer theories, was not the work of the devil or the sign of a forthcoming disaster; it was a puzzle that could be solved rationally. Thus, although showmen offered explanations for their exhibits' conditions, they also encouraged the audience to think and speculate for themselves.

In the nineteenth and early twentieth centuries, medical experts gave opinions on exhibits with glorified presentations, but, as was discussed in Chapter 2, these people were not presented as patients or as being "sick."[5] Before 1900 little was known about genetics and the endocrine system. Teratology was primarily a science of classification. The causes of the exhibits' conditions were therefore open for crowd speculation, with theories of maternal impression dominating both presentations and explanations (Jessup 1888). With the rediscovery of Mendel's genetic principles, the development of the eugenics movement, and advanced understanding of the thyroid and pituitary glands, freaks increasingly became the subject of newspaper articles which described them as being "sick" and as belonging in the domain of physicians, not of public speculation. This medical takeover, together with the eugenics movement (Haller 1963; Ludmerer 1972), began in the first three decades of the century to undermine the tradition of enhancing exhibits' status ("Circus and Museum Freaks" 1908; Lees 1937; "Amusements at the Abnormal" 1908; Stanley 1914; Johnston 1934c). Presentations became less embellished, explanations of cause more straightforward.

Although the aggrandized mode became well developed, rivaling the exotic mode in the frequency with which it was employed, this mode allowed fewer possibilities for variety than the exotic.

Characteristics of People and Modes of Presentation

What factors determined the mode, exotic or aggrandized, in which a would-be freak would be cast? To some extent particular kinds of anomalies typed the person within one mode or the other. People with microcephaly, for example, a condition associated with mental retardation and characterized by a very small, pointed head and small overall stature, were cast as "missing links" or as atavistic specimens of an extinct race. Hypopituitary dwarfs (commonly referred to as midgets), who tend to be well proportioned and physically attractive, were cast as lofty. Achondroplastic dwarfs, whose head and limbs tend to be out of proportion to their trunk, were cast in the exotic mode. Armless, legless, and limbless people were regularly cast as exalted, although occasionally they would appear in the exotic as animal-people (the "snake man," the "seal man"). While a person with a particular disability might more likely be cast in one mode than another, one's physical anomaly was not always the crucial factor. A very tall person, for example, might have the option of being a warrior from a lost civilization or a European prince (Figs. 33 and 34) (*Aaron Moore* c. 1899).

The potential freak's background, appearance, and other personal characteristics, together with the manager's judgment of audience responsiveness, were crucial in deciding a person's presentation. Promoters chose the particulars of the story as well as the general mode of presentation so as to be somewhat compatible with the characteristics of the person to be exhibited. A slovenly, inarticulate, slow, socially inept person, for instance, would not likely be cast as a prince.

Skin color was also an important consideration. Blacks tended to be cast as missing links or savages (Lindfors 1983a). Caucasian native-born Americans were cast within the exotic mode less frequently than blacks, and when they were, they were said to be from the South Sea Islands or South America. Although the presentation and the characteristics of the person exhibited often were congruent, promoters employed much creativity with their tales: "exotic" caucasians might be presented as having lived among or been raised by or tortured by non-Western people following their capture, kidnapping, or being washed ashore after a shipwreck. The standard presentation of "human art galleries" involved tattooing as a torture inflicted on an exhibit by a barbaric people (Parry 1933). Topping the list of blatant fabrication and audacity is the 1930s presentation of a young man and woman, both white Americans with microcephaly, as albinos from a head-binding tribe in Africa (Holtman 1968).

If managers were able to secure potential freaks as children, they could train them to fit the mode most advantageous to their careers. Some of the most famous exhibits in the flaunting status pattern were carefully groomed and trained for exhibit. Millie and Christine, black

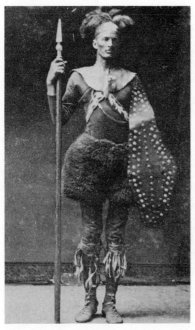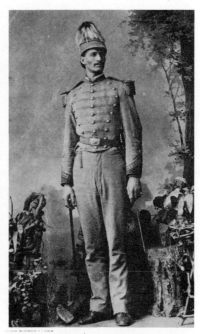

Figs. 33 and 34. Two ways of presenting a giant. In the photograph on the left, a very tall black man is shown as an exotic Zulu. On the right, the same man is cast as an aggrandized military figure. Photos by Charles Eisenmann, c. 1880. (Becker Coll., Syracuse University.)

Siamese twins born in slavery, became the celebrated Victorian "singing nightingales." Similarly, the Hilton Sisters, twentieth-century Siamese twins, were trained to sing in harmony and play musical instruments as part of their high-status presentation; the publicity had them as well-mannered, properly raised, well-adjusted young women. Barnum carefully prepared Charles Stratton, a man born to a family of modest means, to hobnob with society's elite as General Tom Thumb.

A less drastic case of the preparation of a person for the freak role was that of the very tall Texas Jack Shields, one of four brothers who became giants. In 1880 a reporter quoted his manager as saying:

> we are training him to be a giant, and we think that he
> will grow to be the tallest man in the business. He needs
> watching having been accustomed all his life to lower
> himself to talk to his companions, and to allow his arms
> to hang loosely by his side, and to spread out his legs, he
> is yet raw and awkward for the giant business; but now he
> is getting to hold his head up and keep his feet together

and throw his shoulders back, to keep himself in shape, to take flesh and get more height (Source unknown, Hertzberg Coll.)

Complexity in the Modes of Presentation

The exotic and aggrandized modes of presentation represent clear patterns, but they do not capture the entire range of freak images nor do they suggest the complexity in the imagery of many exhibits. In many cases, especially in the mid–nineteenth century, the presentations were played straight—that is, the exhibit was presented with the serious intent that the audience should believe the facade. With other exhibits, and increasingly toward the last decade of the nineteenth and into the twentieth century, the presentation was more whimsical, containing elements of farce, mockery, ridicule, and humor.

The presentation of extremely obese exhibits came closest to a purely mocking mode. People who weighed over five hundred pounds took on such names as "Tiny Brown, "Baby Ruth," "Alpine," Jolly Trixie," and "Dolly Dimples." Huge women wore dainty, little girl's outfits, danced soft shoe, and chuckled. Although a few exhibits were dressed as clowns and cast as fools (such as the 1930's attraction Koo-Koo "The Bird Girl"), the direct presentation of exhibits in a clearly distinguishable humorous mode, separate from the exotic and aggrandized modes, never fully developed. Rather, comic or mocking elements were simply incorporated into the dominant mode, usually as exaggeration. The fabrications, the appearance of the freak, and the overall presentation were so outlandish that both the manager and most of the audience shared a sense of the ridiculous. The lecturer would acknowledge his participation in the farce with asides, humor, and commentary. In some cases he was quite subtle, presenting the exhibit to one segment of the audience, the more worldly, as a farce, but to the more naive, straight. By being able to play this borderline between farce and seriousness, showmen could often avoid confrontations with members of the audience who wanted to yell out and expose the fraud; instead they could have the audience participate in the hoax, much as adults acknowledge Santa's existence in the presence of children.

The exotic and aggrandized modes were not always played in their pure form. Some freaks were presented in a mixed mode, with elements borrowed from each, and interest and sometimes humor derived from the juxtaposition of incongruity.[6] Prince Randian is a good example. This armless and legless man was presented as royalty, together with, very prominently, his wife, Princess Sarah, and his four children. His performance included rolling and lighting a cigarette with his lips and showing the audience how he shaved, unaided. But Randian was also billed as "The Snake Man" or "The Caterpillar Man"; here, wearing a one-piece woolen garment that covered him like a sack, he wiggled his hips and shoulders and moved about like a serpent.

A famous example of a mixed-mode presentation was Krao Farini, a hirsute female from Laos (Howard 1977, 56; Drimmer 1973, 162; Fellows and Freeman 1936, 297). In the 1880s, when still a child, she started her freak career as "Darwin's Missing Link"—halfway between human and monkey—in which she was fraudulently presented as having pouches in her mouth, prehensile toes, cartilage in her nose, and other simian features (Hutchinson, Gregory, and Lydekker c. 1895). Although "Darwin's Missing Link" was part of her presentation all through her life, as she entered her teens she began to be presented as a cultured, intelligent lady who spoke five languages. In the case of Krao, the juxtaposition of the beastly with the refined created novel incongruities that, judging from her long and successful career, had an obvious public appeal.

As Krao's case suggests, some exhibits changed their mode of presentation in the course of their careers. In the early stages of a career, managers often tried different modes to see which appealed to the audience and best fit the person behind the facade. Aaron Moore, a very tall black man from North Carolina, first appeared as a freak dressed in a savage costume and wearing chains, being exhibited in the exotic mode as a wild man (*Aaron Moore* c. 1899). Later in his career he was presented in the aggrandized mode, wearing a fancy military outfit, as Aaron Moore, "The Colored Giant." Eko and Iko, the black albinos who ended being displayed as "ambassadors from Mars," were earlier in their careers unsuccessfully promoted as members of a colony of "sheep-headed cannibals" from the South Seas (Robeson 1935, 276; Bradna and Hartzell 1952, 237).

In some cases the mode of presentation changed to fit the changing characteristics of the person or the society. The original "Siamese twins," Chang and Eng, for example, were first displayed with emphasis on their cultural differences, exotic dress, and habits (Hunter 1964): in early publicity drawings they appear in oriental dress and pigtails. Later in their careers, however, after they had been westernized, they wore American suits and ties and flaunted the fact that they were each married and had large families. In a late Currier and Ives advertisement they are depicted in various status-enhancing scenes of dignity (Durant and Durant 1957).

By the early twentieth century the audience was learning to view freaks as people who were sick—who had various genetic and endocrine disorders[7]—and exotic hype lost its appeal. The razzle-dazzle died down, to be replaced by a more staid presentation. The "talker" began using a microphone, and the "true life" booklets became shorter and much less embellished. The carefully posed, professional-quality photographic images that the freaks sold were replaced by poor-quality postcards.

Part One has presented the historical and conceptual background by which we can understand the idea of the freak as a social construction. We traced the development of the practice of exhibiting people for amusement and profit and introduced some of the major personalities, events, organizations, and forces that helped to mold the freak show. In particular we saw how the amusement world—the showman's culture—was created, and how dimensions of that culture contributed to the social construction of freaks. Finally, we explored the methods showmen used to construct freaks, with special attention to the exotic and aggrandized modes of presentation.

The "modes of presentation" approach provides an alternative to the categorization of sideshow exhibits on the basis of physiological characteristics; it therefore helps us avoid the trap of seeing freaks as objective facts. The modes, moreover, reveal the implicit assumptions embodied in the freak show world by allowing us to focus on the institution of exhibiting people and the perspective of those involved.

II Profiles of Presentation

In the five chapters that follow I provide extensive illustrations of freak constructions. Using the background presented in Part One, and in particular the modes of presentation discussed in the Chapter 4, the chapters in Part Two are organized around the exotic and aggrandized modes of presentation. The chapters alternate between illustrations of exotic and the aggrandized presentations. While my concern is with specific examples of the construction of exhibits, I am also interested in general patterns, issues, and concepts illustrated by particular genre of exhibits.

5

The Exhibition of People We Now Call Retarded

ISAAC N. KERLIN, M.D., superintendent of the Pennsylvania Training School for Feebleminded Children, knew that the 1876 Centennial Exposition in Philadelphia would attract prominent
people from all parts of the country. Capitalizing on the event,
he invited representatives of the handful of American institutions for the "idiotic and feebleminded" to meet in the small
town of Mead, outside Philadelphia. There the American Association on Mental Deficiency, an organization that grew to be
the largest and most influential professional association concerned with mental retardation in America, was born (Sloan and
Stevens 1976, 1).

No complete record of the group's activities exists, but given
the location of the conference and the participants' interests, it
is reasonable to presume that they toured the exposition. It is
also probable that the founders of this prestigious association
visited the "Wild Australian Children," whom showmen were
exhibiting as freaks on Elm Street.

If alive today, these fraudulently presented "wild" humans
would be classified as mentally retarded. In 1876, however,
showmen could take advantage of the fact that even scientists
were confused about the origin and cause of the exhibits' unusual
condition. Continuing a pattern that had begun over twenty-five
years earlier and that would not end until the demise of the freak
show, showmen constructed exhibits using people we would now
call mentally retarded by casting them in an extreme form of the
exotic mode.

The "Wild Australian Children," whose presentation contained numerous elements of the developing stylized pattern,
are a prime example of this type of manufactured exhibit. They
were described by showmen as members of a near-extinct can-

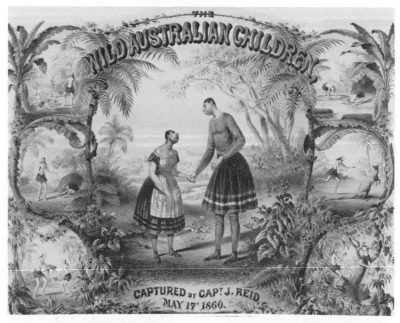

FIG. 35. "The Wild Australian Children." The scenes to the sides depict their exotic "precapture" environment. 1860 lithographic advertisement. (Harvard Theater Collection, Cambridge, Massachusetts.)

nibal tribe from the interior of Australia who had been captured by the explorer-adventurer Captain Reid (Fig. 35). Concocted publicity pamphlets, which were for sale at their appearances, emphasized that "phrenologists and other scientific men" were of the opinion that they were "neither idiots, lusus naturae, nor any other abortion of humanity, but belonged to a distinct race hitherto unknown to civilization" (*Adventures of the Three Australian Travelers* 1864; *Adventures of an Australian Traveler* 1872). Their small and "most curiously shaped heads of any human being ever seen" are described as adapting them "for creeping through the tall, rank grass of their native plains, and springing upon the sleeping game or unsuspecting foe" (*Adventures of an Australian Traveler* 1872).

Actually, the "Wild Australian Children" were Tom and Hettie, severely retarded microcephalic siblings from Circleville, Ohio—a secret known only to people in the amusement world (Coup 1901). They were, in the vernacular of showmen, "pinheads." First exhibited in 1860 (poster, Harvard Coll.), they were a popular exhibit for over thirty years.[1]

PORTRAITS OF PRESENTATION

There is no evidence from the writings or recorded statements of the founders of the American Association on Mental Deficiency that they would have shunned such an exhibit. No scientist or professional of the nineteenth century is on record as calling any freak show distasteful. In fact, as will be seen in the chapters that follow and particularly in this one, scientists and medical practitioners aided and abetted such displays by visiting, examining, and commenting on exhibits (G. Gould and Pyle 1896). They made reference to them in their learned writings.[2] "Human curiosities" were the object of scientific speculation, and although scientists often disagreed with the explanations showmen provided to the public, these explanations paralleled scientific theories about human variation.

In this chapter we trace the careers of five exhibits, mentally retarded in modern terms, who began appearing on freak show platforms in the mid–nineteenth century.[3] These five are important because they had long careers, were seen by millions, and their presentations became the prototypes for later exhibits. They are: Hiram and Barney Davis, brothers who were exhibited as "The Wild Men of Borneo"; Maximo and Bartola, "The Aztec Children"; and William Henry Johnson, who soloed as "What Is It?" or "Zip." The chapter concludes with a discussion of patterns and trends in the exhibition of people we would now call retarded and relationships between exhibits and scientific writings.

Hiram and Barney Davis

In the Mount View Cemetery at Mount Vernon, Ohio, stands a headstone that reads:

<blockquote>
Little Men
Hiram Davis 1825–1905
Barney Davis 1827–1912
</blockquote>

Hiram and his parents, David and Catherine, were born in England and lived there until 1827 when they migrated to the United States, where Barney was born on Long Island, New York.[4] The boys grew up on a farm in Ohio with the other Davis children, two daughters and a son.

Their parents and brother and sisters were of normal stature and intelligence. Hiram and Barney, however, each approximately three and one-half feet tall, were referred to as "dwarfs."[5] One official court record lists them as "imbeciles" ("Wild Men of Borneo" 1973), and people who met them described them as "mentally deficient" or "mentally defective." Their small, thin (they weighed approximately forty pounds each), straight bodies were accented by strong, wiry muscles. Their fair skin, light silky hair, and blue eyes gave them a Scandinavian appearance—not that of natives from far-off Borneo (for pictures, see Roth and Cromie 1980).

The boys' father died, and Mrs. Davis married a Mr. Porter, with whom she had one other normal child. Around 1852, when the brothers were in their mid twenties, a showman, Lyman Warner, visited the Porters and offered to exhibit the pair. By then the demand for unusual exhibits to fill circus and museum freak show platforms was beginning to grow. The family, however, could not bear to part with the boys. Warner left, but he came back and this time emptied a washpan filled with money—gold and silver—into the mother's lap. "She felt if there was that much money for the boys she should let them go" (Randall 1937; "Barnum's Wild Men" 1937).

Warner took them, changed their names—Hiram to Waino and Barney to Plutano—and began exhibiting them, first in rooms and halls, then in dime museums, and later in sideshows at major circuses.

Most stories fabricated as part of exotic presentations were based on real contemporary events—scientific expeditions, colonial struggles, and general exploration of the non-Western world. The placement of Barney and Hiram in Borneo is an early example. In the mid 1800s Britain and the Netherlands were jockeying for control of Borneo. People's minds were frequently drawn to the "mysterious islands" by news accounts and travelogues of Western explorers penetrating the interior. Natural scientists' reports of the "orang-outang," or "man of the woods," were the subject of scientific as well as popular speculation about this creature's place in "the great chain of being" (Morris and Morris 1966). Warner used these reports and the interest they generated as the backdrop to the exotic story fabricated for the Davis brothers.

In an 1860 handbill, Barney and Hiram are presented as "The Astonishing Wild Men, From the Island of Borneo, . . . 2 of the greatest living Curiosities seen by man." Thus Warner launched the Davis brothers' career as freaks, a career that would bring him much money and result ultimately in the "The Wild Men of Borneo"—a phrase that in the American vernacular came to signify the unruly and unkempt.

The Davis brothers were the main attractions in the dime museum of Ezra Stephens, a showman from New England and one of Barnum's principal competitors. Stephens displayed the brothers against a brightly painted jungle scene (Roth and Cromie 1980, 16). Their platform antics, which became standard for later "wild men," included Barney and Hiram talking strange gibberish and scurrying about the platform snapping and snarling, adorned with chains. But this ferocious facade did not fit well with their true character, which was gentle and reserved. As time went on, then, their exhibition began to emphasize their great strength. Using volunteers from the audience, Barney and Hiram would display their strength, lifting even the heaviest of them off the ground.

After Lyman Warner's death in 1871, his son, Hanford A. Warner, took over as the brothers' manager and exhibitor.[6] They, along with the "Wild Australian Children," were there on Elm Street at the Centennial Exposition in 1876. The exhibition gradually evolved to include an incredibly elaborate story about the origin of the "Wild Men." In 1878, for a nickel, one could buy a sixteen-page pamphlet describing in great detail "What We Know About Waino and Plutano, the Wild Men of Borneo" (c. 1878). In a tale paralleling that of the "Wild Australian Children," the capture of Barney and Hiram by Captain Hammond on the rocky coast of Borneo in 1848 was described in vivid detail; they put up quite a struggle, fighting violently, even "with the force of four stout men."

If people wondered how the ferocious men described in the tale could be the mild men before them, they were assured that, "in the course of time, under patient kindness humanity subdued savageism." Hiram, Barney, and other exhibits with the condition we now call mental retardation were always extremely cooperative and well mannered. Not all people with mental retardation are so subservient and well behaved, however. Yet because aggressive and unruly exhibits were difficult to take care of and did not exhibit well, only docile and cooperative attractions were cast as freaks (Mannix 1976, 138). By the 1870s the explanation that kind treatment and training had tamed the "wild men" exhibits had become the standard way of resolving the apparent contradiction between the stories of their capture and their docile platform demeanor.

The booklet also provided an introduction to Borneo and its people. Typical of the descriptions accompanying the exotic mode, it contained accurate and detailed information about climate, geography, flora, and fauna but outlandishly embellished tales of the indigenous people. The reader was told that the interior of the island was so dense and inhabited by such a lost race of humanity that no one knew them: "Yellowish in color, and undersized, they hold no intercourse with semi civilized tribes."

When the "Wild Men" were first found, the pamphlet said, they were literally "wild animals full of monkey antics, ugly in temper and hard to manage." The description picked up on popularized versions of Darwin's ideas by suggesting that they were part human and part ape, and when they were found "no ourang-outang could climb a tree with more agility than they displayed. If you examine their little fingers you will find that conformation such as to afford them astonishing prehensile power, enabling them to grip an object and retain their hold. Either of them can lift his entire body by his little finger, and so swing to and fro, in the manner of a Borneo gorilla."

While our "Wild Men" were becoming famous, relatives in Ohio lost touch with them, and in 1880 a suit was instituted to declare them legally dead. Far from dead, they were about to get an engagement with the Barnum and London Circus. In a courier advertisement from 1882, Barney and Hiram are pictured fighting the crew of the ship that allegedly captured them, with a brief description: "when found they spoke no intelligible tongue and uttered a strange mixture of gibberish and guttural howls; so wild and ferocious were they that they could easily subdue tigers" (Durant and Durant 1957).

During the 1870s and 1880s Hiram, Barney, and Hanford A. Warner posed together for Bowery photographers (Fig. 36) (M. Mitchell 1978). In the nineties, the brothers returned with Henry D. Warner, Hanford's son, to have Eisenmann's successor, Frank Wendt, take the picture. The poses they struck are almost identical—only their age and dress had changed. In the photos their silky hair reaches almost to their waists, and each has a straggly goatee, which became gray with age. Sometimes they wear striped leotards with short pants and overalls; in other pictures they sport serapelike vests (M. Mitchell 1978; Roth and Cromie 1980, 32).

Although their presentation as "Wild Men" appears outrageous to us, the nineteenth-century public apparently approved. Wherever the brothers went, crowds greeted them enthusiastically. They toured the United States for nearly fifty years, passing through every state and large city several times, and they were exhibited in nearly every country of Europe.

In 1903, shortly before the brothers' return from a European tour, Hiram became "infirm" with what was described as general symptoms

PORTRAITS OF PRESENTATION

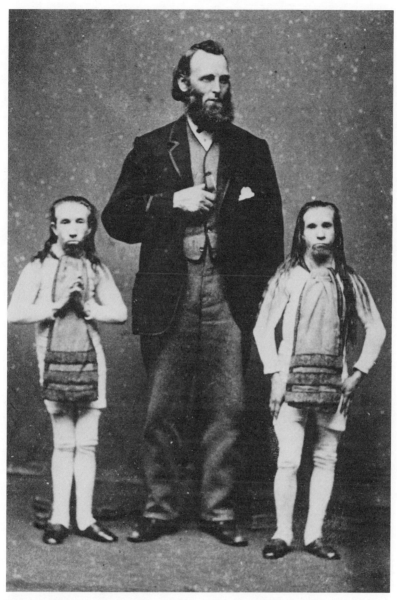

FIG. 36. Hiram and Barney Davis, "The Wild Men of Borneo." The brothers are shown with Hanford Lyman, their manager and exhibitor. Photo by Warren, c. 1876. (Becker Coll., Syracuse University.)

of old age. They settled in Waltham, Massachusetts, with Hanford Warner, Warner's son, Henry, and Henry's wife (Stanley 1914). In 1905 Hiram died, and Barney quit the platform forever. Hanford Warner, who had become their legal guardian, was not in good health. Before Hiram's death he had begun to lose his sight and had stopped accompanying the brothers on tour. He lived his last years, blind, with Barney as a companion.

Barney took his brother's death hard, becoming ill and despondent. But he recovered and, when visited by a reporter in 1906 ("Wild Man of Borneo" 1906), was described as spirited and of remarkable vigor. He behaved for the reporter in a way that showed off his training for the freak show role: "Plutaino [sic] greets you after the manner of the circus attraction—with a half-salute, half wave of the hand, a mechanical smile and a mechanical bow from the hips. Then he straightens up and stands before you, conscious of your scrutiny, but composed."

Barney died in Waltham on May 31, 1912, at age eighty-five. His Ohio funeral, like his brother's, was conducted from the home of Mrs. Workman, Hiram and Barney's niece. She wanted to make clear to the mourners the difference between her uncle the person and her uncle the freak. Although the "boys" had been described as being monkey-like and having paws, their hands and feet were perfectly formed. Similarly, other relatives said that the gibberish they used in the side-show was an act and that they spoke good English. Large crowds filed through the Workman home for the funerals. Thinking back on the two events, Mrs. Workman said: "I wanted people to see they were not freaks. Wouldn't you have done that for them?" (Randall 1937).

Unlike the "Wild Australian Children," the other exhibits discussed in this chapter, and the great preponderance of exhibits who, in modern terms, were mentally retarded, the Davis brothers *did not* have microcephaly. Microcephaly is, in the present taxonomy of mental retardation, a syndrome characterized by a small head with a sloping forehead; large, protruding ears and nose; unusually small stature, in general; and moderate to severe subnormal intellectual functioning. Although there are numerous causes of the condition, microcephaly is usually the result of an autosomal recessive genetic condition. Individuals with the syndrome often have a strikingly unusual appearance.

Although Barney and Hiram did not have microcephaly, their short stature, wiry bodies, and great strength, together with their subnormal intellectual functioning, provided the attributes that Warner could

126

capitalize on in making them freaks. But their physical characteristics were merely the start. The concoction and enactment of the exotic presentation with its amusement world flair is what launched and sustained the brothers' careers and made "The Wild Men of Borneo" a household name and an amusement world legend.

The Davis brothers became extremely well known, and other minor exhibits used "The Wild Men of Borneo" title; they did not, however, instigate a specific lookalike prototype, probably because their appearance was so singular that it was difficult to copy. "Wild Men of Borneo" became a general term that people without demonstrable physical and mental differences used to capitalize on the fame the brothers had achieved in publicizing their more mundane freak show constructions. These "self-made" wild man exhibits are discussed in Chapter 9.

Sam Gumpertz, the Coney Island freak show czar, famous for his importation of sideshow exhibits, was well aware of the drawing power of the phrase "Wild Men of Borneo." In the 1920s, when many second-rate sideshow acts were using the label as a ploy, he imported 150 natives from Borneo and billed them as the "authentic wild men from Borneo" (Butler 1936).

Maximo and Bartola

Looking at the publicity photographs taken in the 1880s of these light-brown-skinned, diminutive, primary microcephalic Central Americans, it is difficult to imagine how the hoax that launched and sustained their freak show careers, as well as those of two later generations of copies, could have been believed by so many (Fig. 37). Fashioned to look "Aztec," Maximo, in a shirt with an Aztec sun sewed on the front, and Bartola, in a dress scalloped with Aztec sun rays, give the appearance of people dressed for a costume party with a prize for the most ridiculous attire. But, for many who viewed them, they were the remnants of an ancient civilization—"The Last of the Ancient Aztecs of Mexico."

When they first appeared, in 1849, three years before the Davis brothers, they were mere children recently taken from their birthplace in the village of Decora, province of San Miguel, St. Salvador (Wood 1868). Because secrecy was part of the showmen's strategy, the true facts of the early life of many exhibits in the exotic mode are obscure; but Maximo and Bartola are believed to be the children of peasants, Innocente Burgos and Marina Espina. Because of their interesting

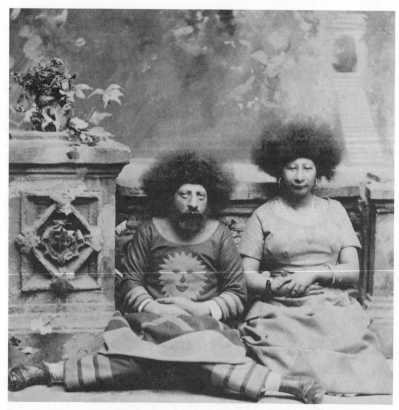

Fig. 37. Maximo and Bartola, "The Last of the Ancient Aztecs." Note the Aztec sun design on their costumes. Photo by Charles Eisenmann, c. 1885. (Becker Coll., Syracuse University.)

"dwarfish and idiotic" appearance, a Spanish trader named Ramón Selva heard of them and proposed to their mother to take them to the United States (Clair 1968). He wanted to sell them, which he did—to an American named Morris, who became their owner-manager. But he told their mother they were going away to be cured of their "imbecility" (Wood 1868, 437).

At mid-century Americans were moderately interested in the wilds of Borneo, but they thirsted for more information about the natural history of their own continent. One two-volume travelogue, written by John Lloyd Stephens (1841, 1843), a well-known New York lawyer turned Central American explorer and archeologist, sold extraordinarily well (Predmore 1949, xvii). These books contained detailed drawings of the ruins of the Mayan civilization, in which relief sculptures on stone altars depicted human forms with elongated heads much like Maximo and Bartola's. In his book, Stephens recalls meeting a Spanish Catholic priest who described a great walled city far back in the jungle that no nonnative had ever entered. These tidbits set the stage and provided the background for the story that showmen fabricated to explain Maximo and Bartola to their audiences.

Maximo and Bartola's manager sold a forty-eight-page booklet in conjunction with their appearances. *Life of the Living Aztec Children* (1860) gave, in elaborate detail, the fabricated "true story" of the discovery of Maximo and Bartola in the temple in the ancient Aztec kingdom about which the priest had told Stephens. As the tale went, three adventurers set out for the lost city of Iximaya, but only Pedro Velásquez managed to escape with the children after his companions were killed. The children were said to have been found squatting on an altar as idols. They were, it was claimed, members of a sacred race worshipped by the city's inhabitants, descendants of the ancient Aztecs who had remained pure because they were only allowed to marry among themselves.

The public as well as the scientific community flocked to see the boy Maximo and the girl Bartola when they first appeared in the early 1850s in Boston. The showmen who exhibited them publicized clergymen's and doctors' endorsements. Even the mayor was brought into the promotion campaign: he presented the two with a gold watch and chain valued at $90 as a token of admiration ("The Aztec Children" c. 1851).

Key to the showmen's success was getting the scientific community interested in the specimens and involved in a debate concerning their origin. Although we do not know whether Maximo and Bartola's manager, Mr. Knox, was instrumental in making the arrangements or whether their appearance was solicited, in any case, in 1851 they were brought before the Boston society of Natural History where, placed "upon a table, the members sitting around, [they] amused all by their interesting and lively movements" (Bouvé 1880).

That they were of serious scientific interest is beyond doubt (Howard 1977, 70). In April 1851 J. Mason Warren, M.D., published a paper in the *American Journal of the Medical Sciences* describing the pair in great detail (Warren 1851). Although Warren was unequivocal in stating his belief that the children did not belong to a race of dwarfs, his article is illustrated with drawings of the children in "Aztec" costumes complete with feathers. The attention of the Boston

Society increased interest and debate regarding the origin and nature of these now famous exhibits. Horace Greeley, apparently enamored of the two, commented, "To the moralist, the student, the physiologist, they are subjects deserving of careful scrutiny and thoughtful observation; while to those whose highest motive is the gratification of curiosity, especially children, they must be objects of vivid interest" ("Aztecs of the Society Library" 1931). One journalist observer of the curiosities provides a sense of the degree to which the hoax was believed:

> Mr. Knox, the exhibitor, has a small carved stone image
> once used as an idol in Mexico, and which was brought to
> this city from Chapultepec, by Lieut. Gibbs of the U.S.
> Army. The features of this image strikingly resemble
> those of the Aztecs; and whenever the latter see it they
> caress and fondle it in a manner which plainly indicates
> that they have seen something of the kind before. When
> it was first shown by the lady who presented it to Mr.
> Knox, the boy, Maximo, danced with delight, and when it
> was taken from him he wept and mourned most piteously.
> This strongly corroborates a portion of their history as set
> forth in the pamphlet. ("The Aztec Children" c. 1851)

The acceleration of these "ethnological curiosities" to stardom occurred quickly, and in the early 1850s they were received by members of the Senate and House of Representatives and were the guests of President Fillmore at the White House (E. Wood 1868, 435). The viewing of exotic exhibits by such prestigious officials was publicized as an endorsement—and part of the making of a successful freak was getting as many such endorsements from the rich and famous as possible. Maximo and Bartola's promoter set the standard.

Mr. Morris, their owner-manager, took them to England in 1853, where they created quite a stir as the "Aztec Lilliputians" (Altick 1978). They were exhibited before the Ethnological Society and summoned to Buckingham Palace to meet the royal family. Exhibited first at the Hanover-Square Rooms, they drew three thousand people in the first two days. They were exhibited later in the Adelaide Gallery and in other places in London and the outlying districts.

One of the observers was the distinguished anatomist Professor Richard Owen. Although skeptical that they were ancient Aztecs, he was impressed with the dwarfs. Soon he, other scientists, and the London press were embroiled in a debate regarding the true nature of

Maximo and Bartola's condition, a debate that further fanned interest and attendance.

The pair toured the Continent, appearing before the Emperor Napoleon and his imperial family in Paris; the emperor of Russia and his family; the kings and queens of Prussia, Bavaria, Holland, Hanover, and Denmark; the emperor of Austria and his family; the king of Belgium; the count of Flanders; the duchess of Brabant; and other members of royal families and noted natural scientists and philosophers.

When they returned to the United States they were engaged for exhibition at Barnum's American Museum. Barnum capitalized on the attention they had received in Europe by lavishly quoting famous people who had commented on the "Aztec Wonders." In a Currier and Ives lithograph advertising the "Aztec Children at Barnum's American Museum," the scientist Baron Von Humboldt is quoted as saying, "They [Maximo and Bartola] appear to offer a worthy study to those who seriously occupy themselves with types of human organization and with the laws respecting them" (Hertzberg Coll.). The press responded with praise and wonder:

> The Aztec children are still the most remarkable attractions in the city, and are daily visited by large audiences. They are certainly the greatest curiosities of the human race ever seen in this country. The boy, about twenty years old, weighs twenty pounds; the girl is thirteen years old and weighs seventeen pounds. They are of a race which has but few surviving members. That they are human beings there can be no doubt; and they are not freaks of nature, but specimens of a dwindled, minikin race, who almost realize in bodily form our idea of "brownies," "bogies," and other fanciful creations of a more superstitious age.[7]

Interest and press coverage faded as Maximo and Bartola got older, making it difficult to trace their careers. They next appear on January 7, 1867, in London, where they got married at the registrar's office. This event, likely a publicity device to stir up business, raises the question of whether they were really brother and sister or whether the wedding was a farce. The extension of the "ancient Aztec" story, of course, would allow them to marry, for in that culture marrying relatives was the rule—although it is doubtful that English law would see it that way. They were married under the names of Señor Máximo Váldez Núñez and Señora Bartola Velásquez, and a crowd attended a wedding breakfast in Willis's Rooms. The groom wore evening dress, the bride a white satin dress (E. Wood 1868, 138; M. Mitchell 1979, 60).

Although they were reported to have been exhibited up to 1901 (M. Mitchell 1979, 60), there are few written accounts of them after the wedding. Photographs of them in the 1880s and 1890s do exist, and they are listed in the Barnum and Bailey Circus route books for the seasons 1888, 1889, and 1890—the last record of them.[8] At that time. Mrs. Nellie March, their sixth "owner" (Buchanan-Taylor 1943), was listed as the "matron of the Aztecs." There is no record of their death. Through imitation and scientific records only did they live on.

Of all the early exhibits of people we would now call mentally retarded, Maximo and Bartola, "The Original Aztec Children," generated the greatest scientific interest and were imitated the most. During their lifetime and after their deaths a host of other people with microcephaly and below-normal intellectual functions were exhibited by showmen as "Aztecs." All borrowed their presentations—their costumes as well as their stories—from the fabrications that had created the celebrated Maximo and Bartola. In typical showman fashion, a number of such copies even claimed to be the original.

Even while Maximo and Bartola were still appearing, a man and a woman with microcephaly were displayed together in the 1880s as the "Estics" (M. Mitchell 1979, 79). Whether the spelling was a mistake or merely an attempt to be original is not clear, but they traveled with the Cooper and Jackson Circus as Hutty and Tain, wearing serapes and indigenous South American–style clothing. A woman with microcephaly was exhibited in the 1880s as Rosi, "The Wild Girl of the Yucatan." Another nineteenth-century "Aztec"-derived exhibit was a young man with microcephaly who traveled with the Wallace circus and was presented as the "Mexican Wild Boy" (G. Gould and Pyle 1896, 248).

At the turn of the twentieth century many people with microcephaly were being exhibited as "Aztecs." By this time people in the amusement world used the term *pinhead* to advertise such people (Gresham 1948)—the Ringling Circus, for example, had one exhibit called "Tik Tak, the Aztec Pinhead." Several turn-of-the-century photographs show children with microcephaly (Pfening Coll.). One group of four children was presented as "The Original Aztec Indian Midgets from Old Mexico." In 1910 the sideshow of the Sells Floto Circus exhibited two children who were referred to as "Aurora and Natali, the Aztec

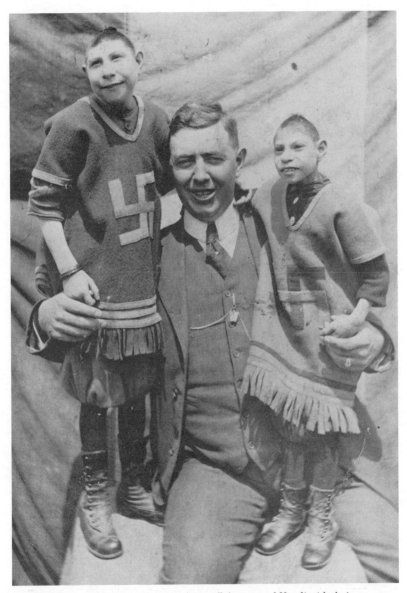

Fig. 38. Twentieth-century "Ancient Aztecs." Aurora and Natali with their manager, Max Klass. They traveled with the Sells-Floto Circus Sideshow in 1910. Photographer unknown. (Ringling Museum of the Circus, Sarasota, Florida.)

Pinheads." Prophetically, their manager, Max Klass, dressed them in loose-fitting serapes Central American—style, with the indigenous religious symbol, the swastika, on the front (Fig. 38). Another person exhibited as an Aztec was a woman called Schlitzie who appeared in the motion picture *Freaks* in 1932.[9] Forty years old at the time, she had been exhibited as "Maggie, the Last of the Aztecs" (Drimmer 1973).

William Henry Johnson

William Henry Johnson's career as a freak spans the period of approximately 1860 to 1926. A black man born about 1840 in the eastern United States, probably in Liberty Corners, near Bound Brook, New Jersey ("Circus Freak Buried Here" 1926; Leech 1926; Fellows and Freeman 1936),[10] Johnson was short, between four and five feet tall.[11] His large, long nose connected with the top of his small head without the interruption of a forehead. His head thus appeared to come to a point. This effect was a result in part of his physiology and in part of the fact that, for the purpose of exhibition, his head was shaved except for a patch about two inches in diameter at the top.

While opinions on the level of Johnson's intelligence are varied, there is little doubt that if he were alive today he would be diagnosed as mentally retarded, with microcephaly.[12] But Johnson was more intellectually competent than the other exhibits discussed in this chapter. He was verbal and apparently an active participant in the construction of his freak role. Those who knew Johnson describe him as an amusement world mascot. He was exhibited in freak shows until his death in Bellevue Hospital, New York City, in 1926.

Johnson became a celebrity at Barnum's American Museum. He played various well-known museums, was a regular at Coney Island, and continued to appear with Ringling Brothers, Barnum and Bailey Circus through the 1920s. Referred to as the "dean of freaks," he had the longest successful career of any of the sideshow attractions. He is best known by his stage name, "Zip," although his original title, "What Is It?" was closely associated with him until his death.

Johnson's story is of particular interest because his career as a freak spans the decades of the freak show's greatest popularity and both pre- and post—Civil War America. (For secondary sources on Johnson, see Drimmer 1973, 351; M. Mitchell 1979, 76; Carmichael 1971, 275; Durant and Durant 1957, 114; E. McCullogh 1957, 269; Fellows and Freeman 1936, 308; and Lindfors 1983, 1984). In all

PORTRAITS OF PRESENTATION

freak constructions in the exotic mode, showmen exploited the public's stereotypes, prejudices, and hatred toward people of color. This tendency was especially apparent in exhibitions in the African motif. Johnson's presentation reveals the patterns of white America's deep disdain and contempt for the black.

The truth of Johnson's origins and of his recruitment into the freak show was very effectively suppressed.[13] In an article written soon after his death, a woman who is reported to be his sister said that Johnson was recruited by a representative of the Van Amburgh Circus when he was four years old and from there taken to Barnum's museum. Although Johnson did talk behind the scenes, he was not very coherent and he never revealed the details of his background. Whether Johnson lacked the information or was purposely kept quiet is unclear. According to one story, Barnum told him that he would pay him a dollar a day for not talking. Others say that he understood that his career as a "missing link" would be severely curtailed if it was discovered he could speak (Teel c. 1930).

The confusion regarding his early life is further complicated by the fact that there was more than one "What Is It?"—at least one prior to Johnson's debut, and Johnson's own success spawned many imitations. The one before was advertised and exhibited by Barnum at the Egyptian Hall in London in 1846 (Altick 1978). The description in the advertisement for that exhibit is somewhat similar to the publicity releases for the "What Is Its?" of our concern. The London exhibit was definitely not Henry Johnson, though. To Barnum's embarrassment, the London public discovered the freak to be Harvey Leech, sometimes known as Hervio Nano, a "small deformed" American actor known to London theater-goers as "The Gnome-Fly."

Advertisements and other literature put out by Barnum describe a "What Is It?" fitting Johnson's description being exhibited first in 1860 (Odell 1931, 254).[14] In a letter to an old friend dated April 4, 1860, Barnum indicates that Johnson had earlier been exhibited in Philadelphia, and Barnum had heard of him through these appearances. In Barnum's words: "I have since secured it, and we call it 'What is it?'" (Saxon 1983, 104).

Victorian America was fascinated by primates, but little was known about them. Even well into the century, people were not clear on the difference between chimpanzees, baboons, monkeys, orangutans, and gorillas (Morris and Morris 1966). The mysterious and elusive gorilla of Africa was not revealed to the scientific world until 1847 (Savage and Wyman 1847). Yet people were not interested only in apes. For years people had been concerned with various forms of man in the great chain of life, but now, with the publication of Darwin's *The Origin of Species* (1859), and, later, *The Descent of Man* (1871), the relationship between various categories took on new significance. Darwin and gorillas were the talk of the day.

In an 1860 publication for the American Museum, showmen took advantage of the public's interest in primates and introduced Johnson as "What Is It? or The Man-Monkey!" describing him as "a most singular animal, which though it has many of the features and characteristics of both the human and brute, is not, apparently, either, but, in appearance, a mixture of both—the connecting link between humanity and brute creation" (*Life of the Living Aztec Children* 1860, 46).

Mr. Flower, who was Mr. Johnson's first "keeper" and who lectured on the "true life" and circumstances of "What Is It?" told the crowds that the "nondescript" (a commonly used phrase for animals not yet classified or described by science) was captured by a group of adventurers who were exploring the River Gambia in search of the gorilla. The men came upon a group of this race which had never before been seen. All were in a "perfectly nude state," roving through the trees like the monkey and the orangutan. The men succeeded in capturing three, two of whom died on the voyage to the United States.

In describing the physical condition of the exhibit, the keeper is quoted as saying:

> When first received here, his natural position was on all
> fours; and it has required the exercise of the greatest care
> and patience to teach him to stand perfectly erect, as you
> behold him at the present moment. But a few weeks have
> elapsed, in fact, since he first assumed this attitude and
> walked about upon his feet. If you notice, you will per-
> ceive that the walk of the What Is It is very awkward,
> like that of a child beginning to acquire that accomplish-
> ment. When he first came his only food was raw meat,
> sweet apples, oranges, nuts, etc., of all of which he was
> very fond; but he will not eat bread, cake, and similar
> things, . . . the formation of the head and face combines
> both that of the native African and of the Orang Outang
> . . . he has been examined by some of the most scientific
> men we have, and pronounced by them to be a CONNECT-

ING LINK BETWEEN THE WILD NATIVE AFRICAN AND THE
BRUTE CREATION. (*Life of the Living Aztec Children*
1860, 47)

An advertisement for the American Museum that appeared in the *New York Leader* of November 5, 1860, contains endorsements for the exhibit from the *New York Tribune:* "It seems to be a sort of cross between an ape species and a Negro"; *The Sunday Times:* "It is an animal which would seem to supply the links supposed by philosophers to exist between the human race and brutes"; and *The New York Herald:* "The formation of its hands, arms and head are those of a orangutan, but its movements are those of a human being."

In the earliest publicity drawings of Johnson, he is presented in a fur cover, with long nails, and against a jungle backdrop (Lindfors 1983a). Early photographs taken by Mathew Brady have him posing in a fur jumpsuit with a long stick in his hands, the stick and the poses closely resembling drawings found in natural history taxonomies of gorillas, chimpanzees, and orangutans (Fig. 39). On and off until 1878 Johnson was presented in a cage ("Zip Back in Circus" c. 1910).

Sometime in the early 1870s Johnson was dubbed "Zip." The origin of the name is probably "Zip Coon," an early minstrel show character who came to personify, for whites, the stereotypically dumb but dapper black (Toll 1976; Wittke 1968).[15] While Johnson continued to appear as "What Is It?" "The Monkey-Man," and "The Missing Link" throughout his life, after twenty years of being on display his presentation increasingly took the form of farce. Photographs of him from the 1880s show him posed in mock boxing matches with other exhibits (Fig. 40). Around the turn of the century the fiddle became one of his trademarks (Leech 1926); all he could manage, however, were loud screeching noises, and there was a circus joke that the money he made as a fiddler came from people paying him not to play ("Fiddle Boosts Zip's Earnings" 1921). In a picture from around 1910 he is on the bally platform in front of Barnum and Bailey's sideshow, fiddle in hand, as a come-on for the show inside (Fig. 41).

He became a favorite object of press mockery and of circus publicity stunts. At the turn of the century his mock marriage to a midget was staged in Madison Square Garden, with Alf T. Ringling as best man (Bradna and Hartzell 1952). In 1914 Dexter Fellows, press agent for Barnum and Bailey, arranged a birthday dinner for Johnson which

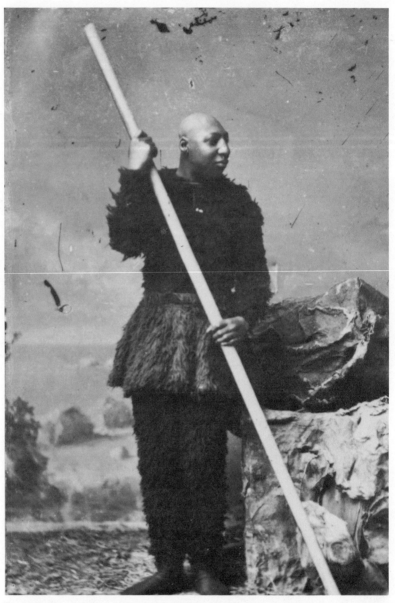

Fig. 39. Henry Johnson, Barnum's "What Is It?" Note the monkey suit, stick in hands, and the shaved head. Photo by Mathew Brady, c. 1872. (Meserve Coll., National Portrait Gallery, Smithsonian Institution, Washington, D.C.)

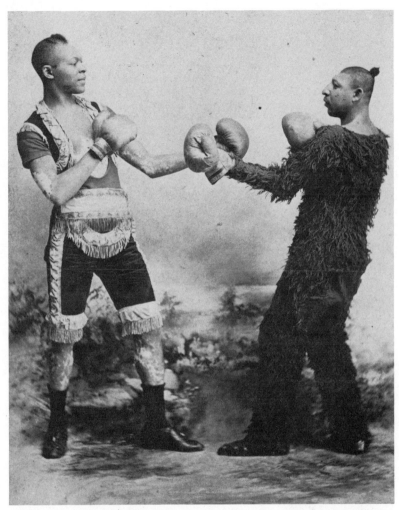

FIG. 40. Henry Johnson as "Zip" in a mock boxing match. Note the tuft of hair on Johnson's head. His boxing partner is Benjamin Ash, a teenager exhibited as the "spotted boy." Photo by Swords Brothers, c. 1887. (Becker Coll., Syracuse University.)

was covered as the "feast of freaks" ("Zip, Pride at "B & B Circus" 1914). Attended by both members of the press and an entourage from the sideshow, the event found its way into many papers ("High Social Set in Freakdom" 1914; "Zip the 'What Is It?' Plays Host" 1914; "Circus Freaks Dine Out" 1914). In one article Johnson's speech of thanks was reported as being "Ugh, Ugh, Ugh" ("Zip, Pride at B & B Circus" 1914). Later publicity photos show him dancing with the lady sword

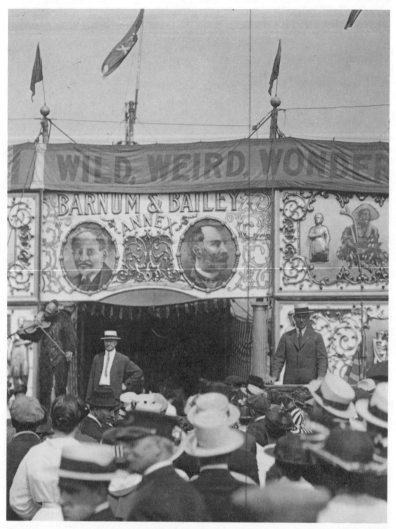

Fig. 41. Henry Johnson on bally. In this rare picture Johnson plays the fiddle, flanked by a lecturer and two ticket sellers. Photo by Fred Glasier. (Ringling Museum of the Circus, Sarasota, Florida.)

swallower. His last press-release photo depicts him playing golf on the beach at Coney Island dressed in a suit jacket, shirt, tie, and knickers and using Coney Island sideshow giant Mlle. Londy as the teeing-off mound (Sarasota Coll.).

Johnson was alleged to have jealously guarded the number-one platform in the Ringling Brothers, Barnum and Bailey sideshow, a place awarded him by virtue of his seniority with the show. One report has him guarding his spot with a pop gun. In the 1920s he was portrayed as believing he was the boss of the circus, walking around the grounds with a large cigar in his mouth giving orders (Teel c. 1930).

Johnson died of acute bronchitis on April 24, 1926. He was in his eighties. Funeral services were held at Campbell's Funeral Church on Broadway and Sixty-sixth in New York City ("Many Circus Folk" 1926). His fellow Ringling Brothers, Barnum and Bailey Sideshow colleagues were there, together with other circus and Coney Island people and a score of newspaper reporters.[16]

For the last thirty-five years of his life Zip was managed by "Captain" O. K. White. White collapsed at the funeral and was taken to his quarters behind the Dreamland Sideshow at Coney Island, which he had shared with Johnson for fourteen years. (Johnson had given up traveling with the Ringling circus but was under a lifetime contract to be exhibited during the summer at the seaside amusement park.) Two months later, Captain White, age seventy-five, died at Coney Island Hospital of what the press described as a "broken heart" ("Manager of Zip" 1926). According to friends, White had no financial worries—Johnson had been very profitable ("Zip's Manager Griefstricken" 1926).

According to Ringling Brothers, Johnson was well paid and White had established a fund for him that would have provided for him until his death if he had wished to give up the life of a freak. Johnson is reported to have owned property in New Jersey and a home that Barnum had given him in Connecticut ("Zip's Manager Griefstricken" 1926). Indeed, a few years before his death Johnson did try to retire, but missing the excitement of that way of life, he returned to the circus, dime museums, and midway ("Zip, Circus Freak Dies" 1926). It is estimated that during his long career as an exhibit he was viewed by over a hundred million people (Lindfors 1983a, 13).

As we have seen, Henry Johnson, "The Original What Is It?" was not the first "What Is It?" But those who came before him never reached his level of prominence, and he rather than his predecessors inspired the many facsimiles that followed.

Barnum exhibited a female "What Is It?" at the American Museum after Johnson first appeared. The only information we have about her comes from an unpublished manuscript written in the late 1800s (Dingess c. 1899). As the story goes, when she was located by one of the managers she was locked in an outhouse on Thompson Street in New

York City with only "a rag over its loins." She was described as "an idiotic little negro girl" with "a long thin head," "twisted and stunted limbs and as filthy as any mortal could possibly be not to be all dirt." Presented as "the connecting link between man and beast" (Dingess c. 1899, 919–920), she generated serious interest on the part of the press and the scientific community. She did present one problem for her exhibitors: she had learned to swear from the museum employees and did so in front of visitors.

At the turn of the century a woman with microcephaly traveled with the Barnum and Bailey Circus on its European tour. She was presented as "Delphi," the female "What Is It?" and was one of twenty-three attractions in that sideshow (a poster of her is on display in the Ringling Circus Museum, Sarasota, Florida).

Johnson inspired other imitators in the twentieth century. The typical citizen of the late 1920s was not gullible enough to accept that the people being exhibited were missing links or members of a lost civilization. Thus, for the most part Johnson's successors were presented simply as "pinheads" (E. McCullough 1957). During the first decade of the twentieth century, a mentally retarded black man was exhibited as "Congo, The Ape-Man." He appeared with a chimpanzee known as "Sally, The Woman-Ape." In the twenties two people with microcephaly were exhibited as Pipo and Zipo (E. McCullough 1957, 271); they were sisters, Elvira and Jenny Snow, born in Georgia and exhibited by their brother, Cliff Snow. They played in the film *Freaks* as sisters (Drimmer 1973, 296), but they were also exhibited as Zippo and Flippo, brother and sister, in circus sideshows.[17] In the thirties a man was exhibited as Zup, Zip's brother. He was not Johnson's brother, however (Fielder 1978, 166), and not enough is known about him to determine whether he would be labeled as mentally retarded by current clinical judgment.

Johnson's trademark, the tuft of hair on the top of his pointed head, became a standard for his followers, and many of the props he used— the pop gun, the violin—and antics he engaged in were incorporated into other exhibits. Contemporary "conehead" and "pinhead" comic characters have their origin in freak show farce made popular by Johnson. The camp comic strip "Zippy the Pinhead" (by Bill Griffith) and the craze it has created on college campuses derives directly from Henry Johnson's presentation.[18]

Headbinders

During the 1930s a number of Americans with microcephaly were displayed using some of the elements of presentation introduced by Johnson—the tuft and the African origins—but the explanation of their condition broke from earlier stories. They were not presented as missing links or members of an unknown race; rather, their presentation was borrowed from *National Geographic* stories of people from other cultures with unusual and body-transforming customs. As the tale went, certain African tribes (sometimes called the Ituris, other times the Beola) bound the heads of babies with cloth, the way the Chinese bound girls' feet, to make them small and pointed—in other words, microcephalic (see Fig. 20).

Nate Eagle, a famous showman of the 1930s, hired two blacks, whom he referred to as "pinheads," for the 1934 Chicago World's Fair. Their names, Willy and Sam, and the fact that they were originally from Alabama are all we know of their past. Given the names Illy and Zambezi for purposes of exhibition, they worked out of the African Village on the midway. They were presented as members of the "Ituri" headbinding tribe from the rain forests of Africa (R. Taylor 1958a). In the 1930s a man and a woman from another "headbinding tribe" of Africa, the Beola, were exhibited under the names Ilikuluin and Zanbezi. Zanbezi, the woman, was erroneously said to have a four-inch-long "caudal appendage," better known as a tail.

The most detailed account of the exhibition of people with microcephaly in the twentieth century is in *Freak Show Man*, the candid autobiography of Harry Lewiston (Holtman 1968), who organized and managed sideshows for thirty years starting in 1914. He worked for such notable shows as Hagenbeck-Wallace Circus, Barnes Circus, and Ringling Brothers, Barnum and Bailey Circus, and also played the major state and world fairs. In the 1930s and 1940s Lewiston used the exotic headbinding fabrication extensively. Two of his exhibits were an American-born Caucasian brother and sister with microcephaly whom he displayed as Bobo and Kiki, albino pygmies from the heart of Africa rejected by their fellow headbinding tribesmen because of their albinoism. In his autobiography, Lewiston explained his approach to exhibiting this attraction: "I might note here that none of the things I had said or would be saying about the pinheads was true. They were plain old white American microcephalics, more popularly known as 'pinheads,' but you can't tell people, 'Now, we've got these idiots here; take a good look at them'" (Holtman 1968, 11–12).

Starting in 1929 Lewiston exhibited Effic, Rosie, Nettie, and Willie, the son and daughters of Joe and Buella House, poor blacks from Memphis, Tennessee (see Fig. 14, front row right) (Holtman 1968, 173, 222). Using methods seventy years old, methods that had originated with Johnson, Lewiston, to accentuate their small, long heads, "had their parents shave them all except for a small tuft of hair at the very tops." He outfitted them in imitation leopard-skin costumes and grass skirts. The parents toured with their children, and Lewiston reports that they were the stars of the show for a number of years, being presented as "Iturian Pygmies" from the "Iturian Colony in deepest, darkest Africa." Lewiston told the crowds that their small heads made them more beautiful and less intelligent. Furthermore, in detail reminiscent of the story told in conjunction with the "Wild Men of Borneo," Lewiston told the audience, "These tiny people live among monkeys, apes, chimpanzees, and other creatures of the simian world. To make themselves more at home in this kind of jungle environment, the less intelligence, the less thinking power they have, the better off they feel themselves to be" (Holtman 1968, 12).

Many elements of Lewiston's presentations contain the themes first developed in the mid-nineteenth-century construction of freak exhibits.

The list of people with mental retardation who were exhibited as freaks in the exotic mode has not been exhausted,[19] although the conventions of their construction have been fully presented. With a few exceptions (Barney and Hiram Davis, for instance), the mentally retarded people who were put on display had a condition we now call true or primary microcephaly (Grossman 1983). Why was this condition so favored for exhibition?[20] One reason is that the appearance of people with microcephaly, when accented with shaved heads and the other trappings showmen devised for them, lent itself readily to the exotic presentation, which in turn became part and parcel of the flamboyant humbug on which the world of amusement thrived. In the mid–nineteenth century, the freak show was becoming standardized, developing a set of institutionalized patterns and modes. The early exhibits of Maximo and Bartola and of Henry Johnson established a "type" of exhibit that became a standard feature of the show. As every good show had to have a "legless wonder" and a sword swallower, it also had to have a person with microcephaly or, in the language of the amusement world, a "pinhead." There were imitations of Barney and Hiram Davis, "The Original Wild Men of Borneo," but these heirs were not noted for demonstrably low mental functioning.

It might be difficult to imagine that people actually believed the lies the promoters told them about the nineteenth-century exhibits described in this chapter. If the founders of the American Association on Mental Deficiency had gone to see these sideshow attractions, what might have been their observations?

The state of knowledge in the field we now call mental retardation was at the time rather unsophisticated. In fact, no agreed-upon generic name existed for the amorphous category of people with subnormal intellectual functioning. While various clinical types were beginning to be recognized and named in the 1870s, the experts were in the dark and frequently in error about causation (Scheerenberger 1983, 112; Cranefield 1962, 489). Experts pointed to organic disease, intemperance, and intermarriage as possible causal factors, but they had not abandoned, nor would they for decades (Crookshank 1921; Bernstein 1922), anthropological explanations and ethnographic classification systems (Barr 1896, 1904). Through the latter part of the nineteenth century and even into the twentieth, the theory that certain forms of mental deficiency were a biological throwback to earlier races of humans and even to apes was still widely believed. "Mongoloid idiots" (for whom the term *Down's syndrome* is now preferred) and people with microcephaly were sometimes explained this way (Gould 1981).

Scientists interested in mental retardation observed the early exhibits described here and incorporated them into their thinking and vocabulary. In a paper written in 1887, J. Langdon Down, for whom Down's syndrome is named, refers in his discussion to the "Aztec type" (Down 1887). Both G. Shuttleworth and William Ireland, British doctors whose ideas were influential in the United States, refer to the "so-called Aztecs" in their papers on diagnosis and classification.[21] In the twentieth century, even as late as the 1920s and 1930s, the term *Aztec-like*, as well as atavistic theories of microcephalus, appeared in the professional literature (Bernstein 1922; Carson 1908; Crookshank 1921). As has been illustrated, although the tales showmen told were out-and-out lies and they knew it, the stories fit into contemporary scientific theory.

Over time the exhibition of people with mental retardation moved from straight presentations emphasizing the attraction's scientific merit to more farcical renderings. Exploration of the world and the medicalization of retardation undermined some of the outlandish tales used to explain exhibits. In addition, with exhibits who enjoyed long careers, mockery added a touch of novelty to stale presentations. After the 1930s microcephalic people began to be eliminated from the roster of standard sideshow exhibits. By then mental retardation had become reified as a disease (Bogdan and Taylor 1982), and people with subnormal mental functioning had been "medicalized"—that is, the mystery surrounding their origin, while not solved, had been contained within a medical mold. People pitied these individuals and were offended by their appearance on the freak show platform.

We do not know what happened to many of the exhibits. Showmen report that some were forced off the platform to spend years in large custodial institutions. Schlitzie, for example, one of people with microcephaly discussed earlier who appeared in the film *Freaks*, met this fate (Mannix 1976, 139). But as with Hiram and Barney Davis, "The Aztec Children," together with a number of twentieth-century exhibits, freak show scouts, using large monetary incentives, occasionally managed to lure exhibits away from their families. By claiming to be interested in saving these people from institutionalization, showmen could conveniently justify their participation in a practice that was falling out of fashion.

Being mentally retarded or microcephalic did not make the people discussed here freaks. How we view people with disabilities has less to do with what they are physiologically than with who we are culturally. Understanding the "freak show" can help us not to confuse the role a person plays with who that person really is.

6

Illusions of Grandeur

WE JUMP FROM the darkest jungles of Africa, the mysterious island of Borneo, and the ancient temples of the Aztecs to the opulent palaces of Europe, the somber churches of New York, and the glamor of Broadway and Hollywood. We move from presentations that created missing links, wild men, and atavistic throwbacks to the manufacture of the aristocratic and the glamorous freak.

In this chapter we leave the exotic mode to take up the aggrandized, a mode in which the showmen flaunted, exaggerated, and created prestigious and high-status attributes for exhibits. Titles such as "General," "Princess," and "Count" were freely distributed. Skills and talent were exaggerated and embellished. Showmen proclaimed some exhibits to be rich, famous, illustrious, and distinguished. They regularly endowed exhibits with an abundance of noble characteristics that they either did not have at all or did not have to a degree that matched the claims.

Some exhibits cast in the exotic mode, of course—those with impaired intellectual functioning, for example—might not have been aware of the demeaning way in which they were being presented to the public, and they might not have been able clearly to distinguish who they really were from how they were presented. But, as we shall see when we return to the exotic in the next chapter, many exhibits in the exotic mode clearly understood the difference between their onstage and offstage personas. They did not take their presentations personally, and understandably, they did not aspire to be the person of the presentation.

For those who operated in the aggrandized mode, however, especially when it was played out to its most extravagant extreme, this situation did not always hold. For many of these people, the invented identity was so flattering that they strove to become their stage persona. Some succeeded. The exhibits who were in high demand earned large salaries, which helped them transform their presentations into reality. They bought fancy clothes, even yachts and race horses. They were invited to social affairs where they hobnobbed with statesmen, nobility, and celebrities. They took on the behavior, accoutrements, and mentality of their freak roles, both on and off stage. For some, at least, the gap between presentation and life narrowed. But gnawing questions about the relationship between reality and image remained, and these proved painful for exhibits to resolve.

The melding of person and role characterized various exhibits. The profiles in this chapter will raise confusion as to which was the real person and which the constructed freak. The reader will thus be as bewildered as the exhibits themselves and their audiences were. Do not fret. We will thereby witness the ultimate in humbug: the hoax becoming the fact, the illusion becoming reality. This form of hoax was, for the showman, the finest achievement.

In this chapter we highlight Tom Thumb and his wife, Lavinia Warren, as well as the Hilton Sisters, Siamese twins who were at the height of their fame in the 1930s. These profiles illustrate the construction of exhibits in the "high aggrandized style"—where pretensions were greatest, where incumbents were decked out in the trappings of high society and claimed the glamor of international celebrities. We will see how their presentations almost made them stars—as opposed to freaks—and provided the basis for their illusions of grandeur.

Love in Miniature: Mr. and Mrs. "Tom Thumb"

In 1863 America was embroiled in the bloody Civil War. President Lincoln had just signed the Emancipation Proclamation. The war was not going well for the North, and Americans had a lot on their minds. But despite all that, and as a testimonial to the manipulative powers of the great showman P. T. Barnum, on February 10 the nation's attention focused on, of all things, a wedding between two dwarfs. (In the language of the post-1865 amusement world, the bride and groom were "midgets." The generic medical term for short people—those under four feet ten inches—however, is *dwarf* [Ablon 1984]. "Midget" appeared in the language as a designation for dwarfs who were well proportioned—men and women in miniature, which the bride and groom were.)

The wedding diverted the public's attention from the war, if only for a day. One full page of the eight-page *New York Times* was devoted to it ("Loving Lilliputians" 1863). Indeed, the lavish wedding, the publicity it generated, and the public's fascination with the couple exemplify P. T. Barnum's finest triumph of freak promotion in the high aggrandized mode.

The groom, twenty-five years old and two feet eleven inches tall, was actually Charles Sherwood Stratton, who had been charming freak show audiences in the United States and Europe for over twenty years. Born in Connecticut on January 4, 1838, Stratton had stopped growing before he was a year old. (Today he would probably be diagnosed as having a pituitary dysfunction.) Barnum, who was recruiting for his American Museum, heard about the boy, visited him, and liked what he saw, stating that he "was not two feet high" (Barnum 1871, 163). The boy's parents were of modest means—his father was a carpenter and his mother worked at the local inn—and Barnum convinced them to bring him to New York.

Yet when his mother arrived with her son, she was incredulous to find that, on handbills promoting Charles, Barnum had taken the liberty of changing his age from four (he was about to turn five) to eleven, his place of birth from Bridgeport to London, and his name to General Tom Thumb. Barnum explained to her the logic of his showman's mind: "had I announced him as only five years of age it would have been impossible to excite the interest or awaken the curiosity of the public" (Barnum 1855, 243). Audiences might not readily believe that the four-year-old was truly a dwarf. The rationale for changing the place of birth was that Barnum had observed, and in the past had taken advantage of, American's fancy for European attractions. If Americans had such a "disgraceful preference for foreigners," Barnum's self-serving logic argued, it was their offense, not his (Barnum 1855, 244). Stratton's incongruous title, "General," added a nice twist to the elevated presentation. "Tom Thumb" was borrowed from the legendary dwarf knight in King Arthur's court.

Barnum did not fabricate just the boy's title, age, and place of origin, however. Barnum recognized in Charles a physical specimen he could make something of. In addition to his small size, Stratton was a "bright-eyed little fellow, with light hair and ruddy cheeks, was perfectly healthy, and as symmetrical as an Apollo" (Barnum 1855, 243). Barnum emphasized these attributes in the publicity: Tom Thumb was a perfect man in miniature, not an ill-formed, offensive-to-look-at dwarf (*Sketch of the Life of General Tom Thumb* 1847).

Barnum's molding of Tom represents the classic case of freak craft-ing. When Barnum met his future star, Thumb was exceedingly bash-ful, so much so in fact that he had to be coaxed into telling his name. So, prior to his exhibition, Barnum took great pains to train his "di-minutive prodigy, devoting many hours to that purpose, day and by night" (Barnum 1855, 244). In a week Charles Stratton had learned proper manners and would patter with adults. Barnum encouraged him to take on regal airs (Wallace 1959, 75) and began coaching him in stage routines. In addition, as became the pattern with exhibits in the aggrandized mode, Barnum enhanced the status of the little Strat-ton by introducing him to influential New Yorkers and playing on these associations in publicity releases.

In his early appearances Tom did imitations of Napoleon Bonaparte, Cupid, and a Revolutionary War soldier, dressing up in appropriate costumes. Mock battles were staged between him, posing as the bib-lical David, and the museum's giants, representing Goliaths. He marched around the stage dressed as a soldier waving a ten-inch sword and performing military drills. He was a fantastic hit, the talk of New York. Twice a day he performed his routine in the museum's lecture room, and between shows he was displayed along with giants, mammoth children, and armless wonders in the Hall of Living Curi-osities. On and off stage, he presented the appearance of a well-mannered gentleman of status, greeting guests with a handshake and a cordial "How d'ye do."

As Charles Stratton's fame grew, so did his salary and the distance he traveled from his home. He appeared for six weeks at Kimball's Museum in Boston and did a similar stint in Philadelphia. Barnum advertised extensively, using "true life" stories, handbills, and litho-graphs that were printed by the thousands and distributed in cities where Stratton was shown (Harris 1973, 52)—all trumpeting the tal-ents and demeanor of Tom Thumb, the gentleman in miniature.

In 1844, Barnum and Tom Thumb left for an immensely successful European tour which opened in London and lasted three years, with visits to France, Belgium, the English provinces, Scotland, and Ire-land. Displayed in a slightly refined version of the presentation used in the United States, Tom was a sensation. From the beginning of Strattons' career, Barnum had embellished Tom Thumb's status with endorsements from dignitaries. Now Barnum used Stratton's appear-ances before European kings and queens to fuel the fire of fame. Queen Victoria saw the little prodigy three times and presented him with gifts which he ostentatiously displayed when on exhibit. To promote his appearances he would drive about in an ornate miniature carriage pulled by matching ponies. The marine-blue, crimson, and white carriage, a gift from Barnum, had been made by the queen's carriage maker.[1]

In 1847, General Tom Thumb returned to the United States after an absence of more than three years. Capitalizing on the publicity generated by his stunning European accomplishments and his visits with royalty, he promptly caused a new American Museum attendance record to be set.

In keeping with the standard framework for all exhibits, assessments of scientific significance were supplied for Tom Thumb as well. The parents' explanation for the birth of their unusual son rested on the theory of maternal impression: shortly before Tom's birth the family's black-and-tan puppy had drowned in the river that flowed behind their house. The mother had been distraught and wept hysterically, causing the baby to be "marked" (Desmond 1954, 5). This story was not emphasized in the presentation of the young man, however. Neither were the comments and observations of physicians and scientists. In the high aggrandized mode, the exhibit's demonstrable difference was not dwelt upon. Although his medical description was not central to the advertising, as was the case with other exhibits, physicians' comments were contained in "true life" pamphlets. An 1854 pamphlet sold in conjunction with Stratton's appearance (*Sketch of the Life . . . of General Tom Thumb* 1854) quotes Dr. J.V.C. Smith, editor of the *Boston Medical and Surgical Journal*, as saying: "Of all dwarfs we have examined this excels the whole in littleness."

During the period when Stratton appeared craniometry was on the rise (S. Gould 1981). One of the most cherished tenets of this science was that the size of the brain is directly related to intelligence. The 1854 pamphlet confronts this view directly by stating that although it might be natural to suppose that the smallness of the general's brain should limit his intellectual facilities, this clearly is not so. His mental abilities, the pamphlet stressed, were quite exceptional—as sharp as those of any big-brained person who came to see him.

We need not go on with Tom Thumb. He is one of the most written-about celebrities of the nineteenth century. His fame is a testimony to Barnum's showmanship and the presentation he developed for the little man. No one who saw or commented on Charles Stratton suggests that he was an immensely talented performer—or even talented enough that people would have paid to see him if he had not been a dwarf. Stratton's talents were those of a showman, not a performer. Barnum took the raw material, an attractive dwarf in whom he saw star potential, developed a clever aggrandized presentation, got Stratton to go along with it, and launched an unprecedented freak show career.

Charles Stratton's presentation, with its costumed finery, snobbish European appeal, and use of various status symbols, is obviously in the aggrandized mode. Aggrandized it is, but there is also a strong current of farce. This farce/mockery characterized many showmen's aggrandized-mode presentations of dwarfs throughout the nineteenth and twentieth centuries. As we shall see, the degree and nature of the farce varied considerably from exhibit to exhibit. In Stratton's case, what made him so charming as a young man was that he played his presentation so as to reveal to the audience that he was as aware of the ludicrous poses he struck as they were. In this way they were not laughing at him; rather, they all laughed together. But as he rose in prominence his airs grew to be increasingly in sync with what he was off stage. In contrast with Henry Johnson, who endured ever more mockery as his career progressed, with Stratton the farce declined as he aged. Tom Thumb became a serious Charles Stratton, a person who wanted others to respect him because of what he had achieved and to ignore how he might have achieved it, the basis of his fame.

By the time of his wedding Charles Stratton was a wealthy man. He owned property in Bridgeport, pedigreed horses, a yacht which he sailed on Long Island Sound, and an elaborate wardrobe. He also became a Knight Templar and a thirty-second-degree Mason, all of which he flaunted when on tour—that is, when he toured. As time went on he was able to spend more time in leisure activities and less time on the road. When Barnum lost all his money in an ill-fated business deal, Tom Thumb rescued him by volunteering for another lucrative European tour. Yet Tom's generosity and his display of wealth did not mean that he had the control and skill to manage his small fortune. He looked like a millionaire because he spent like one, not because he invested wisely.

Mercy Lavinia Warren Bump was Stratton's bride-to-be. Born on October 31, 1841, in Middleboro, Massachusetts, she was twenty-one years old when they met. Her growth had ceased at the age of ten and the height of thirty-two inches. She came from churchgoing, respectable New England stock and was quick to remember that, on her mother's side, her ancestors could be traced back to the Mayflower (*Sketch of . . . General Tom Thumb and His Wife Lavinia Warren Stratton* 1867). She had been a good student, so good that at age sixteen, when the local school district opened a primary department, she was asked to step in; there she successfully performed a school-teacher's duties.

A visit from her cousin, Colonel Wood, changed her life.[2] He owned a dime museum that traveled up and down the Mississippi and Ohio rivers—she referred to it in her autobiography as "a floating palace of curiosities" (Saxon 1979, 39). She and the colonel, with the promise that he would keep her under his careful supervision, persuaded her parents to allow her to join the troupe. Thus, in 1858, she started her career as a curiosity, sharing a stateroom with Miss Hardy, "a nearly eight feet tall giantess" (Saxon 1979, 40).

In 1862 Barnum heard of the pretty Miss Bump and sent an agent to interview her. Her parents were reluctant to have their daughter join a humbug like Barnum. Nevertheless, they took her to visit the showman in Bridgeport, and she accepted his offer of employment.[3] Barnum brought Lavinia to New York to ready her for her big-time debut. Thinking that her name was too cumbersome for the public to remember, he shortened it to Lavinia Warren. Barnun (1871, 584) describes his preparations for her debut: "I purchased a very splendid wardrobe for Miss Warren, including scores of the richest dresses that could be procured, costly jewels, and in fact everything that could add to the charms of her naturally charming little person." Shrewdly, and in a manner befitting the high aggrandized mode, he rented rooms for her at the swank St. Nicholas Hotel and extended an invitation to both members of the press and the city elite to attend a reception. Thus she gained her first press exposure. She then left for Boston where, at the Parker House, she received the elite of that city, including Governor Andrews. Back in New York she held another reception, this time hosting Civil War generals, the Astors, and the Vanderbilts. And all this was before she ever appeared on the Barnum stage.

On January 2, 1863, she gave her first "levee"[4] at the American Museum. It was during the first few weeks of her appearances that she got to know Charles Stratton who, although not employed by Barnum, dropped by the museum when he was in town to hobnob with his old friends.

Prior to Tom Thumb's romantic interest in Lavinia, Barnum had encouraged another man of small stature who was on exhibit at the museum, Commodore Nutt, to pursue her. Although Barnum had been accused of setting up the Thumb/Warren romance, the couple's involvement, and the rivalry between Thumb and Nutt, were unplanned publicity bonanzas which the showman merely exploited.

How much of the marriage and the wedding arrangements were Barnum's doing, and how much of his involvement was motivated by pure showmanship, is unknown. Lavinia is defensive about the question in her autobiography. While acknowledging that Barnum reaped untold publicity from the wedding and the surrounding ceremonies, she is adamant that her and Tom's motives were not mercenary. Lavinia's parents first opposed the union because they saw it as a publicity stunt, but eventually they were persuaded that the couple's intentions were genuine.

A year before Lavinia's first appearance at the American Museum, Barnum had hired George Washington Morrison Nutt, whom he named Commodore Nutt, to be exhibited at the museum in a naval uniform as the "$30,000 Nutt." This billing was Barnum's way of publicizing the dwarf's salary: $30,000 on a three-year contract. Barnum soon learned that Lavinia had a sister, Minnie, who was seven years her junior and similar in stature; he hired her too. Prior to any hints of a wedding, then, Barnum had already thought about re-engaging Tom Thumb so that, as Barnum expressed it, he could "present to the public a quartette of the most wonderful, intelligent and perfectly formed ladies and gentlemen in miniature the world has ever produced" (Saxon 1979, 57). As Lavinia tells it, the idea of them forming a touring foursome prompted the choice of Minnie as bridesmaid and Commodore Nutt as "groomsman." The wedding was a preliminary, "that the public might have a glimpse of us together" (Saxon 1979, 57).

The announcement of the engagement and wedding plans created immense excitement, which Barnum capitalized on. Lavinia's presentations at the American Museum were "crowded to suffocation" (Barnum 1871, 601). Barnum reported in his autobiography that she sold more than $300 worth of her cartes de visite photographs daily, and museum receipts were frequently in excess of $3,000 a day.

Barnum engaged General Tom Thumb to appear with his financée, help to sell her photos, and add his own to the inventory. They remained on exhibit until three days before the wedding. As the wedding approached, the billing became more flamboyant. "Now or Never" read one ad; another, "The 6,000 years of the world's existence has never produced her equal before" (James 1975). Barnum was so intent on his money interests that he offered the couple $15,000 to postpone their marriage for one month and continue the exhibitions at the museum. They refused. But Barnum made so much money that, as he put it, "I could therefore afford to give them a fine wedding and I did so" (Barnum 1871, 601). Barnum reports that it had been suggested that he hold the wedding in the grand hall of the Academy of Music and charge a large admission, but, although he was sure he could get $25 dollars a ticket easily, he "had promised . . . the couple a genteel and graceful wedding, and I kept my word" (Barnum 1871, 603).

And what a wedding it was (Fig. 42)! Held on February 10, 1863, at the Grace Church, it was described by one observer as a pageant. The ceremony was originally to have taken place at Trinity Church, but after a controversy over the propriety of the event and the degree to which it was a showman's extravaganza, the rector refused ("Loving Lilliputians" 1863). Barnum controlled the invitation list and stacked the audience with governors, members of Congress, generals, and New York's richest and most distinguished citizens—"a gay assemblage of youth, beauty, wealth, and worth of the metropolis" (*Sketch of . . . General Tom Thumb and His Wife Lavinia Warren Stratton* 1867). Attendance was limited to two thousand guests.

Although one of the parishioners of Grace Church who had been displaced from her pew on the nuptial day referred to the ceremony as a "marriage of mountebanks, which I would not take trouble to cross the street to witness" (Barnum 1871, 604), crowds jammed the streets. Broadway between 9th and 12th had been blocked, the police setting up barricades to contain the gathered throngs. At noon the miniature wedding carriage approached the church.

The bride wore a snowy white satin dress with a flowing train decorated with point lace flounce, which a publicity booklet revealed cost "half a hundred a yard" (*Sketch of . . . General Tom Thumb and His Wife Lavinia Warren Stratton* 1867). Her veil was woven into her hair, and above her brow sparkled a diamond star. Her bouquet was roses and camellias. Her white satin slippers werre covered with rosettes and seed pearls. As wedding gifts, her husband had given her a diamond necklace and diamond pins, which she wore. Tom wore all the finery of an elite gentleman: a full dress suit of the finest dark broadcloth, a vest of white corded silk, a blue silk undervest, white gloves, and shiny boots.

The reception was held at the Metropolitan Hotel, its spacious parlors thrown open to invited guests. The couple had a difficult time

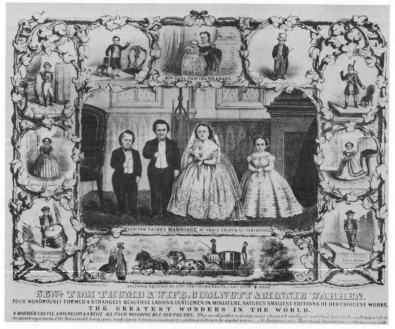

FIG. 42. Tom Thumb and Lavinia Warren's wedding. The wedding party is at the center of this Currier and Ives print, with scenes from their careers around the outside. C. 1863. (Becker Coll., Syracuse University.)

fighting the crowds that mobbed the streets. The bride's presents, which were on display, included a coral leaf brooch and earrings with a diamond center from Mrs. Astor, magnificent pearls from Mrs. Cornelius Vanderbilt, a set of silver goblets from Mrs. Livingston, and a Tuscan gold necklace from Mrs. Belmont. Tiffany presented a silver horse and chariot decorated with rubies. President and Mrs. Lincoln, who were unable to attend, sent a spectacular set of Chinese fire screens, which the couple thanked them for personally when, on their honeymoon tour, they attended a reception given in their honor by the president and first lady in Washington. Their costumes, the wedding, the reception, their honeymoon tour, were all described in flowery and elaborate detail in publicity materials promoting their postwedding appearances. Carte de visite portraits sold by the thousands, with details of the wedding and reception printed on the back of some.

To top off the magnificent aggrandized presentation of Mr. and Mrs. General Tom Thumb, the young couple needed only one more thing: a little Thumb. Whether mainly Barnum's doing or a conspiracy of equals, it was publicized that the couple had given birth to a daughter on December 5, 1863.[5] Photographs of the child taken at the Brady studio with the parents were clearly captioned "Tom Thumb, Wife and Child," and they sold widely (Fig. 43). Lavinia and Tom appeared with "their" daughter on exhibit. Pictures of Lavinia smiling with the child and other indicators show that she was comfortable going along with the charade. Although other authors have been misled into believing the couple actually had a child (Werner 1926, 271) in an interview in 1901 Lavina revealed the truth: "I never had a baby." The child shown with them was borrowed from a foundling home and exchanged for a smaller one when it grew too large. On tour in Europe in the 1860s they "exhibited English babies in England; French babies in France; and German babies in Germany" ("Tom Thumb's Baby" 1901). The display was merely a status-enhancing hoax (Desmond 1954, 232; Saxon 1979, 184). Apparently realizing that the fiction would be difficult to maintain, the showmen milked the baby charade for the publicity and then announced that the child had died of inflammation of the brain. This humanizing touch of tragedy, on top of the whole "Tom Thumb's baby" humbug, illustrates the aggrandized mode at its most daring heights.

Compounding the drama of the little Thumb incident is the mystery surrounding the couple's childlessness. Lavinia never mentioned the stand-in child in her autobiography or the fact that she was childless. Desmond says she grieved because she was not a mother, but whether they were infertile or chose to be childless is unknown. The dangers inherent in a woman of Lavinia's size delivering a child were substantial. Adding a note of tragic irony to the earlier hoax, Lavinia's dwarf sister died in 1878 immediately after the painful delivery of a baby girl weighing five pounds ten ounces. The baby died shortly after birth.

Following their wedding Tom Thumb and his wife, under the title of "General Tom Thumb Company," toured the world. The principal original members consisted of Lavinia, her diminutive sister Minnie, Tom Thumb, Commodore Nutt, and their manager. Their entourage was a full-blown entertainment consisting of impersonations, songs, dances, and skits, all executed in glamorous attire. Their manager appeared on stage so that the audience could keep the performers' size in perspective.

Near his death in 1883, Charles Stratton climbed the stairs to Eisenmann's studio to sit for a portrait with his wife. Although he was only in his forties, he looked old, portly, and tired. In the later years

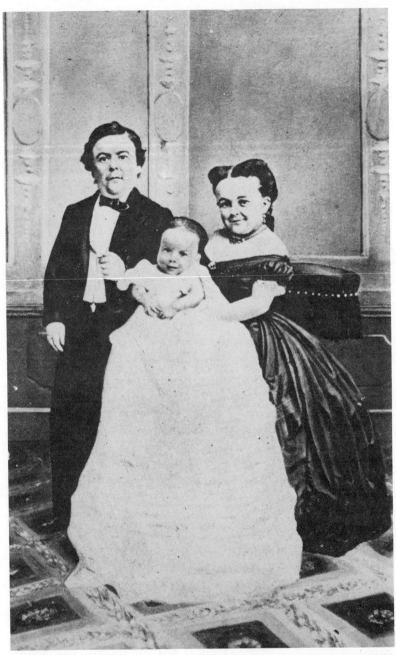

Fig. 43. "Gen. Tom Thumb, wife, and child." Although they never had a child, the couple was exhibited with a little Thumb. Photo by Mathew Brady. (Author's collection.)

of his life he had grown,[6] and he now stood forty inches tall and weighed seventy-five pounds. He had a thin mustache and goatee and smoked cigars, a habit of his for almost as long as he had been on exhibit—since age five. He continued to make public appearances, but the dancing and the farcical elements were gone. On the morning of July 15, 1883, Charles Stratton suffered a stroke and died.

When we think "midget," we think Tom Thumb. His name and fame epitomize the status-enhanced presentation. Bodin and Hershey (1934, 192) remind us that he had no real outstanding talent or qualities—except perhaps those of an amusement world showman, and Barnum certainly outdid him in that arena. Many small people before and after him surpassed him in talent, skills, and even diminutiveness. His fame was manufactured. It was the product of ballyhoo.

Through a combination of frivolous spending, poor management, and the financial climate of the time, the immense fortune Tom and Lavinia had earned—the jewels and horses, the yacht and properties—dissipated. Lavinia was left with an estate valued at only $16,000, plus modest real estate holdings.

Two years after Tom's death, Lavinia married Count Primo Magri, another high-rolling small person exhibit/performer (Fig. 44). She and her husband, together with his dwarf brother, the Baron Ernesto Magri, formed the Lilliputian Opera Company and took to the road. At first they did quite well. They enlarged their troupe to include some of the most famous midgets of the day, performing such operas as *Pocahontas*. As the opera troupe became less popular, Lavinia and the brothers formed their own act. Lavinia sang, the count warbled Italian operatic selections, and the baron whistled. Dime museums employed them most frequently, but they continued to work with traveling vaudeville companies as well. Financially, Lavinia continued to slide, and she gradually looted her home of the valuable memorabilia of her life with the general. In private and public life she remained fashionable, although in this period of her life her gowns were local creations rather than those of Parisian dressmakers (Saxon 1979).

Facing the twentieth century at a stout sixty was not easy for her. The romantic parts she played in skits and her girlish singing were incongruous with her appearance. The glamor was gone. She signed the souvenir photographs as "Countess M. Lavinia Magri," but almost always added "Mrs. Genl. Tom Thumb"; in a letter to her brother in 1915 she noted that the troupe's business was poor but that the old name still drew a crowd (Saxon 1979, 18). When Sam Gumpertz

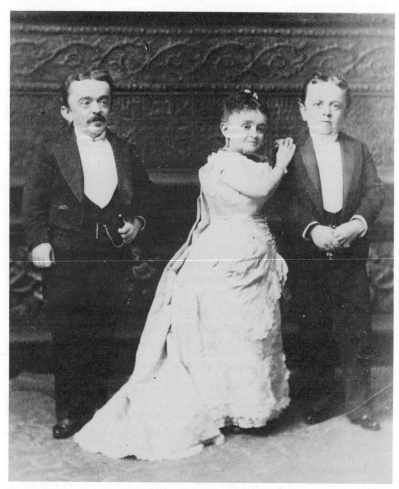

FIG. 44. Lavinia with her second husband, Count Primo Magri. Primo's brother, Baron Ernesto Magri, is on the left. Photo by Charles Eisenmann. (Author's collection.)

opened "Midget City" at Coney Island's Dreamland, he hired Count and Countess Magri, and they became its most famous residents. In the last years of their lives they continued to exhibit while running a general store in Lavinia's hometown. Needless to say, their store offered, in addition to the usual items, a good stock of signed and properly posed photographs.

Lavinia Warren died in her home in Middleboro, Massachusetts, in 1919 at the age of seventy-eight. In her later years, when asked the question "Don't you get tired of this public life?" she would respond, "I belong to the public. The appearing before audiences has been my life. I've hardly known any other." At her request, she was buried next to Tom Thumb in Bridgeport, where a large crowd of mourners, including many showmen from the amusement world, attended the funeral. In their coverage of the funeral the *Bridgeport Post* described Lavinia as "one of the world's most famous dwarfs" (Saxon 1979, 19). At the height of her fame, she thought she was much more than that.

Other Grand Little People

General Tom Thumb was not the first exhibited dwarf to be dressed up, decked out in jewels, and given a fancy title, nor was he the last. There was General Mite, General Carver, General Totman, Great Peter the Small, Admiral Dot, Colonel Small, Colonel Speck, Eliza Nestel (Fair Queen), Major Stevens, Princess Ida, Princess Winnie Wee, Baron Littlefinger, Count Rosebud, Little Lord Robert, Prince Ludwig, King Rector, Princess Wee Wee, Commodore Foote, Baroness Simone, Duchess Leona, Jennie Quigley the Scottish Queen, Prince Nicholi, General Grant, Jr., and many others.

And, while Tom Thumb's touring troupe of performing midgets was one of the first, it definitely wasn't the last traveling high-aggrandized dwarf review to sing, dance, and in other ways perform before crowds. Dressed in tuxedos and evening dresses, smoking cigars and cigarettes in holders, carrying walking canes and parasols, many troupes danced their way across America through the last decade of the nineteenth century and first four of the twentieth.

The famous Horvath Midgets, in addition to appearing in the Barnum and Bailey Sideshow, did independent tours of the United States in the late nineteenth and early twentieth centuries (Fig. 45). Their description in a 1903 courier for the Barnum and Bailey Circus rivals the aggrandized flamboyance of Tom Thumb and Company:

> Five of the smallest, most diminutive Human Beings ever
> brought together since the days of Adam and Eve. Highly
> accomplished operatic singers, terpsichorean, artists,
> pantomimists, prestidigitateurs, comiques, burlesquers
> and mimics, out rivaling the world in a wonderful reper-
> tory of their own devising, embracing every kind of per-
> formance or exhibition. Artists of the most marvelous
> versatility imaginable.

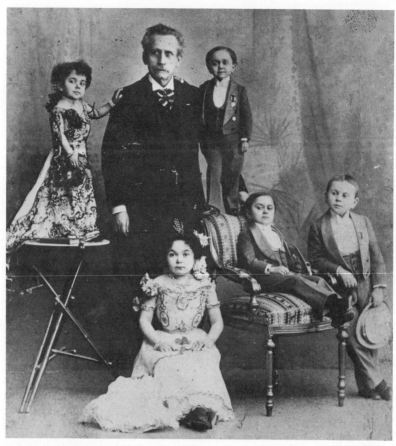

FIG. 45. The Horvath Midgets, "Smallest People in the World." Horvath with Miss Rossie, Miss Anna, Mr. Paul, Mr. Ferry, and Mr. Ernesto. Photo by Frank Wendt, c. 1900. (Becker Coll., Syracuse University.)

Many twentieth-century groups of high-aggrandized little people performed in the United States, including the Ritter Midgets, the Marechal Midgets, Rose's Midgets, Henry Kramer's Midget Starlets, Klinkart's Midgets, the Del Rios, and the Doll Family. Nate Eagle managed many midget troupes, including one with 187 performers (Truzzi 1968).

Of all the managers of midget companies, Leo Singer, the international manager and promoter of Singer's Midgets from 1910 to 1935, stands out most prominently. Their elaborately costumed extravaganzas represented the epitome of the lavish aggrandized mode (Bodin and Hershey 1934, 230). Although the troupe originated in Europe, its members emigrated to the United States and toured this country for years. Their performance of *Lady Godiva* (Fig. 46) was always a favorite, although their high-society nightclub performance was equally popular (Fig. 47).

As Roth and Cromie (1980) point out, many little people worked on stage and screen, but they were not accorded full status as performers. Their talents were treated as secondary to their stature. Although dwarfs played a variety of roles in movies, including Munchkins in the 1938 smash hit *The Wizard of Oz* (Harmetz 1977), the Screen Actors Guild did not admit midget actors until 1970.

In addition to dwarfs in regular freak shows and in touring companies, a series of Midget Villages sprang up around the country. Amusement parks had them—the ones at Mamid Pier in Atlantic City and Coney Island's Dreamland were the most famous and elaborate— as did many of the world's fairs of the twentieth century. The Century of Progress Exposition in Chicago in 1933 had a midget community of sixty, complete with an elected mayor. Billed as a reproduction, reduced to midget scale, of an ancient Bavarian city, it had forty-five buildings, its own police and fire departments, a school, a church, and, as might have been assumed, its own souvenir store (*Official Guide* 1933). For twenty-five cents admission one could visit the village, where, in the theater, glamorous midget stage shows were performed every hour (Roth and Cromie 1980). Typically, midget villages employed the aggrandized mode in their design and stage performances.

Although many midgets were exhibited in groups, there were single exhibits as well, traveling with circuses and appearing at dime museums. The emphasis here was not on a stage performance; rather, the uniqueness of the particular attraction was played up—thus the exhibit might be billed as the smallest man or woman in the world. Occasionally, and in a style similar to the cases reviewed in this chapter, elaborate stories would be told about the attraction's life. These fraudulent stories, then, combined with the dress and other trappings of the aggrandized mode, "made" the exhibit.

One example of a status-enhancing tale is that which accompanied the presentation of "Prince Nicholi, the Russian Prince" early in this century. It was claimed that this exceptionally small person, who appeared either in Russian military dress or in a bemedaled tuxedo, was the offspring of a political prisoner born in the mines of Siberia. The elaborate story ends with the little prince proving to the czar that his father was innocent, thus allowing the whole family to return to their

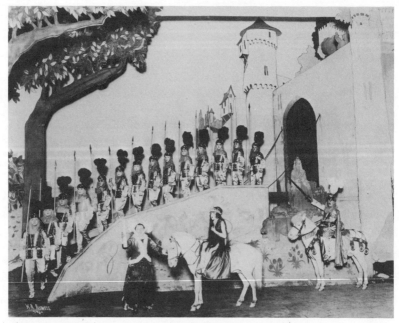

FIG. 46. Singer midgets performing *Lady Godiva*. Publicity photograph by H. A. Atwell, c. 1925. (Becker Coll., Syracuse University.)

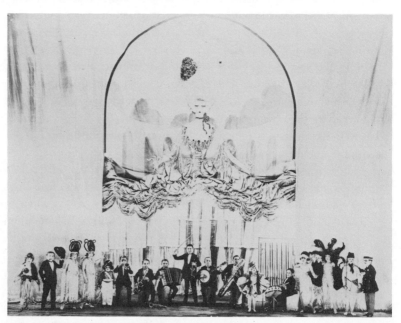

FIG. 47. Singer midgets' high-society musical review. The men wore tuxedos and smoked cigars, the women were adorned with fancy gowns. Photo by H. A. Atwell, c. 1925. (Becker Coll., Syracuse University.)

proper social place in the city of Kiev, whence the prince launched his career.[7] In the detailed fabricated tales of aggrandized-mode exhibits, the freak was not merely a passive character as in the exotic mode. Rather, as the case of Nicholi illustrates, the aggrandized personage is often cast as a hero (*Sketch of the Life of the Russian Prince* c. 1900).

The aggrandized mode was preferred for presenting midgets, but little people were not always "perfect miniatures of Apollo." Those who had physical deformities or misproportioned bodies were often cast in the exotic mode or took jobs as circus clowns.[8] Miss Olaf Krarer, "The Little Esquimaux Lady," who was actually an achondroplastic dwarf, appeared in Eskimo furs against an iceberg background. Similarly, two other achondroplastic dwarfs, "Chief Debro and Wife, The World's Renowned Esquimaux," were presented as being from Greenland and in the exotic mode. Another achondroplastic dwarf was the popular late-nineteenth-century exhibit Che-Mah from China. He appeared in elaborately embroidered Chinese robes and with a queue reported to be thirteen feet long (M. Mitchell 1979). Black dwarfs were cast as exotic pygmies.

At the height of freak show popularity, exhibition was the most common occupation for dwarfs—although apparently not by choice, for as late as 1934 most non–amusement world jobs were closed to them (Truzzi 1968a; Bodin and Hershey 1934). The prevalence of dwarfism among the population is relatively low,[9] but there was a large enough supply that competition among single-attraction dwarfs in standard freak shows became intense. Thus, if one's boasts of being the smallest in the world did not hold up under scrutiny, one could perhaps, as Carrie Akers did, be booked as the dwarf fat lady. Carrie was allegedly thirty-five inches tall and weighed close to three hundred pounds (Durant and Durant 1957, 116). (As with all reports of dwarfs' heights and weights, a few pounds should probably be subtracted from the weight and a few inches added to the height.) Appearing in the 1880s, Carrie had to compete with the thirty-inch Sophia Schultz, another dwarf fat lady. Although Sophia was not as fat, she did boast a straggly goatee (M. Mitchell 1979). In the spirit of one-upmanship, the 1880 Murray's Midgets claimed to be triplets, and Dolletta, an early-1900s exhibit, was featured in her advertising as the mother of three living normal children, all born by the hazardous Caesarean operation. Not only did she boast of being the smallest mother "on medical record," but the smallest grandmother as well.

We have digressed somewhat from our focus on high aggrandized presentations. While midgets represent the best examples of this mode in full bloom, and enjoyed maximum success, other sorts of exhibits employed it as well. The Hilton Sisters exemplify another brand of exalted exhibit.

Violet and Daisy Hilton

The life and career of the "The Hilton Sisters, San Antonio's Siamese Twins," provide an illustration from the 1920s and 1930s of the "high" aggrandized mode. Rather than using the Victorian aristocratic motif, which Tom and Lavinia Thumb exploited so well, Daisy and Violet Hilton were packaged in the twentieth-century wrappings of glamorous stage and screen idols. Their story demonstrates how their fraudulent presentation created a front that became the sisters' reality.

As is typical of presentations in the aggrandized mode, the Hilton Sisters were presented as attractive, engaging celebrities who were exceptionally talented, charming, happy, and normal in every way except for one physical inconvenience: in their case, being born joined at the buttocks. (Joined, or Siamese, twins are identical twins in which the fertilized egg has failed to divide completely, producing siblings of the same sex who are attached. Their attachment can be almost anywhere, but those who were exhibited were most often attached at the chest, back, or buttock.) Although their presentation downplayed the difference that made them an attraction—their attachment—and flaunted their normal attributes, for their patrons as well as the rest of society their difference was what defined them.

The twins were born in 1908 in the resort town of Brighton, England, to a poor, unmarried barmaid, Kate Skinner, and an unknown father ("Pygopagus Marriage" 1934). For reasons not explicit but easily imagined, the mother gave her infant daughters to Mary Hilton, who was the proprietor of the bar where she worked and who had served as midwife at the girls' birth. The details of the transaction are fuzzy, but Mary Hilton gave Kate money in exchange for the children. Whether what transpired was considered an adoption or a sale, Mary Hilton thought she owned the twins, and was intent on exhibiting them. By the time they were three years old they were on the road, appearing at circuses, carnivals, and fairs. They traveled with Mary Hilton, whom the twins were forced to call "Auntie," her husband, whom they were required to call "Sir," and their daughter Edith. At the age of four they toured Germany, and at five, Australia. Long trips

PORTRAITS OF PRESENTATION

in crowded compartments and short stays in various towns character-ized the sisters' preteen life.

They remembered their early years as a nightmare, with whippings on the back and shoulders from the buckle end of a belt that their guardian wore about her waist. According to the sisters, their keeper showed them no affection and constantly reminded them that she was not their mother—their mother had abandoned them. They recalled Mary Hilton's fifth husband, "Sir Green," telling them that they would never be hit in the face because "the public will not be so glad to pay to look at little Siamese twins with scarred faces" (Hilton and Hilton c. 1942). They said that they had been confined to one room and regu-larly schooled and trained.

Their mistreatment shows their keepers' lack of care, but it also reveals a plan. Mary Hilton believed that the girls would be less valu-able if regularly exposed to public view. As the sisters remember it, "She argued that people would not pay to look at us if they could see us for nothing" (Hilton and Hilton c. 1942). In addition, she operated on the assumption that they would be more attractive and have more drawing power if they could play musical instruments, sing, and dance. From an early age she trained them for their careers, paying for lessons in violin, piano, clarinet, voice, and dance. In addition, their manners and dress were carefully monitored as she forced them to work on their public presentation. In fact, they had little else in their lives.

When the twins were in their teens, and while appearing with a circus in Australia, Mary Hilton's daughter met and married Meyer Rothbaum, a showman who ran a balloon and candy concession on the circus grounds. "Auntie," who had lost her fifth husband and needed a man to travel with, went along with the marriage on the con-dition that Rothbaum, who changed his name to Meyer Meyers, joined them. Mary Hilton was then close to sixty years old and was having health problems, so Mr. and Mrs. Meyers took over the book-ing, travel, training, and promotion of the twins.

The Meyerses had big ideas for the girls and their future. They em-phasized the sisters' musical talents, had them take up the saxophone and the ukulele, and traveled with them to the United States. "Auntie" died in Birmingham, Alabama, while on tour. The twins did not grieve, but they did experience considerable fear. Mary Hilton may have been cruel, but she had, the twins felt, protected them from the Meyerses, whom they distrusted as potentially even more controlling than Mary Hilton had been. The night of the funeral Edith and Meyer came to the sisters' rooms to announce that Mrs. Hilton had bequeathed them, along with her jewelry and other belongings, to her daughter Edith (Hilton and Hilton c. 1942).

Meyer became quite a showman, revamping the promotion and management of the twins, who were then in their late teens. His goal was to move them out of the circus and carnival and into vaudeville, which in 1925 was in its heyday. A prestigious and profitable career in vaudevile outshone any carnival or traveling circus possibilities. Working up elaborate publicity materials, he promoted a series of highly lucrative U.S. and world tours. Their first tour on the prestigious "Orpheum Circuit" included appearances with Eddie Cantor and Charlotte Greenward ("Show Family Album" 1938).

Meyer's promotion of the twins exemplifies the aggrandized mode. By the mid 1920s, teratology had grown stale as a framework for exhibiting people with physical anomalies. Increasingly, human differences were seen as diseases, and people who had them, as patients. Presentations were hailed as medical exhibits, but the physiological aspects of the conditions were not highlighted in the elaborate and blatant way they once had been. Nevertheless, the twins' being joined together is what gave them their appeal, and approximately one-quarter of *The Life Story and Facts of the San Antonio Siamese Twins* (c. 1925), the booklet sold in conjunction with their appearance, was devoted to the science behind their condition. The pamphlet used the word *handicapped* in reference to the exhibit, and it even included "an artist's drawings made from X-Ray Photographs" showing where the two spines were attached. As a measure of the increased scientific status of psychology, psychologists' opinions are cited. The introduction contains an overt pitch to frame the exhibit as scientific:

TO SCIENTIFIC COLLEAGUES AND THE
APPRECIATIVE PUBLIC
In placing this booklet before the public the writers desire to thank numerous scientific colleagues and authorities for their courteous and valued cooperation in clinical research dealing with the anatomical problems relating to twin-born progeny.

While the scientific basis was there, the high aggrandized mode of presentation stood out most prominently. A pamphlet sent out to publicity agents to help advertise their tour described the twins as

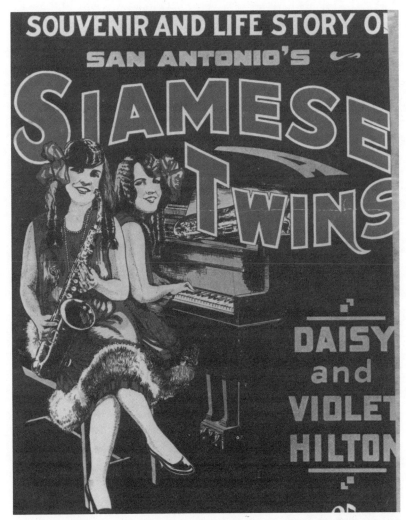

FIG. 48. "San Antonio's Siamese Twins." A publicity pamphlet with this cover was sold in the mid 1920s promoting the Hilton Sisters, who were then in their teens. (Hertzberg Coll., San Antonio Public Library.)

thus: "These Lovely Girls Happy and Vivacious in Their Inseparably Linked Lives Have Perfected Natural Talents Which Make Them One of the Greatest and Most Meritorious Attractions in the World" ("San Antonio's Siamese Twins" 1926).

In a publicity pamphlet sold at their appearances (Fig. 48), the life attributed to the twins is startlingly different from the one they lived.

Rather than being born out of wedlock and unwanted, the "Life Story and Facts" booklet states that they were "the daughters of an English Army Officer. Their mother died a year after their birth. Their father was killed in Belgium in 1914. They were adopted by their uncle and aunt, Mr. and Mrs. Myer Myers, who devote their entire time to the girls and their activities" (*Life Story and Facts of the San Antonio Siamese Twins* 1926). The same pamphlet informs us of their interest and activities in the kitchen, how they love to sew, get meals, cook, sing, practice the piano, romp, raise pets, play tennis, golf, handball, go to the theater and the movies, read good books, and converse with "cultured people" (Fig. 49).

> Their minds are supplied with those things that stimulate the mind and body with high ideals and healthful thoughts. If a young unfortunate jazz-crazed girl kills her mother there is every effort made to keep this sordid story from lodging in the minds of these little innocent girls. But instead of rehearsing all these tales of woe that make such fat fodder for mental morons, these girls have their ideals stimulated by higher ideals and nobler aspirations.

The propaganda went on to quote a recent interview with the girls and their guardians:

> Aunt Lou, as Mrs. Myers is affectionately called, said, "We have tried to show the girls every care and devotion and have been paid back with every ounce of love their little bodies hold." Then with a sort of hushed tone she said, "That in itself is enough." The girls radiate happiness for they say, "We have all the good things in life that other girls enjoy, so what more could we ask."

One thing they could ask for was freedom. Their tours brought a fortune to the Meyerses, but the twins met only with unhappiness. Although they lived in a mansion in San Antonio, Texas, they were miserable. Confined, held in bondage, and completely controlled by the Meyerses, they were isolated from the rest of the world and longed for normal life. Although the publicity photos showed them smiling while dancing with handsome beaux, beautifully dressed, and deeply involved with the joys of music, they were actually slaves.

One day they chanced to be alone with a lawyer and took the opportunity to confide in him. Their servitude was quickly brought before the 94th District Court in San Antonio in a trial that won them their

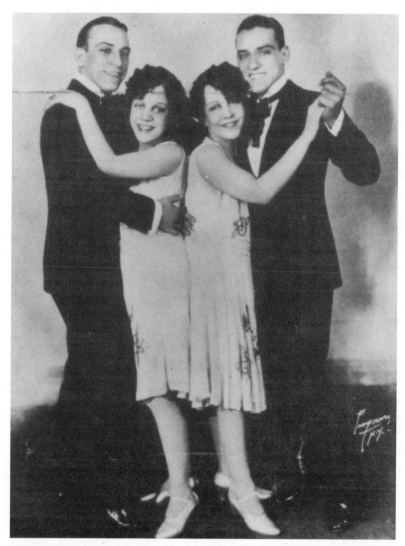

FIG. 49. Hilton Sisters with dates. This picture is taken from 1926 publicity material in which the twins were depicted as happy, well-adjusted, superior teenagers. (Hertzberg Coll., San Antonio Public Library.)

freedom. Thus, in 1931 at the age of twenty-three, they found themselves free, wealthy, and still in demand for stage appearances ("Siamese Twins 'Bondage' Trial" 1969). They played in vaudeville and films and attempted to live the life of glamorous, high-status show personalities. But they were never able to sustain the image; there were too many contradictions and barriers. For example, in their movies they were cast either as freaks (as in Tod Browning's *Freaks*) or as Siamese twins who suffered tragic romances—relationships that paralleled their own experience.

When they went back on the road free of the Meyerses, they called their act the "Hilton Sisters Revue." Promotional material listed their weight at 166 pounds, their height at four feet nine inches. while they claimed to be just like everyone else, with the same feelings and desires, this view of them was not universally accepted. After Daisy had two awkward engagements with eager suitors, Violet became engaged to their orchestra leader, Maurice Lambert. Maurice and the twins apparently worked out the interpersonal difficulties that such a romance would entail, but when they went to obtain a marriage license they encountered even greater problems: their request was repeatedly refused in no less than twenty-one states. As William Chanler, Manhattan corporation counsel speaking for the city, exclaimed, "The very idea of such a marriage is quite immoral and indecent. I feel that a publicity stunt is involved" ("Pygopagus Marriage" 1934). Interestingly, the coverage of their frustrated attempts to get a license was covered by *Time* magazine, not in the "Entertainment" section, but in "Medicine." Maurice and Violet gave up.

Another suitor, James Moore, was more successful in obtaining a license. He and Violet Hilton were married in 1936 before one hundred thousand onlookers at the Texas Centennial Exposition. But the marriage was not what she had hoped for, having been carried out, it seems, as much for publicity as anything else. It was, Violet said later, in name only (Drimmer 1973, 77), and it ended in annulment. In 1941 Daisy finally had her chance to live the life she said she dreamed of, that of a married woman. She wed a dancer, Harold Estep, who appeared on stage as Buddy Sawyer. But her marriage worked out no better than Violet's, ending quickly in divorce.

Their career reached it height in the thirties but soon went downhill. Although they continued to tour, they often ended up stranded and out of money ("Twins Were Popular" 1969). Finally the public lost interest in the dancing of aging Siamese twins, and they settled in Miami and opened a hamburger stand, which they called the Hilton Sisters' Snack Bar. When that too failed, they tried the stage again, this time not on the high-status theater circuit but back with a traveling carnival sideshow.[10] Their last appearance was in 1962 in Charlotte, North Carolina, at a drive-in movie theater to publicize the reissuing of the film *Freaks*. The agent who arranged their appearance brought them there and promised to pick them up, but he never returned. Stranded, out of money, and out of dreams, they settled in Charlotte. Through the kindness of a supermarket owner, they landed a job as checkout clerks. The manager of the market had to buy them dresses to start the job, for they had only show clothes ("Siamese Twins Found Dead" 1969). Until their death in 1967 they led reclusive lives.

They were found dead in their apartment by a neighbor—victims of the flu. Sixty at the time, they left no will, diary, or relatives. They had seldom talked to their acquaintances at work and in the neighborhood about life in the sideshow or the glamor of vaudeville. While their friends were few, many people came to the funeral. The minister asked, "How many of you came here to grieve?" and stated that "they [Daisy and Violet] were always looked upon as freaks" ("Twins Were Popular" 1969). Although they thought it was in their grasp, the image of the happy, exceptionally talented, and capable celebrities that their publicity campaigns painted never really materialized.[11]

It is easy to see the Hilton Sisters' lives as a tragedy and to picture them as victims of unscrupulous showmen. Interestingly, they did not view their situation that way. In their autobiography they identify with the amusement world and see their life on the stage as saving them from, of all things, the medical profession. In their words, they "loathed the very tone of the medical man's voice" and feared that "Auntie" would "stop showing us on stage and let the doctors have us—to punch and pinch and take our pictures always" (Hilton and Hilton c. 1942). Indeed, most exhibits preferred being presented as freaks to being cast as "pathological."

Charles Stratton, Lavinia Warren, Daisy and Violet Hilton, and other freak show attractions presented in the high aggrandized mode did obtain a certain degree of status. To some measure, at least at the height of their careers, they were what they were presented to be. This uniting of pretension and reality was the epitome of their and their managers' success—the showmen's day in the sun.

But ultimately they were forced to separate pretense from reality—and so must we. How were people in the high aggrandized mode actually perceived? How did they think about themselves? What problems did they and their managers have with their presentation?

At first glance, the high aggrandized mode, when it was executed successfully, seemed to serve the interests and concerns of the exhibits and their managers quite well. Fortunes were made through its employment. It pleased and amused. This mode of presentation also seemed to relieve some of the anxieties exhibits had. From what we know about small people of this period (1840–1940), they resented being taken for and related to as children (Truzzi 1968b; Bodin and Hershey 1934); rather, they strove to be viewed as adults. Similarly, given the difficult and sequestered early life of attractions like the Hilton Sisters, it is likely (and evidence in their stories supports the proposition) that they strove too to dissociate themselves from childhood. The high aggrandized mode, with its use of such adult-associated items as suits and ties, cigars, canes, diamond rings, and elaborate makeup and hairdos, the black-tie public appearances, and the hobnobbing with celebrities, provided the superficial trappings of high-status adulthood (Truzzi 1968b). [12]

The high aggrandized mode encouraged the construction of a preferred self-image, with emphasis on exhibits' theatrical or musical talents rather than their demonstrable physical differences. The high aggrandized performers who were of significantly small stature or joined together at the buttocks could certainly feel the stares and knew that they were attractions because they were blatantly different, but they minimized the importance of their physical anomaly as a factor in making them stars.

The content of their presentations served to reinforce this self-image, but other factors helped. Those exhibits who met with great success using the high aggrandized mode became physically dissociated from other freak attractions. Whenever possible, managers purposely separated high aggrandized performers from the sideshow proper as a way of enhancing the attraction's status. Moreover, the high-status performers themselves tended to distance themselves physically and psychologically from other curiosities. While almost all high aggrandized exhibits had careers that intertwined with circuses, dime museums, amusement parks, and carnivals, and at some time during their careers all appeared alongside other freak attractions, they tended to mask these associations with euphemisms such as "levees" to talk about their exhibitions. They played up their vaudeville, moving picture, and theater appearances and downplayed their employment in the amusement world.

The dissociation of high aggrandized exhibits from other exhibits, especially from those more deformed than they, was evident in the "dwarf"/"midget" distinction that existed among little-people per-

174   PORTRAITS OF PRESENTATION

formers. The terms *midget* and *dwarf* had important social meaning in the amusement world. Small people who were well proportioned—"perfect humans in miniature"—in particular coveted the term *midget* for themselves as a way of disaffiliating from the more physically deformed "dwarf" exhibits (Truzzi 1968b). For midgets, who were typically cast in the high aggrandized mode, to be called a "dwarf" was like being called a "child": it was an insult. "Dwarfs" were associated with exotic freak or circus clown roles, and these roles "midgets" shunned.

It is easy to see how the aggrandized mode fit into the exhibits' preferred self-image. But being cast in that mode also wrought problems for these people, and sometimes for their managers as well. Although high aggrandized attractions preferred to see themselves as very talented high-status adults who happened to be small or fused together, they were haunted by another view. Their fear—a fear continually fueled by press coverage, audience reaction, and a host of other indicators—was that they were not what they preferred and were presented to be. One nineteenth-century dramatic-theatrical critique pointed out that Tom Thumb, Lavinia Warren, and all the other performing human oddities "occupy the same position in regard to the drama that the armless youth who cuts paper pictures with his toes occupies in regard to pictorial art" (Hutton 1891, 221). People saw them as caricatures of elite adults, as freaks first and performers second. High aggrandized exhibits may have developed ways of insulating themselves from this view, but it remained their constant plague.

The conflict led some to become what their managers called prima donnas. Managers had to live with their stars' egotism and still be sensitive enough to treat them with the dignity they sought. They had to overlook their pretensions and, at the same time, take care of them and their affairs as managers are supposed to do.

Age played the devil on these exhibits' illusions of grandeur. Their youthful form, which served as the basis for their claims to attractiveness, deteriorated. With prolonged public exposure came declining audiences and downward mobility. The large salaries they commanded, and which they spent with abandon, declined, leaving them in circumstances too humble to lay any realistic claims to a glamorous life-style.

7

Cannibals and Savages

SHOWMEN LOVED to brag of their trickery and tell of embarrassing moments between them and rubes. George Middleton relates an incident involving an "African" exhibited with the O'Brien Circus in 1884.

> In the side show we had a big negro whom we had
> fitted up with rings in his nose, a leopard skin,
> some assagais and a large shield made out of cow's
> skin. While he was sitting on stage in the side
> show, along came two negro women and remarked,
> "See that nigger over there? He ain't no Zulu, that's
> Bill Jackson. He worked over here at Camden on
> the dock. I seen that nigger often." Poor old Bill
> Jackson was as uneasy as if he was sitting on
> needles, holding the shield between him and the
> two negro women. (Middleton 1913, 69)

Many phony Zulus were exhibited in sideshows. Locals dressed in outrageous costumes and portrayed as authentic representatives of exotic non-Western tribes were particularly common, being easy to hire, cheap, and cooperative. But besides the impostors, there were also more authentic "natives"—exhibits who actually hailed from the part of the world the lecturer claimed they were from.

It was a standard sideshow practice from the days before Barnum through the 1930s for people from the non-Western world to climb on to the freak show platform to be gawked at by Americans. These non-Westerners were not necessarily individuals with disabilities, or who were unusually tall or short, or who performed some novelty act like fire eating. Such unusual people were indeed displayed; but those whose only difference lay in the fact that they belonged to an unfamiliar race and culture had value as show pieces as well. Dexter Fellows, exalted press agent of the amusement world, explained: "The Borneo aborigines, the head-hunters, the Ubangis, and the Somalis were all classified as freaks. From the standpoint of the showman the fact that they were different put them in the category of human oddities" (Fellows and Freeman 1936, 296).

People from Oceania, Asia, Africa, Australia, South America, the Arctic—people from all over the non-Western world—were brought to the United States and soon formed a separate genre of freak show exhibit. They were present in the early museums and circuses and later filled the human exhibit ranks at fairs, amusement parks, and carnivals. Large groups were brought to populate "native villages" along midways; they also came alone and in small groups to take their place in the freak show proper.

Aborigines as exhibits fit well into the nineteenth-century framework in which freak shows doubled as scientific presentations. Explorers took along natural scientists to collect all forms of animal and plant species; in this scheme, native people constituted the living specimens from the human kingdom. Exhibits of "primitive" and "barbaric" people went hand in hand with the cabinets of curiosities.

By 1850 a new science, ethnology, the early cousin of cultural anthropology, had begun to lay claim to the exotics. Yet still, use of the word *primitive* seems as appropriate for these early practitioners of the science as for their subjects. Not until the 1930s and Franz Boas did the idea of cultural relativism—that a culture should be evaluated by its own standards, not by those of another—gain currency in learned circles. Non-Westerners as exhibits fit the early-twentieth-century mentality well. Indeed, belief in inherent racial inferiority and the undisputed superiority of Western culture remained part of the American frame of mind well past the 1930s.

Display of non-Westerners in freak shows was not intended as a cross-cultural experience to provide patrons with real knowledge of the ways of life and thinking of a foreign group of people. Rather, it was a money-making activity that prospered by embellishing exhibits with exaggerated, bogus presentations emphasizing their strange customs and beliefs. Showmen took people who were culturally and ancestrally non-Western and made them freaks by casting them as bizarre and exotic: cannibals, savages, and barbarians.

A lengthy chronicle of non-Westerners as freaks and a myriad of stories associated with particular exhibits could be told, but this chapter does not present the whole story. Rather, it is a sampler, concentrating on exhibits from two areas, the South Sea Islands and Subsaharan Africa.[1] Although I do mention some exhibits presented as natives from Africa who were really local recruits, I do not discuss these in any depth. Nor do I deal with native exhibits whose major claim to fame was a physical anomaly or a unique novelty act.

Obviously, non-Western people were presented in the exotic mode. But exotic is an understatement for what will be discussed. As we shall see, showmen elaborately embellished the exotic and wrapped it with a profusion of creative tales and twists, finally packaging it all within a pseudoanthropological framework.

South Pacific Cannibals

In the sixteenth century both the Spanish sailor Balboa and the Portuguese explorer Magellan sailed through Oceania, or the Pacific Islands. Abel Janszoon Tasman, a Dutch navigator, "discovered" New Zealand in 1642. In the late 1700s Captain James Cook of the British Royal Navy charted the islands of the South Seas. These and other explorers brought home descriptions of a land that was like Eden, where natives lived in utter serenity. To eighteenth- and early-nineteenth-century Westerners, many of the islands' tribal people were synonymous with Rousseau's noble savages. Sailors jumped ship to partake in the splendor of free love and the other fruits of this unspoiled wonderland (Daws 1980).

With the nineteenth century came traders, imperialists, natural scientists, and missionaries, all of whom had more than a passing interest in the islands. They wanted to penetrate its beauty, seize its resources, learn its secrets, and tame its "savages." The factor that helped to upset the romance of the West with the Pacific Islanders was cannibalism. This practice sent chills down the backs of Westerners and, after a boatload of Cook's men were killed and eaten in New Zealand, Americans were bombarded with tales of the most ghastly of human atrocities (Daws 1980).

Joseph Banks, a naturalist traveling with Cook on his first voyage, collected specimens of all sorts, including humans (Daws 1980). He tried to bring a Tahitian back to England with him, but the native died en route. Cook's second expedition was successful in bringing home a live Polynesian in 1774. This man, whose name was Mai, was tattooed, and he was promptly put on public display.

The first record of Oceanian people being exhibited in the United

178

States dates from early September 1831, when "Two Cannibals of the Islands in the South Pacific" were exhibited at Tammany Hall in New York City (Odell, 1927, vol. 3). Later that month Peale's museum engaged them. Another pair, "cannibals" named Sunday and Monday, were exhibited in Northeastern cities starting in 1834. A merchant explorer named Captain Benjamin Morrell had brought them to the United States from the islands near Papua. Sunday was gentle and adapted easily to the new land. Monday, however, became despondent, physically ill, and then died, after which Sunday, in Western dress and carrying many gifts, proudly accompanied a trading vessel back to his native island (Jacobs 1844, 14).

With his keen showman's acumen, Barnum sensed the appeal cannibals might have. In June 1842, one and one-half years after the opening of the American Museum, he exhibited Vendovi, "A Cannibal Chief" (Odell 1928, vol. 4), thus capitalizing on the public interest and helping to make cannibals standard freak show fare.

Of all the countries in the South Pacific, Fiji was perhaps considered the most exotic. Its people had the characteristics of Polynesians, yet they were strongly associated with the more Melanesian custom of eating one's neighbor. In the last decade of the eighteenth century and the first decade of the nineteenth there was increased contact between Islanders and Westerners as a result of sandalwood trading and aggressive missionary interest. In 1838 the United States sponsored an expedition to Fiji, to survey the islands and investigate a massacre of the crew of an American vessel. Americans followed this early imperialist venture carefully. It sparked their imaginations.

While the American exploratory expedition had seen only one incident of cannibalism (an eye had been ceremonially consumed), Americans nevertheless had the impression that human flesh was the mainstay of the Islanders' diet. Yet if the extent of cannibalism had been as great as some reports led people to believe, Fijians would have consumed themselves out of existence. The exaggerated reports did have some basis in reality, however. Prior to 1800 cannibalism had been confined to ceremonial sacrifices, but in the Fijian wars of the early nineteenth century the practice became pervasive in some areas, where a portion of every captive was eaten and raids were undertaken solely to procure human flesh (Thomson 1908). By mid-century, details of cannibalism among the Fijians began to reach America through missionary reports (Hogg 1958; Thomson 1908).

The truth about cannibalism was ghastly enough to Americans, but the embellished tales added another level of horror. One alleged custom involved sending portions of the flesh all over the country for chiefs to sample when a warrior of repute was cooked. The body of a missionary named Baker who was killed in 1860 was allegedly treated in this way, with almost every chief in the area receiving a portion. According to one oft-repeated story, the chief of Mongondro received a leg from which Baker's high leather boot had not been removed. Taking the leather to be the white man's skin, the chief complimented the white race on its toughness (Thomson 1908, 107–108).

In 1872 it was announced that there had arrived in this country, expressly for P. T. Barnum's Great Traveling Exhibition, four Fijians from Na Viti Levu, the largest island in the Fiji group. Three were men, and cannibals through and through. Two of them were of normal stature, but the last was a ferocious warrior dwarf, about four feet tall, named General Ra Biau. The last Fijian was a woman, but no ordinary one: she was a Fiji princess, the granddaughter of Thokambau,[2] king of Fiji Island. She had been educated in the Wesleyan Mission in Mbau (*History of P. T. Barnum's Fiji Cannibals* 1872) and was acting as translator and custodian on the trip to the United States.

The fictitious story behind their capture involved a rebel cannibal chief who had seized two missionaries and threatened that they would be eaten alive piece by piece. The aid of King Thokambau, a real Fiji king who had converted to Christianity and who had helped the missionaries curtail cannibalism, was sought, and he sent several hundred of his bravest warriors to the rescue. The battle was bitter, but Thokambau's men were victorious in the end. They took many prisoners, including the three men we are concerned with here. General Ra Biau had distinguished himself by killing four of Thokambau's valiant warriors with his own hands, even though they were giants compared to him.

According to the Fijian code, the captives were condemned to death by the most cruel and systematic torture: "to have their tongues cut out, their brains eaten and their skulls converted into drinking-cups, while the bones of their bodies were to be made into ornaments to be worn by the vanquishers" (*History of P. T. Barnum's Fiji Cannibals* 1872). The missionaries, not wanting a reversion to cannibalism, sought an alternative to the punishment. At this point an agent showman stepped in and proposed to take the prisoners to the United States for exhibition. The deal involved a three-year rental fee to

Thokambau and a $15,000 bond to insure their safe return home. The princess accepted the job of accompanying them so that she might become familiar with the "modes and customs of civilization" and convert the three savages to Christianity.

The only photographs available of the "Figi Cannibals" were taken at Mathew Brady's studio in New York in 1872.[3] In one picture the three men are standing bare to the waist with the lower part of their bodies wrapped in white sheets (Fig. 50). The woman is sitting in their midst wearing a full-length dress, high on the neck and long sleeved. All four have high teased hair, a style characteristic of Fijians displayed in the United States. Each man has a long spear in the right hand and a thick wooden club in the right. Heavy bone necklaces adorn their necks. General Ra Biau, considerably shorter than the others, has a small mustache, and he, like the others, stares at us as though to tell us that he is outraged at his treatment and at the story concocted about his death.[4]

P. T. Barnum's Museum, Menagerie, and Circus, also known as P. T. Barnum's Great Traveling World's Fair,[5] played York, Pennsylvania, on May 14, 1872. The patrons who came to see the "Figi Cannibals," the feature attraction, were disappointed. Although the museum tent contained a wide assortment of Fijian artifacts, the live "cannibals" were nowhere to be seen. The *Daily York* explained their absence in an article the following day: the "cannibal dwarf" had died. According to the article, the "little Figi," who refused to wear shoes and warm clothing, had fallen ill a few days before. On the day of his death he shivered constantly, and his "keeper" could do nothing to cheer him up. He would not take food and kept mumbling "the only word he pronounced intelligently, 'Figi,'" thus suggesting his preoccupation with home.

The article went on to provide a sensational twist to the otherwise sedate and sad story:

> Shortly after the corpse was placed in the coffin last evening, S. S. Smith, the keeper, locked the door upon the three companions in an adjoining room and left the building for the purpose of consulting the manager at the National Hotel. He states that he was not absent 30 minutes, but that upon returning, a scene presented itself too horrible to detail. The two male associates had gained access to the corpse and were biting and gnawing at the

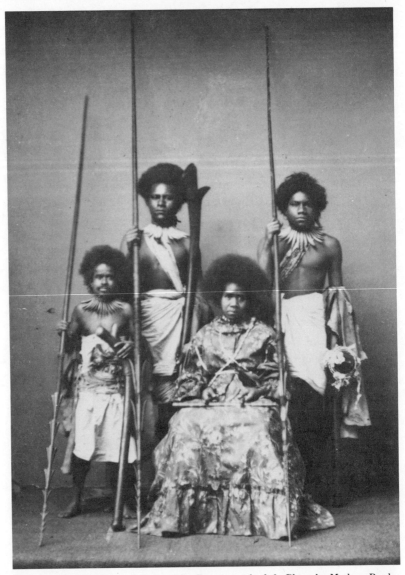

FIG. 50. "Figi Cannibals." General Ra Biau is on the left. Photo by Mathew Brady, 1872. (Meserve Coll., National Portrait Gallery, Smithsonian Institution, Washington, D.C.)

fleshy parts of the body with all the eagerness of their native cannibalism. The female stood aloof in one corner and by sign, word and gesture, was enthralling them to desist. (Shettel 1929, 47)

PORTRAITS OF PRESENTATION

The only item of truth was that the dwarf had died. The rest was a publicity stunt, a press agent's humbug to turn the tragic death into an opportunity to fan interest in the three remaining Fiji Islanders. Or I should say, two Fiji Islanders, for it was discovered that the female member of the "cannibal" troupe was actually a native of Virginia and, prior to joining the show, had been the domestic of a gentleman who resided in Baltimore. At about the same time, a Mr. George Boyne from Sacramento, California, wrote a letter asserting that the "Figis" in question were hardly cannibals. On the contrary, while they may have been born in Fiji, they had been under Christian training for a number of years and had spent a portion of their lives in California (Shettel 1929). Fijians they were, but they must have been showmen as well to have carried out the cannibal farce so effectively.

During the first quarter of the nineteenth century missionaries were not very successful in Christianizing the Fijians and convincing them that they ought to give up their flesh-eating ways. In the second half of the century, however, they had made considerable progress and even claimed to have almost eliminated cannibalism. The "cannibals" exhibited in Barnum's traveling show were presented as the vestiges of the practice. Other Fiji Islanders who were exhibited were said to be reformed cannibals.

Ruto Semm and Annie Semm, better known as "Fiji Jim and Wife," had a twenty-year career in the freak show (Fig. 51). A few pictures, including one with Ruto's February 9, 1897, obituary taped to the back, provide the only evidence of their presentation and background.[6] The Semms were brought from their island home in the Pacific in approximately 1877 by a circus agent, who offered them golden prospects. Inexplicably, however, the agent deserted them shortly after their arrival in the United States. In any case, they apparently became socialized and were integrated into the amusement world by way of Barnum's circus, with which they traveled for eight years. They then joined the dime museum circuit and finally finished their careers on exhibit in New York City amusement parks in the summer and at Huber's Museum in the winter. According to the obituary, "Their life was a constant struggle to obtain sufficient money to return to their island home."[7] Whether this was an accurate description of their circumstances or merely a line from their presentation is impossible to ascertain.

"Fiji Jim" died at the age of fifty of a "cold, which developed into pneumonia and subsequently pleurisy." He was said to have been

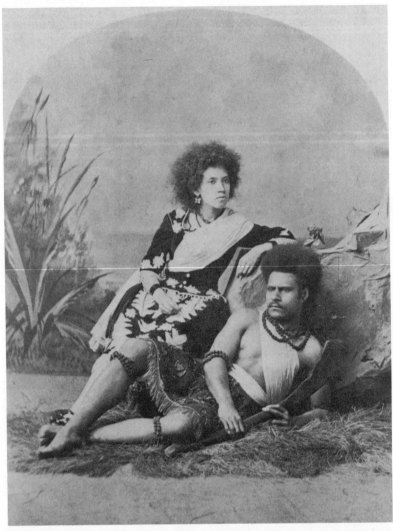

Fɪɢ. 51. Ruto Semm and Annie Semm. The papier-mâché boulders and tropical background complement the exotic presentation of "Fiji Jim and Wife." Photographer unknown, c. 1880. (Hertzberg Coll., San Antonio Public Library.)

born in the island group of Lau, a part of Fiji. He lived his last two years with his wife on the top floor of a New York tenement.

Jim and Annie are striking in their photographs. One shows them both leaning on a papier-mâché boulder, straw scattered on the ground around them, against a background of tropical plants and a South Sea

PORTRAITS OF PRESENTATION

ocean view. Their hair is teased, and Jim stands bare-chested, draped with beads, and holding a club. They look handsome and stoic. We have no "true life" pamphlet or other accounts that would provide the details of their presentation. Whether they were hailed as practicing cannibals or as reformed cannibals is not very important. Even though their picture was undoubtedly purposely posed to evoke a certain dignity, the dignity that comes through almost transcends the embellished exotic presentation.

As discussed in Chapter 2, displays of "native villages" on the midway of Chicago's 1893 Columbian Exposition inspired circuses to enlarge their own displays of tribal people. Although by 1893 the eradication of cannibalism in the Fiji Islands was widely accepted, showmen could still exploit cannibal imagery. Instead of displaying people who actually did eat human flesh, or had once done so, they offered the real sons and daughters of cannibals. Barnum and Bailey's Circus did so in their Great Ethnological Congress, which was the featured attraction of their 1893–1895 show.

In the Ethnological Congress, which Bailey assembled (Barnum had died in 1891), seventy-four non-Western people, some recruited from the Chicago Columbian World's Fair, were displayed in the menagerie tent (Fig. 52). One person exhibited was Memene, a Fijian princess, whose ancestors were claimed to have been cannibals.

The details of her background appear in a human interest story done by a New York Sunday paper ("Around New York with a Cannibal Girl" 1895) in which a reporter took the princess around the city on Easter Sunday:

> Many years ago . . . there dwelt in Laveta, the wildest of the Fiji Islands, a noted savage chief. His name was Komele. It was his playful custom after a particularly successful encounter with a hostile band of natives to sit beneath his own palm trees, and surrounded by his followers, to enjoy a nice roast—the component parts of which were supplied by portions of the anatomy of his recent departed foes.
>
> As time wore on and the white man set foot upon his domain this diet changed, and where once he dined on sun-kissed savages he now partook of the more delicate and toothsome missionary.
>
> Years passed by. A son, Kakela, took up his scepter.

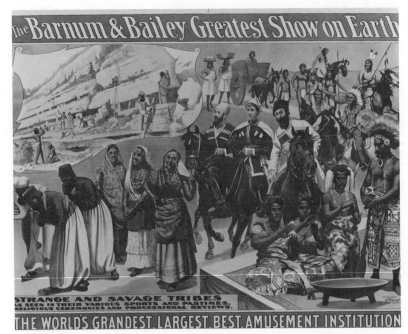

FIG. 52. Poster for 1893 Ethnological Congress. Fiji Islanders are shown on the right. (Richard Coll., Worcester, Massachusetts.)

> He, too, on occasion enjoyed a missionary meal, but
> gradually this custom died out, and when his daughter,
> Memene, the heroine of this tale had grown to maiden-
> hood, cannibalism was but a memory in the islands.

Although the newspaper article treats the progress of the Fijians with sarcasm, it also contains elements suggestive of some progress, however small, in Americans' relations with Third World people. The report does more than supply an outsider's view of Memene's presentation. We visit with her as she sees the Easter parade, and we hear, for the first time and in her own words (albeit reconstructed for us by the reporter), her impressions of the city. As she passed the famous Delmonico's restaurant, for example, she commented: "I should think the people would rather have dinner at home in their beautiful houses." One gets the feeling that Memene is accepted as a human being, a person with a point of view and ideas—a message absent from earlier coverage of such exhibits. But as we shall see, this was an isolated incident rather than the beginning of a significant trend.

The profit in exhibits lay in constructing cannibals and savages, not in humanizing presentations of the inhabitants of the non-Western world.

African Bushmen

The first black landed in the United States in 1619 (W. Jordan 1968, 44). By 1700 black Africans had begun to flood into English America, not as citizens but as slaves. Negroes were thus a common sight in many parts of the United States in the eighteenth and nineteenth centuries; they were certainly not unusual enough to appear in the freak show. But blacks were of great interest to scientists and laypeople alike. Americans were active in the debate concerning the Negro's place in the great chain of being. Some argued that they were a separate species, closer to the ape than to whites (Stanton 1960; W. Jordan 1968). Others held that they were inferior not because they were an inferior species but because they had degenerated owing to climatic conditions.

The nineteenth century also saw numerous Western expeditions into the interior of the African continent. Stories of apelike creatures with strange savage customs and unusual physiology spread among Americans. It was also a time of ferocious battles between the Zulus and the Boers and British. White Americans had no interest in seeing the run-of-the-mill Negro, but they did want to see the warriors, the bestial Africans, and the pygmies. Showmen thus had a mandate to mold the presentations of the Africans they exhibited to justify slavery and colonialism—that is, to confirm Africans' inferiority and primitiveness.

There are hundreds of examples of nineteenth-century African exhibits. Hottentots were displayed as examples of the most primitive people in the world (Lindfors 1983b; S. Gould 1985); Dahoman women warriors, who were referred to as "Amazons," were featured for their size; and ferocious Zulus were commonplace (Lindfors 1983a; M. Mitchell 1979). In fact, "Zulu" came to be the generic name for American circus workers who dressed as Africans (Lindfors 1983a).

But perhaps the most fascinating exhibits for Americans were the South African "Bushmen." For years explorers had spread tales about tribes of pygmies, and in 1860 the public finally had a chance to see an actual pygmy firsthand. The exhibit was not any ordinary Bushman, however; it was a "Troglodyte-Bushman" or "Erdmanniges," also referred to by promoters as an "Earthman." The foreign guest displayed in the United States was a lone woman named Flora. She and her male companion, Martinis, who died before reaching the United States, had had their first showing in England in 1852.[8]

In November of that year the *Illustrated London News* presented an extensive description of them ("Earthmen from Port Natal" 1852). The boy was said to be fourteen and the girl sixteen, yet each stood only thirty-nine inches high. "The origin of the Earthmen at the Cape of Good Hope," it was explained, "is supposed to be analogous to that of the Bushmen and Hottentots; but their habits are totally distinct. The Bushmen build huts and live in little villages; but the Earthmen burrow in the ground, and hence derive their name." The article continues with a clarification: "By burrowing, the reader must not understand that they dig and hide under the surface like rabbits, but that they scratch hollows in the ground to shield them in a measure from the wind."

They, like the other "remarkable varieties of Human Species represented now in London," were the subject of ethnological inquiry and debate by scientists in learned societies (Latham 1856). Flora's first appearance in the United States was probably at Barnum's American Museum in 1860 (*Life of the Living Aztec Children* 1860, 41). While the explanation of the name *Earthmen* that appeared in a Barnum publication[9] resembles that in the *Illustrated London News*, Barnum's provides a wonderful example of American showmen's embellishment:

> The Earthman has no friends. He lives in a large, un-
> varying circle of enemies, from whom his only escape is
> invisibility, and this he accomplishes by burrowing holes
> into the ground, and there finding shelter beyond the
> reach of man or beast. It is this singular habit from which
> the name of "Earthmen" is derived. A colony of them
> resembles a gigantic warren of rabbits. Along the pre-
> cipitous sides of a range of mountains the sunny border of
> which lies by a stream of fresh water, and high up from
> its banks thousands of holes are constructed, which ex-
> tended back into the mountain, sometimes as far as three
> miles, and continuous passages from which penetrate
> from one mountain to another, upwards of twenty miles.
> These holes are so numerous and intricate, that in the
> course of time while mountains become honey-combed,
> and a colony of Earthmen, who have been hunted from

one side of a mountain, will speedily reappear on the other. (*Life of the Living Aztec Children* 1860, 41)

For those who might doubt that such a mammoth system of tunnels could possibly be constructed by such small and primitive people, an explanation was offered:

> Thousands of little figures are constantly busy hewing out new excavations, at which long practice has made them most expert. For this purpose, their toe and finger nails are cultivated in the shape of scoops or shovels, and the arms and legs being worked rapidly together, a fountain of dirt flies from the ground under the efforts of the busy little creature, who penetrates into it like the point of an auger, scattering rocks and dirt in every direction.

The Earthman's sustenance was described as "almost every kind of living creature and creeping thing, lizards, locusts, and grasshoppers not excepted," and "poisonous, as well as innoxious serpents, they roast and eat." In preparing the snakes for feasting, the brochure sold in conjunction with Flora's exhibition relates: "They separate the head from the body with a knife, or, for want of that, bite it off!" With regard to their language, the pamphlet states: "The Earthmen have no recognized language beyond the simple and almost unintelligible patois which designates their simple wants." Filling out the description, the pamphlet explains that Earthmen have "no knowledge of the Supreme Being," and "they know no marriage state and make no distinction of girl, maiden or wife." Flora was a Bushman from South Africa all right, but the description of her tribe and their customs was outrageously inaccurate.

Flora was not the last of the Earthmen presentations in American freak shows. G. A. Farini, an active showman who managed a number of stellar attractions to stardom, imported a family of South African Bushmen in the 1880s who he said were Earthmen or "Yellow Dwarfs" (Fig. 53). Using the original fabrications as the basis for his presentation, he made adjustments for the people he displayed by saying that their lighter, yellowish skin resulted from long periods of living underground. As the picture of the family shows, the four children and parents were displayed in leopard-skin briefs, with the males holding bows and arrows—in stark contrast to tuxedo-clad W. A. Healey, their manager.[10]

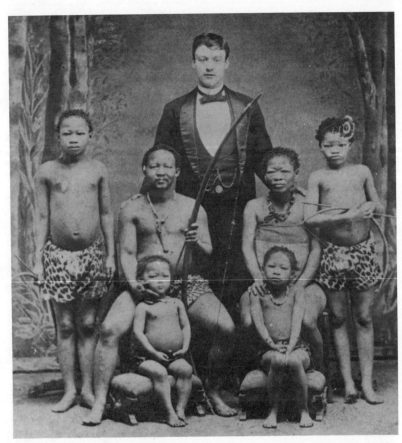

Fig. 53. Farini's "Earthmen." Photographer unknown, c. 1884. (Circus World Museum, Baraboo, Wisconsin.)

We have to move into the twentieth century to meet the person with the longest and most successful career as an "African Bushman." Presented as Clicko (or Clico), "The Wild Dancing South African Bushman,"[11] his real name was Franz Taibosh (Fig. 54). He was brought to the United States from Europe in 1912 (Clicko obituary 1940) by Frank A. Cook, a lawyer for the Ringling Circus. Cook, who at the time managed the importation of all Ringling's international attractions, became Clicko's guardian (Cook, private correspondence, 1984). Clicko was a regular and featured attraction of the Ringling Brothers, Barnum and Bailey Sideshow in the 1920s and 1930s. He also appeared at Coney Island for Sam Gumpertz and traveled with various dime museums. When he died in 1940 he was being advertised as 115 years

PORTRAITS OF PRESENTATION

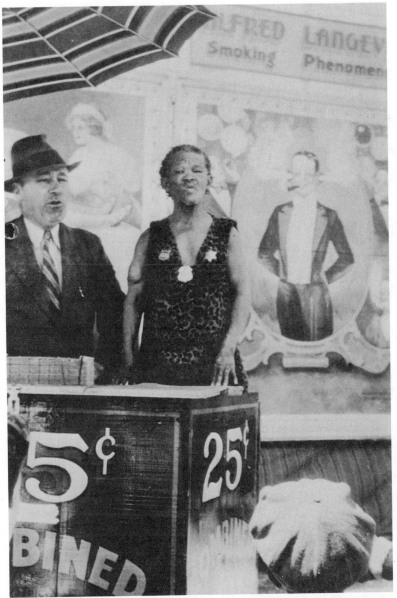

FIG. 54. Clicko, "The Wild Dancing South African Bushman." Postcard of Clicko with a ticket seller in front of the bannerline at Ringling Brothers, Barnum and Bailey Sideshow, c. 1930. (Pfening Coll., Columbus, Ohio.)

old and the only African Bushman ever to enter the United States (Clicko obituary 1940; Holtman 1968, 199). Although the story of his discovery and other aspects of his presentation were wild exaggerations, all evidence indicates that Clicko actually was a South African.[12]

In his presentatioin, Clicko, who was often used as the bally, wore a leopard-skin robe that draped over his shoulders and came down to above the knees. Shoeless, he would dance about the platform emitting "ungodly yells" (Tucker 1973). In conjunction with his appearances he sold a pamphlet, *The Life History of Clicko: The Dancing Bushman of Africa.* The 1922 version described his capture by a Captain Du Barry. The captain, hunting in the Kalahari Desert and having wounded several ostriches, was riding up to secure his prey when he noticed what looked to be one of the birds running away. He gave chase, only to capture Clicko wearing an ostrich hide. The pamphlet concludes with this description of Clicko: "He is as near like the ape as he is like the human. He has a good understanding of things, but with the mind that would correspond favorably with that of a two-year-old child, and we cannot help but wonder if Captain Du Barry has not brought Darwin's missing link to civilization."

When Frank Cook died in 1937, his wife Evelyn took over Clicko's care. Apparently he had become an accepted part of the Cook family. During the off season he lived with them in their New York apartment. People who knew Clicko and his situation are unanimous in pointing to his positive adjustment to circus life and his overall happiness. "Always cheerful and seemingly happy, he was the pet of many of the circus executives, who were always bringing him his favorite smokes, or a bottle of beer, his favorite refreshment" (Holtman 1968, 199). He developed a fondness for large black cigars, and these became his trademark. In his own way he was part of the amusement world—a showman of sorts.

Ubangi Savages

"Genuine Monster-mouthed Ubangi Savages World's Most Weird Living Humans from Africa's Darkest Depths," the circus ad proclaimed. Although the late nineteenth and early twentieth centuries saw the most extensive exhibition of non-Western peoples, as well as the greatest amount of hyperbole regarding their character, this ad publicized an early-1930s attraction that some showmen consider the greatest freak exhibit of the century (Fig. 55).

PORTRAITS OF PRESENTATION

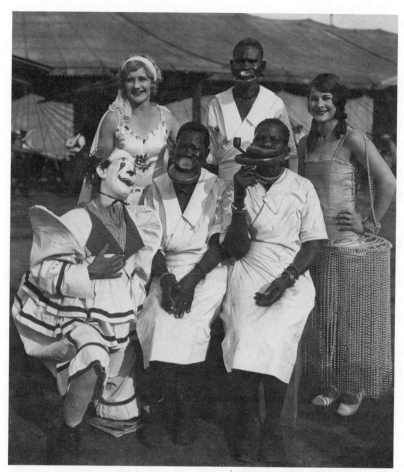

FIG. 55. "Monster-mouthed Ubangi Savages." Shown here with a clown and two other circus performers, this attraction was featured in 1930 with the Ringling Brothers, Barnum and Bailey Circus. Photographer unknown. (Circus World Museum, Baraboo, Wisconsin.)

The story of how this exhibit reached the United States and became a featured attraction of the Ringling Brothers, Barnum and Bailey Circus has several variants.[13] The issue is merely complicated by the many gaffs and other troupes of Africans who, in the promoters' chase after the success of the "original" exhibit, were displayed as Ubangis.

According to Fred Bradna, who spent forty years with the "big one," the original "Ubangi Savages" were procured by a circus agent, Ludwig Bergonnier, after seeing people from this tribe at a Paris fair (Bradna and Hartzell 1952). They were from the Congo, and they could be distinguished from other people in the world by a peculiar custom: the women beautified themselves by enlarging their lips. This effect was accomplished by slitting female babies' lips and inserting wooden disks, with the one in the bottom lip larger than in the top. By increasing the size of the disks as the child grew, the lips could be extended to huge proportions—mature women had lips that extended ten inches or more, giving them a duckbill appearance.

Realizing the potential of such an attraction, Bergonnier went to the French Congo where, with promises of wealth, he persuaded a chief to allow him to take thirteen women and two men with him on tour.[14] For two years he displayed them in Europe, and then John Ringling booked them for their U.S. appearance in the Ringling freak show. Bradna says that Ringling paid $1,500 a week for the exhibit; Bergonnier took all and let the Congolese make what they could by selling souvenir postcards at five cents a piece.

They arrived by boat in the spring of 1930 after the circus had opened. Mr. Cook, the same circus lawyer who had imported Clicko, cleared them through customs and brought them right to the show. They were an immediate sensation; according to Bradna, at first the women's being bare above the waist attracted as much attention as their lips. In addition to appearing in the sideshow prior to the circus performance, they paraded around the arena during each main big-top show. Sideshow manager Clyde Ingalls made the introduction: "Ladies and Gentlemen, from the deepest depths of darkest Africa we present the world's most astounding Aborigines—the 'Crocodile Lipped Women From the Congo'—the Ubangis" (Tucker 1973, 2). Then, from the far end of the arena, they would slowly walk in, single file—the men in loincloths carrying spears, and the barefoot women wearing sacks for skirts and little else.

When the Congolese arrived in this country, they were not called Ubangis. In fact, the tribal name was made up for the purposes of presentation. According to Robert Taylor, Roland Butler, press agent for Ringling Brothers Circus, was studying maps of Africa and encountered an obscure district, named Ubangi, several hundred miles from the tribe's true location. It had the proper exotic ring, and so, as Butler put it, "I resettled them" (Taylor 1956).

The drawings for the poster advertisements extended the lips far in excess of reality: in some they appear as if they have turkey platter inserts. One poster referred to them as the "greatest educational feature of all time," while on the next line they are described—with a lie—as having "mouths and lips as large as those of full-grown croco-diles!" Another poster hails them as being "New to Civilization" and a "Tribe of Genuine Ubangi Savages."

The booklet sold in conjunction with their exhibition was entitled *Saucer Lips, Ubangi Savages, French Equatorial Africa, Historical Sketch, Origins, Habits and Customs* (1930). Emphasizing the remote-ness of their village, their strange marriage and funeral customs, it was richly illustrated with pictures of women bare to the waist.

Darkest Africa at the Century of Progress World's Fair

The Congolese women just discussed were embellished by showmen to conform to a distorted exotic presentation. But their story does not reveal the extremes that could go into fabricating an "authentic" ethnographic educational exhibit. For that I turn to the 1933–1934 "Darkest Africa" exhibit and accounts by three showmen who orga-nized and worked it: Harry Lewiston, Nate Eagle, and Lou Dufour (Holtman 1968; Taylor 1958a; Dufour 1977).[15]

This exhibit at the Century of Progress World's Fair in Chicago was enclosed by a "stockade" of large bamboo stalks and occupied approxi-mately forty thousand square feet of midway space. Harry Lewiston described the facade: "Out front, we had large banners depicting life in Africa in its most primitive form—of course, highly exaggerated. In other words, the men's G-strings were as minimal as possible, and the dear African ladies wore nothing above the waists" (Holtman 1968, 186). A large sign announced to midway strollers that this "Darkest African Village" was "Presented by Buck, Who Brings 'Em Back Alive" (Taylor 1958a). The 1930s were in fact the heyday of Frank Buck, the famous animal trainer, but Frank Buck had nothing to do with the attraction. The Buck on the sign was actually Warren Buck, an obscure animal importer who provided the monkeys for the display. In front, the sound of drums echoed constantly across the midway, interrupted by an occasional gunshot. To add to the exotic draw, on the bally were two microcephalic black men from Alabama. Their real names were Willy and Sam, but they were renamed Illy and Zambezi and the crowd was informed that they were representatives of the Ituri headbinding tribe. In describing the come-on, Lewiston commented that those who heard the pitch "were subjected to 'fact' which had no relation whatsoever to the truth" (Holtman 1968, 190).

Where did the "natives" inside come from, and how were they pro-cured? Lewiston provides one account: "First of all, there was a group of Ashantis from the Gold Coast of West Africa. These were the only 'authentic' part of the show, and even there you had to stretch the meaning of the word a little. Dufour and Rogers rounded them up in New York, which, if you look hard enough, harbors little pockets or colonies of people from all over the world" (Holtman 1968, 186). Despite elaborate "African" costumes purchased at Brooks Costume Company in New York and consisting of "ostrich plumes, leopard sarongs, clubs, spears, zebra hide shields, nose bones and matching accessories" (Taylor 1958a), the fourteen Ashantis proved to be "too dull." The producers needed something to liven up the scene: "For this we hired a tall, handsome New York Negro by the name of Charles Lucas, who became the leader of the rest of the 'African' population" (Holtman 1968, 188). He was decked out in the most elaborate ostrich-feathered costume, and protruding "through" his nose was an ivory decoration (which was actually clamped on). Called Wu Foo, he cultivated a gibberish "language." He could do such side-show feats as eating fire and spouting flames, swallowing hot swords and walking on burning embers. Charlie was the chief, and another flamboyant black American played the medicine man, who chanted mumbo jumbo through performances of dancing, fire eating, and hot coal walking.

The rest of the "natives" in the African Village were recruited from Chicago pool halls (Taylor 1958a). The managers did not worry that the crowd-grabbing novelty acts had nothing to do with the cultures they were supposed to be depicting. As one of them put it, the African lore was "pure hokum" anyway (Holtman 1968, 190).

The show's blow-off was "Captain Callahan," an old seaman who allegedly had been castrated by African savages. As Lou Dufour, the exhibit owner, tells it, Callahan was not advertised outside the village; rather, he was displayed in a thatched hut in the rear. After meandering through the village patronizing the concessions and observing the animal exhibits and native performances, the rubes wound up facing Callahan's hut. The village manager, Nate Eagle, dressed in a safari outfit complete with pith helmet, riding breeches, and boots, spieled from an elevated platform:

> Ladies and gentlemen, on the inside of this enclosure you
> will see and hear Captain Callahan, that brave and du-
> rable man who was so horribly tortured by a ferocious
> group of savages in the Cameroons, who were about to
> fling his ravished body into a steaming pot of boiling

water, after a sadist beast had decapitated his penis and testicles. Please, please, just stop to think—what a terrible, despicable crime! On the inside you will hear from the very lips of Captain Callahan how he was rescued from those ruthless cannibals. (Dufour 1977, 68)

The "Darkest Africa" exhibit was booked as an educational display.

It is difficult not to feel disapproval or even incredulity when confronting the presentation of non-Western people in the nineteenth- and twentieth-century freak show. The exhibition of foreigners as freaks is certainly incongruent with our current perspective: not only is the idea repugnant in itself, but the host of specific practices of presentation violate our sense of propriety. These presentations, of course, all took place before World War II and before modern communication systems brought us into wide contact with people from extremely different cultures. They were also before UNICEF, the Experiment in International Living, and the Peace Corps, organizations that have shaped the more enlightened outlook on the non-Western world that most modern educated Americans share.

At the time, however, Americans viewing such displays of non-Western people did not confront their own ethnocentrism. On the contrary, what they saw merely confirmed old prejudices and beliefs regarding the separateness of the "enlightened" and "primitive" worlds; they left the freak show reassured of their own superiority by such proofs of the others' inferiority. These attitudes also provided good support for the United States' exploitation of the non-Western world during the late nineteenth century. Further, freak show depictions of Africans as being inherently inferior and animallike, arising as they did from racist attitudes, helped sustain first the institution of slavery and later systematic, unfair, and unequal treatment of nonwhites.

Sam Gumpertz, freak show czar of Coney Island and perhaps the most active twentieth-century importer of non-Western sideshow attractions, and others engaged in the trade had no feelings of impropriety in what they did. While at Dreamland, Gumpertz, who later managed Ringling Brothers, Barnum and Bailey Circus, traveled extensively throughout the Third World procuring exhibits, whom he paid small amounts for being presented as savages. But Gumpertz clearly saw himself as a friend of these people. Discussing his relationship with a group of Dahomans he had engaged, he said:

as with all other African and Far East peoples, I got along
splendidly with these Dahomey tribesmen. I am lucky
that I seem to understand them. Of course most of them I
have first visited in their native corners of the world, for I
have circled the globe six times, and the primitive tribes
and savage peoples have a fascination for me. I like them
instinctively. They seem to know that. We always get
along. We are in sympathy, as the Latins say. (Butler
1936, 11)

In 1905 Gumpertz imported a group of so-called Bontoc head-
hunters from the Philippine Islands. His relationship with them suggests that his ideas about the ideal relationship with his exhibits were
part of a chauvinistic arrogance, an attitude typical of the times. One
couple that was part of the troupe had a four-year-old daughter whom
Gumpertz described as "one of the prettiest and most lovable children
I have ever known" (Butler 1936, 11). He and his wife, Evie, became
fond of the child and offered the parents the then huge sum of $5,000
to adopt her. To the parents that amount was a fortune. But Evie
and Sam never got their wish, for the parents refused to sell their
daughter.

The presentation of imported non-Westerners was big business.
They were in greatest demand during the last decades of the nineteenth century and the first decade of the twentieth, when they were
featured at world fairs and amusement parks. Major circuses and other
amusement establishments had full-time agents who, like Gumpertz,
combed the globe for cultural curiosities. With the whole non-Western
world as their hunting grounds and sensitivity to exploitation un-
developed, there was a ready supply of exhibits and no opposition to
the use of oppressive tactics to capture specimens.

The legal status of many of the foreign exhibits in the United States
is difficult to determine. Some came to this country under contracts
arranged with the governments of origin. In these cases the period
of service was specified in their contracts. In other cases, when no
such arrangements were made, exhibits were referred to as being
"owned by" their exhibitors, and they remained indefinitely in the
United States.

As illustrated by the case of Sunday and Monday (see above) adjustment to amusement world life varied considerably. Freak show exploitation caused the most suffering for non-Western natives, but
nevertheless, some of these exhibits adjusted quickly and even be-

came "showmen." Those who did not, like the "Ubangis," lived miserable lives. But these matters did not seem to concern pre-1940s American audiences or the exhibitors—after all, the people being exhibited really were cannibals, savages, and barbarians. Through costuming, staging, advertising pictures, and "true life" booklets, showmen fabricated a conception of "natives" that accurately captured—or, rather, reflected—what they were to U.S. citizens. The presentations reinforced pictures already in the American mind.

Insensitivity to the feelings of non-Western people, as well as ethnocentrism, with its resultant exaggeration and fabrication of the odd and eccentric in other cultures, made the exhibitions we have seen in this chapter not only acceptable but also popular. The non-Western world was an important source of exhibits for the expanding freak market. Showmen needed to produce exhibits that drew crowds, and presentations emphasizing cultural peculiarities did just that. Freak show organizers responded to popular demand with gross and wildly imaginative presentations of anthropological humbug. We should not be surprised—after all, they were interested in taking in dimes, in getting rubes, in putting on a good show.

8

Respectable Freaks

CHAPTER 6 FOCUSED on freaks manufactured in the high aggrandized mode who were plagued by illusions of grandeur. We now
return to status-enhancing freak presentations, only the exhibits
in this chapter are more down-to-earth, less pretentious about
who they were and where they had been. Yet by no means could
they be considered modest, nor were their presentations free
of hype. But these presentations relied on more conventional
status concerns: acceptance, normality, respectability. The incumbents had no problem separating themselves from their freak
show role.

Many were presented as "human wonders," but they did not
sing opera or claim heroic feats; rather, they merely performed
pedestrian tasks which the marks assumed were too difficult for
them given their physical disabilities. They brandished such
mundane achievements as finding a spouse and giving birth. Exhibits without arms delighted audiences by signing their names
and cutting out silhouettes with their toes. Legless freaks exhibited their ambulatory abilities. In short, their claims to fame
were quite commonplace. While high aggrandized exhibits really
were full of grandeur, with respectable freaks the mundane was
exploited as amazing and ordinary people were made into human wonders.

We pick up where we left off in chapter six—with the exhibition of fused twins.

Chang and Eng: The Original Siamese Twins

Daisy and Violet Hilton were one of the last sets of joined twins
to receive national prominence as aggrandized exhibits. Other
Siamese twins appeared in freak shows later in the century
("Weeping Mother Puts Her Siamese Twins in the Circus" 1951;

Shipley n.d.), but their popularity was curtailed by declining public interest in the exhibition of human oddities. By then over 120 years had passed since Chang and Eng, "The Original Siamese Twins," were first exhibited in the United States.

Part of the fascination of joined twins was the puzzle of how they performed such normal activities as walking and sitting. While people born with this condition never seemed to have any problem functioning fully in daily life, and their friends and relatives took their competence for granted, it was difficult for most unjoined people to imagine how a normal life was possible. Further, the general public was curious about how "as one" they were. Did they feel the same emotions? When one was touched, did the other sense it? How similar were they in personality and taste? How did they achieve privacy? How intertwined were their bodies? Could they be separated?

These questions, as well as the general mystery surrounding joined twins, were brought into focus when people contemplated their marriage. As we saw with the Hilton Sisters, for joined twins marriage was a constant issue in full public view. Indeed, it led to much of the publicity they received, for it titillated the general public. Being normal meant establishing nuptial ties, yet the intimacies of marriage were allowed only under the most private circumstances—to which, of course, joined twins had no access.

In Chang and Eng's presentation, the questions concerning their accomplishment of mundane tasks were answered on stage. Although they were not professional acrobats, they performed physical feats that boggled the minds of patrons, who expected them to have basic mobility problems. In addition, they imparted an aura of confidence and competency that challenged the basic notions of those who came to see them.

Chang and Eng were the vanguard of joined twins. They were the first put on display in this country, and it is to them we can attribute the term *Siamese twins*. Their story has been told many times, and told well, so there is no need to repeat it at length here (Wallace and Wallace 1978; Hunter 1964), but a number of interesting and revealing aspects of their lives and of their presentation as respectable folks deserve mention.

The first truly nationally known and universally popular "curiosities" in the United States, they traveled throughout the settled part of the country, playing to large audiences. Their long career spans both the period when curiosities traveled alone and the period when they were integrated into amusement organizations. They started as an individual exhibit touring with a showman, and gradually became absorbed into dime museums and circus sideshows. They also moved in their careers from being controlled and exploited by their managers to administering and promoting their own lives.

Chang and Eng, who were joined at the chest, were born in Siam (now Thailand) in 1811 and brought to this country in 1829. Their first public exhibitions were in a low exotic mode. In handbill pictures and publicity pamphlets as well as in person they appeared in native dress, barefoot, with their hair in long queues tied in a ring about their heads. As they got older and took control of their own management, their presentation gradually became more aggrandized, incorporating a view of the pair as respectable Americans. They adopted the name Bunker, became American citizens, married, had children, and, as part of their presentation, flaunted their American ways, their wives, and their children—their normal life-style.

Lithographic advertisements from the 1850s and 1860s show them in well-tailored suits and ties, accompanied by their devoted wives and talented children, and engaged in such status-enhancing activities as violin playing, reading, rowing, hunting, and riding in a coach (Fig. 56). In their later appearances they toured and appeared on stage with their children (Fig. 57). They and their families posed for Mathew Brady, and their cartes de visite likenesses were popular collector's items.[1]

The controversy that enveloped their entire lives revolved around the question whether Chang and Eng could be separated and whether they would pursue a surgical end to their two-ness. After all, the difficulties inherent in such an uncommon union might best be resolved by the knife. Physicians' opinions on the matter were sought at every opportunity, and the twins' visits to learned medical societies to obtain information were cited profusely in their publicity. The matter was especially debated at the time of their marriage. This question of separation became a major promotional focus not only for Chang and Eng but for all Siamese twins displayed after them. Their lack of privacy and the potential freedom an operation could offer were reservoirs of "human interest" which showmen exploited from Chang and Eng through the Hilton Sisters.

Chang and Eng Bunker did not die in poverty. They settled in rural North Carolina and led a rich and prosperous life as plantation own-

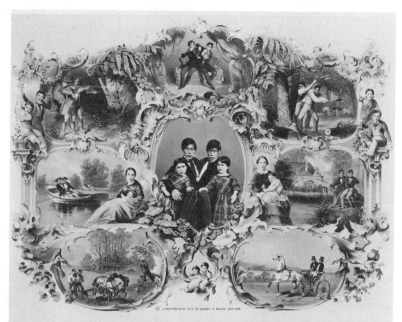

CHANG AND ENG THE WORLD RENOWNED SIAMESE TWINS, THEIR WIVES AND CHILDREN,

FROM DAGUERREOTYPES BY BRADY, 205 BROADWAY & HOLMES, 289 BROADWAY NEW YORK, TOGETHER WITH A REPRESENTATION OF THEIR RURAL EMPLOYMENTS AT THEIR RESIDENCE IN NORTH CAROLINA.

FIG. 56. Chang and Eng. In this lithograph from about 1855, the twins are surrounded by pictures of their wives, children, and scenes of them participating in status-enhancing activities. It epitomizes the aggrandized mode of presentation. (Harvard Theater Collection, Cambridge, Massachusetts.)

ers, respected citizens, husbands, and the fathers of twenty-three children. Yet the question remained: could two people joined together really live lives approaching normal? Their presentation took pains to dangle before the eyes of their patrons evidence that they indeed could. Part of their act exaggerated their identical appearance, their unity of thought and action, and the harmony in their lives (Robertson 1952). But whereas their publicity pamphlets presented them as being close partners, in real life they did not get along. It was this discord, then—not exploitive showmen, their presentation, or life on the road—that plagued them. They were proud and flaunted their attainments, but they had no illusions that people came to see them for any reason other than that they were joined together and that people were skeptical about their ability to live normal lives.

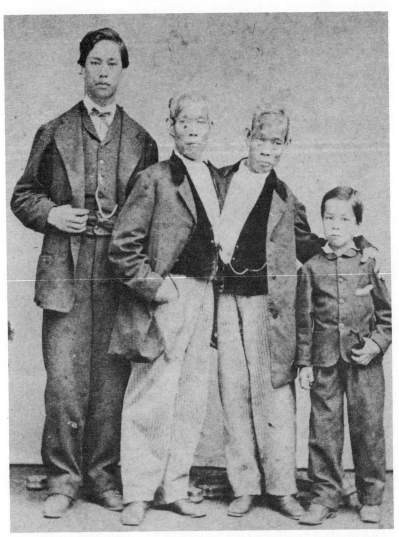

FIG. 57. Chang and Eng with sons. This picture of, on the left, James with his father, Eng, and on the right, Albert with his father, was taken after the twins came out of retirement. James was twenty-one years old at the time; Albert was twelve. Photo by Masury, c. 1870. (Becker Coll., Syracuse University.)

Love and Marriage

Although marriage was a theme in the presentation of Chang and Eng Bunker, their marriage itself was not a public event. The grand marriage of Tom Thumb and Lavinia Warren was an extravaganza. Exhibits in more modest status-enhancing presentations, however, used weddings and marriage to flaunt normality and to capture audience attention. Some of the marriages were staged merely for publicity purposes, others were short-lived frivolous affairs, but some were real and serious unions.

Mr. Chauncey Morlan and Miss Annie Bell were married in Huber's Dime Museum in New York City on November 30, 1892. The event was a masterpiece of showmanship (FitzGerald 1897c). Hundreds of well-wishers were unable to purchase tickets, the building was so crowded. Of course, Mr. and Mrs. Morlan were no ordinary couple: they were booked as the heaviest couple alive, with an alleged combined weight of 1,148 pounds. As we have seen, exhibits, whether giants, dwarfs, or obese persons, were forever claiming the ultimate in size. With marriages between like exhibits, bragging about composite superiority became possible.

Frank Wendt, the photographer who took over Eisenmann's business, took the large couple's wedding pictures, she in a flowing wedding gown and he in his tux before a formal parlor backdrop. While she was four inches taller than her spouse (she measured six feet two inches), he outweighed her by sixteen pounds.

The colossal couple held receptions at Huber's daily for six weeks, and the museum was packed day and night. Mr. and Mrs. Morlan received many fine gifts from customers. Their honeymoon trip, which they spent touring dime museums around the country celebrated as "the newlyweds," was a business boom (FitzGerald 1897c).

Chauncey and Annie made no claims to European nobility. Rather, they were presented as just the ordinary boy and girl next door—well mannered, respectable, nothing out of the ordinary except a few hundred extra pounds. She, born in Columbus, Ohio, in 1873, was known as "The Ohio Giantess." Extremely tall and obese exhibits often included the names of states (or, in the case of nonnatives, countries) in their titles. They could thus claim to be emissaries of their place of birth. Chauncey, from Indianapolis, was a few years older.[2] He became a professional fat man in 1884 and was the leading attraction with the Adam Forepaugh shows later in that decade (M. Mitchell 1979).

Their careers are difficult to trace, making it impossible to ascertain the seriousness and duration of their relationship. Their marriage was likely a showman's ploy to convince audiences of the normalcy of this peculiar union. When Morlan died in his home state of Indiana in 1912 he was married to a different woman (M. Mitchell 1979).

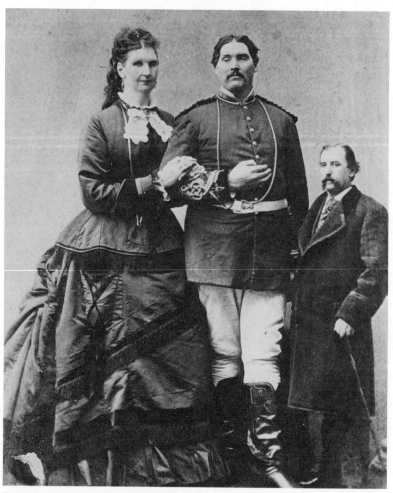

FIG. 58. Captain and Mrs. Bates, "The tallest couple alive." Mrs. Bates, the former Anna Swan, died in 1888. Giants and dwarfs commonly appeared in photos and on stage with typical-sized persons to provide a gauge for proportion. Photo by Charles Eisenmann, c. 1882. (Becker Coll., Syracuse University.)

On July 29, 1871, *Harper's Bazaar* reported the marriage of Martin Van Buren Bates to Anna Hanen Swan, the famous North American–born and–bred "giants" (Fig. 58) ("The Giants' Wedding" 1871). Published along with the story was a large etching depicting the ceremony. The bride and groom, whose combined height was alleged to be fifteen feet eleven inches[3]—"The Tallest Couple Alive"—appear in

PORTRAITS OF PRESENTATION

the finest of wedding apparel before the distinguished Rev. W. Rupert Cochrane. The etching shows the couple towering over both the reverend and the crowd of well-dressed guests. On the left side can be seen Millie and Christine, "The Two Headed Nightingale" (actually black joined twins who sang their way across America with a patriotic presentation that fell between high aggrandized and respectable on the continuum), with whom Bates and Swan were frequently exhibited.

Anna, born in Canada, was billed as "The Nova Scotia Giantess"; Martin, who had served in the Civil War, was presented as "Captain Bates, The Kentucky Giant." Both had been featured by Barnum early in their careers. At the time of their wedding they were touring Europe with a company organized by Judge H. P. Ingalls. In typical aggrandized style, when the troupe arrived in London their manager rented accommodations in a plush setting, held a reception exclusively for editors, physicians, and a few dignitaries, and announced the wedding. A day later, after publicity had circulated, a public reception was held.

Queen Victoria summoned the pair to Buckingham Palace. The queen gave the bride-to-be a cluster diamond ring and a wedding dress (Lee 1979; Bernard 1932). In a well-publicized ceremony, the two were married on June 17, 1871, in one of London's oldest sanctuaries. A few days after the wedding a private reception was given at the Masonic Hall for the benefit of the Prince of Wales and other dignitaries. All this attention, a direct result of their marriage, was of tremendous value in drawing crowds to their appearances both in England and, later, at home.

Whether because they could not be seduced into believing they were anything other than curiosities to their audiences, or whether because of the tragic death at birth of their child, they never engaged in the glamorous life that Charles Stratton and Lavinia Warren did. After they returned from their European tour they settled on a farm in Seville, Ohio, having built a house to match their size. Apparently the neighbors soon accepted them into the community. The local Baptist church even installed a large, specially built pew to accommodate the couple. Although they were occasionally lured away from their subdued life of farming to tour as curiosities, for the most part they lived their lives unpretentiously as respectable American citizens (Jennings 1882).

Other famous married giants exhibited together as the "largest couple alive." Toward the end of the nineteenth century, for example, Captain S. A. Shields—who, when younger, had toured with three brothers as the "Texas Giants"—married a woman billed as "The German Giantess," and they promptly declared themselves "The Tallest Married Couple on Earth." On the back of one publicity photo the captain is listed as being seven feet seven inches, his wife, seven feet eight; also printed are the names and numbers of the two Masonic lodges of which Shields was a member. He, like Tom Thumb and other exhibits in the aggrandized mode, commonly flaunted Masonic affiliations. Women exhibits were name-droppers as well, flaunting involvement in the Daughters of the American Revolution and church-sponsored associations.

Another giant couple of note appeared right after the Shieldses. They billed themselves as Patrick and Annie (Mr. and Mrs.) O'Brien, "The Irish Giant and Giantess." The name O'Brien was borrowed from a giant of the past, another common ploy showmen used in inventing catchy names for freaks. The pictures reveal that Mrs. O'Brien, the "Irish giantess," was none other than Mrs. Shields, the "German giantess." Whether we have here an early case of spouse swapping, mere name swapping, or remarriage is difficult to determine. Her change in nationality does, however, show that some form of showmen's skulduggery was at play.

In the 1930s a Mr. and Mrs. Fisher paraded about in cowhand outfits, calling themselves the "biggest married couple in the world" (Fig. 59). Mr. Fisher was claimed to be eight feet one inch tall, his wife, seven feet eleven—figures that must be adjusted for showmen's exaggeration. The pair traveled with the Ringling Brothers, Barnum and Bailey Circus.

A whole line of dwarf marriages were solemnized after Tom and Lavinia. For example, Count and Countess Phil-Nicole, "King and Queen of All Midgets," claimed to be the smallest married couple on earth, "barring none." These Lilliputians were united in matrimony in 1906 at St. Joseph's Catholic Church, Lowell, Massachusetts.

In the late 1920s Ray Marsh Brydon, a real showman's showman, arranged a marriage between two midgets that was a publicity bonanza. The groom was Ike, an identical twin whom Brydon was managing along with his brother Mike. Ike married "Princess Marguerite" in Forsyth Amusement Park, Savannah, Georgia, in a wedding that attracted a huge crowd (Pfening 1983). Later Brydon claimed that

PORTRAITS OF PRESENTATION

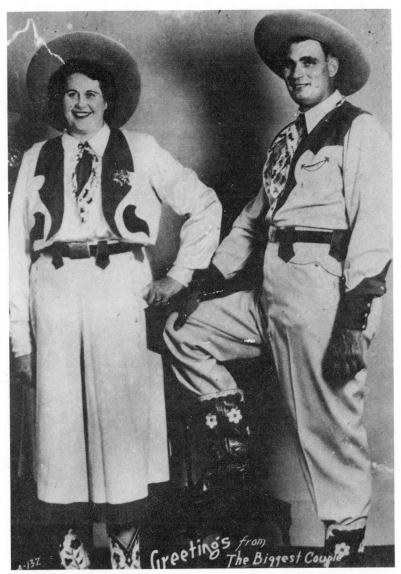

FIG. 59. Mrs. and Mrs. Fisher, another "tallest couple." As in this postcard, "giants" often wore high hats and boots to augment their height. C. 1938. (Becker Coll., Syracuse University.)

newspapers throughout the world printed 1,250,000 column inches of free publicity on the wedding. Mike and Ike were twice the breakfast guests of President Calvin Coolidge at the White House.

The marriage of dwarfs, giants, and fat people to each other was a stock promotional strategy, but romantic matches between opposites was another twist showmen employed to generate interest in freak attractions. Most of these unions were part of aggrandized presentations; often, though, the wedding and the marriage were presented with a comic twist that, through use of stereotypic images, made fun of domestic tranquillity. The marriage of Pete Robinson and Bunny Smith is a good example of this ploy. When they married in a large ceremony at Madison Square Garden, he was Ringling's "Living Skeleton," being of normal height but weighing only 58 pounds. Bunny, in contrast, weighed 467 pounds—at least according to promotional releases. In a publicity photograph taken at the couple's honeymoon breakfast in their apartment, Robinson is pictured trying to get his arms around Smith. In another he is holding a dish and she is feeding him, stereotypically trying to do what any good wife was expected to do—fatten him up. The couple's wedding and their striking outward incongruity served their careers well. Other couples, too, profited from the union of fat and skinny (Fig. 60). One 1870 marriage united 40-pound John Battersby with 688-pound Hannah Perkins. They exhibited together for years.

Not all weddings between human oddities were publicity affairs besieged by reporters. Some couples slipped away for private ceremonies, only to return to the stage as a team. Even though such couples lost out on the advertising advantage of public weddings, their promoters used the marriages to enhance the exhibits' respectable aggrandized presentations. Such was the case of Mr. and Mrs. Al Tomaini, "The World's Strangest Couple," who appeared in various freak shows throughout the 1930s. Al claimed to be eight feet four and one-half inches tall (he was actually closer to seven feet six; Lifson 1983); Jeanie, his wife, would have been of normal height except that she was born with no legs. She was advertised as the "Half-Girl," a standard amusement world expression for exhibits with that condition. In the "true life" booklet sold in conjunction with their postnuptial appearances (*Life Story of Mr. and Mrs. Al Tomaini* c. 1939), the term *handicap* is used with reference to Mrs. Tomaini, and an explanation of Mr. Tomaini's pituitary problem is provided. In addition, the booklet offers glimpses into their domestic life; for instance, Al is

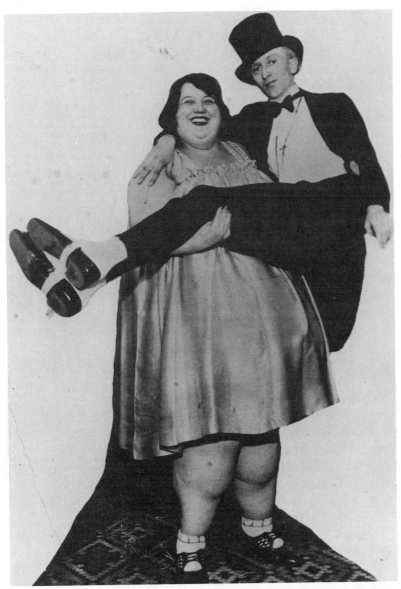

Fig. 60. "Living skeleton marries fat lady. Postcard showing unknown "fat lady" carrying her unknown thin man across the threshold. C. 1930. (Goldman Coll., Baltimore, Maryland.)

quoted as saying that his wife does all her own housework and cooking. The couple may have been odd, but they were presented as not being any different in their housekeeping arrangements than other newlyweds of the day. Al and Jeanie owned and managed their own sideshow (Mannix 1976).[4]

Legless Wonders

Jeanie Tomaini's low-keyed aggrandized presentation, although it flaunted certain aspects of her domestic skills and of the normal relationship she enjoyed with her husband, did not highly embellish who she was behind the scenes of the freak show. What made her stage appearance a "presentation" was the exaggerated importance that was assigned to her normal accomplishments. Key to the success of such presentations was the commonsense notion that a person with missing limbs could not be expected to do mundane tasks. Thus, Jeanie Tomaini and other legless and armless sideshow exhibits were "wonders" not so much for what they did as for the simple fact that they violated people's expectations of what they could do. While neither armless and legless wonders nor those who fawned over their achievements apparently considered such praise condescending, in retrospect, it was. But even if showmen—exhibits and promoters alike—had understood the patronizing quality of what they did, it would have changed nothing. Playing to the public's stereotypes was part of the game.

Jeanie Tomaini was probably unaware of it—tradition often exists only in the shape of our lives, not in our knowledge of it—but she was a participant in a long history of the exhibition of people without legs. In her modest aggrandized presentation, her normal accomplishments were flaunted just as the normal accomplishments of countless other legless persons had been flaunted in the past.

Perhaps the best known of the legless wonders was Eli Bowen, a man whose career spanned over half a century of freak show history. With the exception of the fame he achieved with his freak show career, however, the life accomplishments of Bowen, "Wonder of the Wide, Wide World!" (1880), were modest. He was born in 1844 in Ohio, without legs but with two feet, each a different size, growing where a leg should be. Starting in infancy, Bowen used his arms to accomplish the work of legs. He furthered his mobility with the aid of wooden blocks held in his hands, which elevated his hips enough that he could swing his body between his arms. Like other people with

PORTRAITS OF PRESENTATION

similar conditions, Bowen achieved a normal degree of mobility. In addition, because he used his upper body so extensively, his arms and shoulders grew extremely powerful and agile. He capitalized on this physical strength by training himself to tumble and do stunts on a long pole; he then incorporated these acrobatics into his presentation.

Bowen started as an exhibitionist at the age of thirteen, traveling with early circus wagon shows throughout the Midwest. By the 1870s he had toured with a number of major circuses and had appeared in the country's premier dime museums. He eventually teamed up with the Barnum and Bailey Sideshow, of which he was a part when it made its famous turn-of-the-century European tour.

When Bowen was twenty-six he married the attractive sixteen-year-old Mattie Haight, with whom he had four children. His marriage and growing family were flaunted in his presentation. A 1903 courier for the Barnum and Bailey tour of the United States informs us that one of his sons is a judge and the other a successful merchant.

Bowen's posed photographic images provide a complete chronicle of the growth and maturation of his family. In an 1867 carte we see the curly-haired young bachelor (Fig. 61). A few years later, in about 1873, he sits with his wife and young child (Fig. 62). Still later, around 1880, he is shown with his wife and three children (Fig. 63). The final family shot, from about 1890, includes Bowen with his wife and four children, the oldest of whom are now young adults (Fig. 64). The family pictures are all formal arrangements shot against a respectable Victorian parlor backdrop, with Bowen in the center and his family arranged about him. His wife typically stands in back, her hand on his shoulder, and the children are to his side and in front; like their father, they hold their arms crooked over their chests, with part of the hand tucked in their tailored outer garments.

It must be remembered that, as with the thousands of other photo portraits of freaks, a showman's scheme lay behind the elegant, complimentary poses taken of Bowen and his family. But even though the "legless wonder" presentation was patronizing, the pictures do portray dignity and independence. Some popular exhibits such as Bowen actually did give up the ways of the showman, marrying outside the amusement world and having attractive families. They made enough money to dress well and settle down comfortably in typical communities—Bowen, for example, retired to Ogden, California.

Back to Mr. Eli Bowen, at least to the aggrandized presentation described in an 1880 pamphlet he sold while on exhibit at Bunnell's Mu-

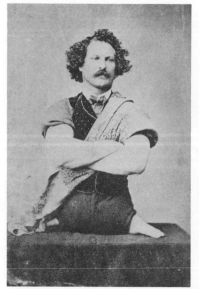 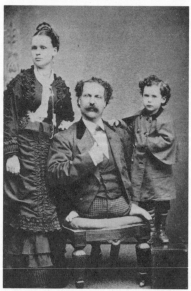

61 62
63 64

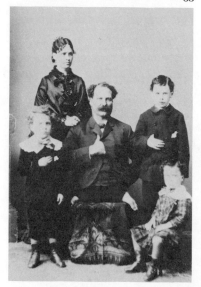 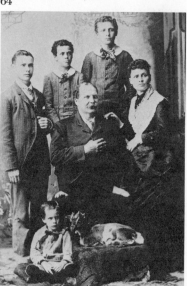

FIGS. 61–64. Eli Bowen at different points in his career. Fig. 61: Photo by Atkinson, 1867. Fig. 62: Photographer unknown, c. 1873. Fig. 63: Photo by Charles Eisenmann, c. 1880. Fig. 64: Photo by the Sword Brothers, c. 1890. (All from Becker Coll., Syracuse University.)

PORTRAITS OF PRESENTATION

seum in New York City (*Wonder of the Wide, Wide World!* 1880). This pamphlet reveals the intense competition that characterized the freak show world of the 1880s. Early in the narrative Bowen denigrates the competition: others who claim to be legless but really have stumps, those who say they are acrobats but seldom get the same applause Bowen allegedly received. The section ends with a pronouncement:

> Above these and all others of this class of curiosity, Mr. Bowen, the subject of this narrative, rises and towers conspicuously in this—that he has no lower limbs at all—in fact *not a leg to stand on*, and yet is able to move off very swiftly and gracefully to the astonishment of all who witness his dexterous movements—in fact I do not believe any country of any age has ever produced anything like unto him. (emphasis mine)

The passage illustrates the typical boastfulness of showmen's propaganda, but the phrase "not a leg to stand on" points out something else. Bowen and others who used the straight aggrandized presentation occasionally inserted humorous twists in their pamphlets and performances. (Johnny Eck, a legless person whose presentation approached the high aggrandized mode, used to say that he did not miss having legs because if he had them he would have to worry about keeping his pants pressed [Drimmer 1973, 117].) This brand of humor was different from that found in the high aggrandized mode with its exaggeration of status and in the mockery in the exotic. Here, freaks used humor to ease the tension patrons might have felt in the presence of disabled people by indicating that they took their condition lightly. In addition, jokes revealed the exhibits' cleverness and their willingness to relate to the audience as peers, thus reinforcing the aggrandized presentation.

Johnny Eck, "The Only Living Half Boy, Nature's Greatest Mistake," was a popular twentieth-century legless wonder who began traveling with the amusement industry in 1924 (Lifson 1983). One of his hobbies was model building. He built, and displayed for publicity, detailed miniatures of various traveling carnivals with which he had appeared. His sideshow performance consisted of acrobatic and trapeze performances as well as musical numbers. He always appeared in formal attire. His "true life" booklet reports that, in the winters "when show business is dull, he has a twelve-piece orchestra in the city of Baltimore, of which he is the conductor and composer, that he books for Night Clubs, Cabarets, and Dances" (Lifson 1983)— although one interviewer claims that this tale was, at best, an exaggeration. He was a feature attraction in the film *Freaks*.[5]

Armless Wonders

Legless wonders were popular, but armless wonders have a much longer history and were more common in the American sideshow and, even taking Eli Bowen into account, were generally more popular. While legless people could show impressive gross motor moves of their arms and upper bodies, armless people wowed audiences with their ability to do fine motor tasks with their toes. Cutting paper silhouettes, embroidering, writing, whittling, and such mundane tasks as eating, drinking, combing hair, dressing, and shaving were all part of the performance.

Master Sanders K. G. Nellis was probably the first completely armless person to exhibit himself publicly in America. He made his debut in 1830, when he was only thirteen. His career, like that of the original Siamese twins, spanned the period when curiosities were being absorbed into museums and circuses.[6]

Nellis's first appearances were in private halls and rooms, but soon he was appearing in Peale's Museum (Odell 1927, 3:533), and later he became a regular at Barnum's American Museum. His presentation contained many elements of later armless exhibits, including the use of the word *wonder* in his title—"The Wonder of the World." In his performance, he cut paper valentines and profiles with scissors, opened and wound his watch, loaded and discharged a pistol, shot a bow and arrow, and performed on various musical instruments "with great taste and precision" (Odell 1927, 3:534).

Born in Johnstown, New York, in 1817, Nellis was less than five feet tall and weighed 116 pounds. About his performance it was said:

> He executes many other things with his feet, which a vast majority of mankind cannot with their hands, without long and arduous practice. *In him, we have an instance of what can be accomplished by a strong mind, aided by indomitable perseverance and untiring industry*, without the common appliances by which it usually manifests its creative skill and power of adaptation. (emphasis mine)

216

The italicized phrase in the above quotation points to a theme that became prominent in many respectable aggrandized presentations of people with missing limbs and other disabilities. Such phrases suggested to onlookers that the exhibits' accomplishments and their ability to overcome disadvantages were a sign of their moral worth. The "wonder" was not merely physical, it was the work of steadfast courage and perseverance. In other presentations the exhibits' ability to overcome disadvantages and their uplifted spirits are presented as the work of the Lord. Thus, these persons' elevated status is based on moral superiority and their religiosity rather than on glamor, a title, or wealth.

In considering moral superiority as part of the presentation of human oddities, Ann E. Leak Thompson stands out.[7] This popular nineteenth-century "armless lady" would certainly win the prize for most pious. A carte de visite or cabinet photograph with her signature accompanied by a short message on the back was a sought-after souvenir. Although while she did write nonreligious jottings—"So you perceive it's really true, when hands are lacking, toes will do" (Koste Coll.)—homilies were more characteristic: "Indolence and ease are the rust of the mind" (Becker Coll.). Ann E. Leak Thompson was proud of her Southern background as well; she concluded many of her autographed cards with the message "Born in Georgia December 23, 1839." As she got older she stopped giving the date of birth and simply reported her age, minus a few years (Koste Coll.).

The first available pictures of her date from the early 1870s and are rather plain. Pictures Eisenmann took of her in 1884 show her sitting on a box draped with samples of her crocheting and embroidery, which are decorated with religious symbols—the cross, the Bible—and the symbol of her father's Masonic affiliation, Meridian Sun Lodge, No. 26, F.A.M. Griffin, Georgia (Fig. 65).[8] In addition, there are embroidered phrases from the scripture: "Holiness to the Lord," "To thee I Cling," and "A Lamp unto My Feet" (M. Mitchell 1979). In some poses her husband, William R. Thompson, stands behind and her six-year-old son beside her. (Ann either had the boy when she was in her late forties or she was the child's stepmother.) The images are the pinnacle of Victorian respectability.

In the preface to her 1871 autobiography, which she sold in conjunction with her appearances, the showman/publisher cleverly undercuts any sentiment against the incongruous idea that such a re-

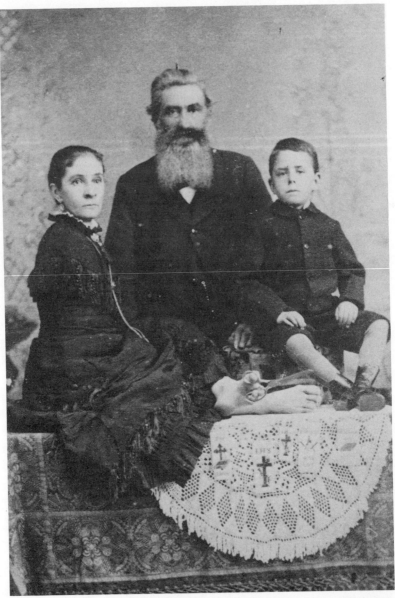

FIG. 65. Ann E. Leak Thompson, armless wonder. Ann is shown here with her husband, William R. Thompson, and her son. Photo by Charles Eisenmann, 1884. (Becker Coll., Syracuse University.)

spectable and pious women should ostentatiously show herself in circuses and dime museums:

> Miss Leak, in presenting this, her autobiography, to the
> public, feels no little delicacy at seeking, to make the
> deprivation which she suffers in the entire absence of
> arms at her birth, the occasion of gain to her, by gratify-
> ing the eye, oftentimes, of a curious public; though
> averse to it at first, and till circumstances, changing,
> necessitated such a course. She can, in this way, nev-
> erthelsss, best meet the obligations which she owes to
> herself and to her aged parents, in a measure dependent
> on her endeavors, and confidently trusts that the motive
> which thus actuates her will stay any cold look of in-
> difference, and draw forth the sympathy and considera-
> tion of every heart that witnesses her operations, or to
> whom this little volume many come. (*Autobiography of
> Miss Ann E. Leak* 1871, 1)

In this introduction, as well as in the pamphlet's body, we are lam-basted with examples of and references to her respectable religiosity. Although the theme of her superiority clearly puts her presentation in the aggrandized mode, her autobiography comes closer than any other presentation to an appeal based on sympathy or pity. But the appeal is not for a handout; she does not seek that form of charity. Rather, she is presented as a talented, self-sufficient, and pious "armless wonder" who merely wants the equally pious segment of the community to let her earn her living in this manner.

Ann's explanation for having been born armless suggests that her piousness grew out of adversity. Her father, she said, drank a great deal and quarreled with his friends. "Her mother learned of his being in a scrap down in the town, and when she saw him coming home, he had his overcoat thrown over his shoulders without his arms in the sleeves" (Middleton 1913, 70). Thus she used the theory of maternal impression to explain her armlessness.

Of all the many armless wonders, none was better known or had a longer life of exhibition that Charles Tripp. Born in Woodstock, Can-ada, completely without arms, he was quick to master all the tasks people normally do with their hands. His writing, accomplished by holding a pen between his toes, was well formed and easily legible. In 1872, at the age of seventeen, Charles ventured to New York in search of P.T. Barnum. As the story goes, Barnum hired the boy on the spot.

Tripp remained an amusement world exhibit for over fifty years, working in Barnum shows and with Ringling Brothers, Barnum and Bailey. In the later years of his career, in the 1920s, he traveled with carnivals.

Tripp's performance during his more than fifty years as an exhibit did not change much. He neither sang nor played a musical instrument but merely showed patrons what he could do with his feet: carpentry, penmanship, portrait painting, paper cutting, and the like. At the turn of the century he took up photography. Press agents for Barnum and Bailey Circus heralded him as "The Armless Photographer," and in a 1903 Barnum and Bailey Circus courier he was shown beside a camera taking a picture. A photograph of him and Eli Bowen, then in their middle age, riding a bicycle built for two was widely circulated, but there is no clear evidence that the two were an exhibition team.

While we have no "true life" booklets or other written publicity material describing Tripp, he did leave as comprehensive a set of photographic images as any human oddity, with the possibile exception of Henry Johnson ("Zip"). Shortly after his arrival in New York in 1872, Tripp sat for a full-length portrait in Brady's studio. He appears camera shy as, unsmiling, he looks down. Between his toes a pen is poised as though he were writing a letter. Conveniently for Barnum's advertising interests, propped against the box on which Tripp is sitting is "Barnum's Great Menagerie, Museum and Circus" stationery.

In his first picture he is dressed in knickers, a performer's vest, and a white shirt, with a bandannalike tie under his collar. A picture taken in his early twenties shows him in similar attire. After that, all his pictures take on a remarkably similar look, varying only with the telltale signs of aging. The props consist of overstuffed Victorian chairs and other ornate furniture, and there is usually a tea set on a table (Fig. 66). In one picture he is shown holding the cup, in others he is holding a pen. Often a card with the date written on it is displayed, in addition to the paraphernalia of his performance. Typically he appears in a vested businessman's suit with a gold watch chain, a white shirt, and a dark tie—the height of middle-class respectability. Later in his life we see him put on weight and start wearing glasses, and his mustache turns grey. Even after exhibits stopped vending cartes de visite and cabinet photos from the freak platforms, Charles still sold postcard images of himself. The poorer quality of these pictures makes it more difficult to pick out details.

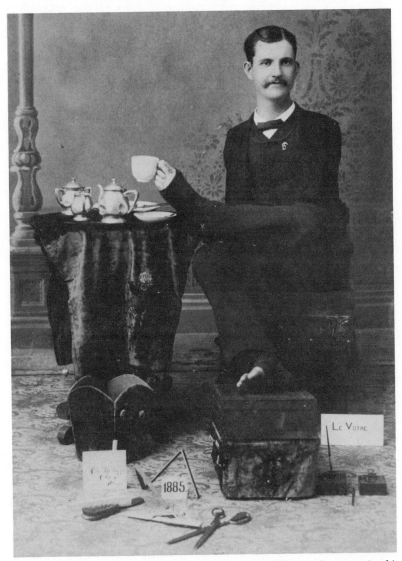

FIG. 66. Charles Tripp, armless wonder. In this picture Tripp is demonstrating his "talents" by drinking from a teacup. On the ground in front of Tripp are the scissors he used to cut paper dolls and the pen he used to sign his autograph. Photo by Charles Eisenmann, 1885. (Author's collection.)

Unlike many of the other aggrandized-mode exhibits, Tripp did not marry until late middle age. For most of his career he was presented as the responsible and prudent bachelor. As far as we know he never had children and was not photographed for commercial purposes with his wife. While still a bachelor he toured the world three times as an exhibit. He died in 1939 at the age of eighty-four. An editorial in the newspaper of his retirement town, Salisbury, North Carolina, picked up on a familiar aggrandized-mode theme when it expatiated on the virtues of Charles Tripp: ". . . and the fine accomplishments and achievements despite handicaps should be a challenge to those of us who possess all our facilities. . . . He was a real hero in every sense of the word and overcame odds in life that would have submerged many a man with less determination and spirit" (quoted in Drimmer 1973, 106).

For the most part, armless and legless wonders acknowledged that their major claim to fame was their anomaly and their presentation, not their performance. A classic exception to this rule was Carl Unthan, born without arms in Germany in 1848, who toured the United States in the last decades of the nineteenth century and first decade of the twentieth. His 1935 autobiography, *The Armless Fiddler: A Pediscript Being of a Vaudeville Man,* is a revealing portrait of a person who refused to define himself as a human oddity regardless of how the audience saw him. Take, for example, the title of his book. He played more circuses, fairs, and traveling shows than vaudeville revues, yet "vaudeville" is what he identifies himself with. Although the title emphasizes fiddling, his act involved not only playing the violin but also shooting a rifle with his toes, swimming in a large tank, and performing mundane tasks before his audience. As part of his violin playing at each performance, he purposely cut a string so the audience could marvel as he repaired it with his agile toes. In one revue, his armless swimmer routine was followed by an act consisting of twelve fox terriers performing a water show.

Unthan's story is full of the tension that characterized those physically unusual exhibits who refused to acknowledge that their performances were not their prime calling card but merely part of their presentation as human oddities. Unthan survived quite well, though. He remained a well-dressed and formal gentleman both on and off stage. He spent his later years visiting amputeed World World I veterans and advocating for people with missing limbs. In regard to armless people, he advised that they avoid every kind of show business. "It has not harmed me, thanks to my stubbornness, but ninety-nine out of a hundred will go to the bad on its slippery side" (Unthan 1935, 272). The "Armless Fiddler" died in 1928 at the age of eighty.

It is important to reiterate, with an example, a point made in Chapter 4, that is, that particular physiological conditions were not inevitably linked to specific types presentation. Although armless and legless wonders were commonly presented in a low aggrandized mode, there were notable exceptions. In the 1890s an armless boy was exhibited in this county in the exotic mode of the "Hand-Footed Indian Hunter" (FitzGerald 1897b, 410). The young man, Warrimeh Boseth, was in his mid teens when he was allegedly "discovered" living with his "tribe" in Vancouver, Canada, by a "ubiquitous freak-finder." As the story went, the boy was a "natural" hunter and shot his prey with a bow and arrow that he held between his feet while lying on his back. One observer saw and described Warrimeh as exhibited in a dime museum in New Orleans: he was dressed in a makeshift "indian outfit," which included beads and a feathered headdress, and included in his presentation was an archery exhibition in which he shot live pigeons on the wing, to the thunderous applause of the audience (FitzGerald 1897b).

The amusement world's supply of armless wonders has been seemingly inexhaustible. Barney Nelson, the black child "Armless Phenomenon," wowed New York dime museum goers in the 1880s with his mundane tricks and winning ways (*Life of Barney Nelson* 1883). John Owens is pictured in a late-nineteenth-century Wendt cabinet photograph—an armless man writing with his toes, while all about him are the musical instruments he apparently played: harpsichord, guitar, and violin. Handsome Freddie Esele, "The Armless Wonder," was seen mainly on the carnival circuit. Joan Whisnant, who played the guitar with her toes, was with the "Believe or Not" show. The most famous of the twentieth-century women aggrandized "armless wonders" was the pretty and, according to her presentation, sophisticated Frances O'Connor. In one postcard photo she strikes a stylish pose, smoking a cigarette held between her toes; in another she holds a teacup. She was a regular with the Ringling Brothers, Barnum and Bailey Sideshow and made an appearance in Browning's film *Freaks*.

Thus far in discussing aggrandized presentations of people with missing parts we have covered only "Half Men" and "Half Women":

armless or legless wonders. Yet some exhibits had neither arms *nor* legs. Amusement world hype billed these people as "human trunks." Although most such individuals were exhibited in the exotic or a mixed exotic/aggrandized mode, some played an aggrandized presentation as well. "Violetta" was a twentieth-century "human torso" featured at the Dreamland Sideshow in Coney Island. Her performance consisted of her singing while perched on a pedestal (Lifson 1983). In the late 1930s, Frieda Pushnik, an "armless and legless wonder," appeared in circus and carnival sideshows accompanied by her mother.

The most successful exhibits had some unusual anomaly plus the attributes needed to pull off the presentation—they were competent and had the manners and appearance of upstanding citizens. The premier "wonders" discussed above were singular enough not to need to bend with the competition. Exhibits such as Eli Bowen and Charles Tripp were remarkable for the consistency in their presentation over many years. But less stellar attractions often made various attempts at novelty. In this regard, one more missing-limb exhibit should be mentioned: Joe Maloney, who lacked a left leg and arm. Performing in carnivals in the 1920s and 1930s as a "half man," he was billed as "The World's Greatest High Diver" and, for his act, plunged from a high platform into a tank of water.

Bearded Ladies

Although some women with excessive hair were presented in the exotic mode as missing links or beasts,[9] the incongruity of whiskers and femininity made the aggrandized mode most popular for these women. Their presentations were never as grand as those of midgets in the high aggrandized mode; instead, hirsute women typically appeared in straightforward status-enhancing motifs—except for the beards, these women represented the quintessence of refined respectable womanhood.

They were typically pictured striking feminine poses in elegant surroundings, wearing fashionable dresses and with their hair done in the latest style. Annie Jones, for example, appears in a number of photos sitting before a mirror, her long hair hanging down her back (Fig. 67). For those who had husbands, and most did, a favorite photographic prop was their spouse. After all, being married and a devoted wife was the epitome of womanhood—which is what bearded women's presentations proclaimed them to be. Some photographs—

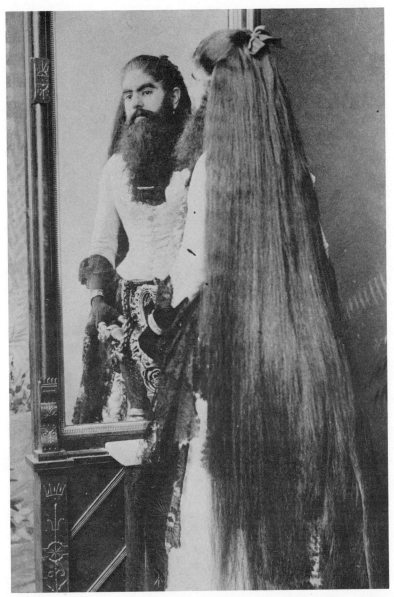

FIG. 67. Annie Jones, "The Bearded Lady." Shown admiring herself in a mirror. Photo by Charles Eisenmann, c. 1888. (Becker Coll., Syracuse University.)

such as one of Mr. and Mrs. Meyers, he sporting a large handlebar mustache and she with her incongruous whiskers and feminine dress— represent the finest examples of formally posed Victorian normalcy (Fig. 68).

These women stocked the sideshow platforms of the United States from the inception of sideshows through the 1930s, and their names— Lady Olga, Madame Devere, Princess Gracie—achieved a certain tone that showmen deliberately sought. Madame Jane Devere was born in Kentucky in 1842 and played with such circuses as Sells Brothers, Campbell Brothers, and finally, in 1908, the Yankee Robinson Show. While midgets boasted about how small they were and giants about how large, bearded ladies bragged about the length of their beards. When the madame's beard was measured in 1884 it was fourteen inches long, which led her and her manager to claim she had set a record (M. Mitchell 1979). Eisenmann photographed her and her husband, Bill, on a number of occasions. The setting is always the ultimate in Victorian respectability, more on the stuffy side than the glamorous.

Publicity for Siamese twins revolved around the question of separation; for bearded ladies authenticity was the issue. Whether the person behind the beard was really a woman was a question that generated much speculation and publicity. (There were many gaffs; I deal here only with authentic bearded women.) "Madam Clofullia, The Bearded Lady of Geneva," was imported from Switzerland and featured by Barnum in the 1850s. Born Josephine Boisdechene Versoix in 1831, she appeared in formal dress and adorned with jewels.

Prior to her first appearances in London Madam Clofullia was extensively examined by W. D. Chowne of Charing Cross Hospital, who declared her hair to be genuine and "her breasts . . . large and fair, and strictly characteristic of the female." In 1851 she gave birth to a normal-haired daughter. At the request of her manager, the physician who delivered the child provided an affidavit of the birth and a statement that the child was indeed hers and that she had a genuine "abundant beard." The child died at eleven months.

When Madam Clofullia made her first appearance at the American Museum, a person in the audience—whom Barnum had paid— charged that she was a fraud, a male disguised as a female. The matter went to court. It was exactly the kind of controversy that Barnum loved to provoke. Three doctors affirmed that she was indeed a woman, as

PORTRAITS OF PRESENTATION

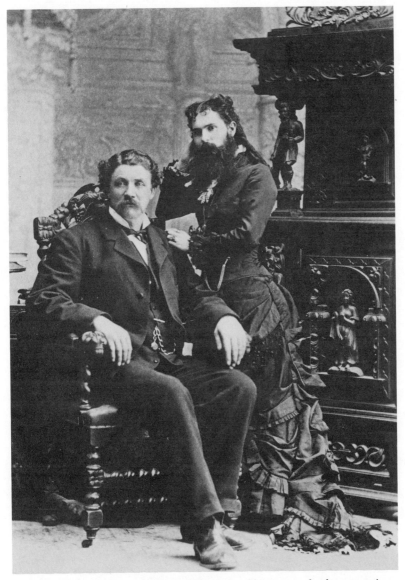

FIG. 68. Bearded lady and husband. Mr. and Mrs. Meyers pose for the camera in an elegant Victorian setting. Photo by Bogardus, c. 1885. (Becker Coll., Syracuse University.)

did her husband, her father, and a doctor employed by the city. The judge dismissed the charge, but not before press reports drew large crowds to the museum.

Annie Jones was a famous bearded lady whom Barnum launched to fame by, as showmen commonly did, using a biblical name, Esau, as her calling card: "The most marvelous specimen of hirsute development known since the days of Esau, 3,700 years ago." [10] When she was first exhibited in 1866, she was twelve months old—"The Infant Esau," a female child with a beard (*History of Miss Annie Jones* 1885).

As Annie matured, so did her billing—from "Esau infant" to "Esau child" to "Esau lady." Her "true life" pamphlets describe her beauty, high moral character, cultured interests, winning personality, and musical ability (she played the mandolin). Her soft voice and stylish feminine wardrobe provided an appealing dimension to her aggrandized presentation. At sixteen she married Richard Elliott, a sideshow talker. When that marriage ended in divorce fifteen years later, she married another showman, William Donovan, who died while accompanying her on a European tour. She died in her mother's home in Brooklyn in 1902; thirty-seven years old, she had known no other life than that of a freak ("Bearded Lady Dead" 1902).

Madam Squires was a favorite on the dime museum circuit in the late 1870s and early 1880s. The publicity booklet sold in conjunction with her exhibition, *Brief History of a Celebrated Lady, Namely, Madam Squires, the Bearded Lady*, illustrates yet another aggrandized presentation of a bearded lady. According to the booklet, Madam Squires was a married woman and the mother of three children, two of them deceased. The living child was a fine son, "handsome, brave, an energetic business young man," "a gentleman who has made his mark on the world." As to Madam Squires:

> She is a woman of extensive travel, great reading, and
> acute, innate perceptive faculties, which give her an al-
> most instantaneous knowledge of the human charac-
> ter. . . . In disposition she is most kind and womanly,
> loving all and hating none. While the wonderful magne-
> tism nature has endowed her with, enables her to exercise
> a magic spell upon all who come within the circle of her
> large and varied acquaintance, and having a large and
> Christian feeling towards all the Master's creatures, she
> looks upon all around her, of whatever condition or reli-
> gion, as her brothers and sisters, and is ready at all times

PORTRAITS OF PRESENTATION

to help the struggling ones on earth with a warm grasp of the hand, a kind, loving word or an assuring smile.

Many other bearded women of elevated status deserve mention. Jane Barnell, a late-nineteenth-, early-twentieth-century phenomenon, was first exhibited when she was four years old and was still appearing in freak shows in the early 1940s, when she was interviewed by a *New Yorker* writer (J. Mitchell 1943). Over the course of her career she changed her name from Princess Olga to Madame Olga to Lady Olga. Once a showman tried to get her to dye her beard blue and appear as "Lady Bluebeard," but she declined, preferring the more sedate presentation of Lady Olga. She appeared in dime museums, amusement parks, and circuses in every state in the union and in many countries around the world. She played the bearded lady in *Freaks*.

Others

The aggrandized mode was used for a great many "respectable freaks" who had a variety of real physical differences. Some but not all of the major categories have been covered here to some degree. Neither obese men and women nor giants are fully described, and omitted entirely are people with cerebral palsy or other conditions that left them with stiff joints and atrophied muscles—the exhibits billed as "Ossified Men."[11] Men with extremely long beards, women with unusually long hair (most notably the Seven Sutherland Sisters), people with skin disorders, elephantiasis, and unusual hornlike growths were standard attractions. A whole genre consisted of exhibits, mostly fakes, that claimed to be of mixed sex—that is, half man and half woman. Other names include Barney Baldwin, "The Broken Neck Wonder"; James Wilson, "The Expansionist"; A. C. Hollis, "The dislocationist"; Ashbury Ben, "The Spotted Boy"; Etta Lake, "The Elastic Skin Woman"; Leonard Perry, "The Popeyed Wonder"; Grace McDaniels, "The Mule-Faced Woman"; Fanny Mills, "Big-Footed Girl"; and Joe,"The Big-Fingered Boy."

The patterns in the presentations soon become redundant. Nevertheless, a few other respectable aggrandized curiosities who won freak show fame need to be mentioned. They are included both because of their prominence and importance in the history of presentations and because their stories further illustrate how respectable freaks were made.

Myrtle Corbin, "The Four-Legged Woman," deserves mention for a number of reasons. For one thing, she represents the aggrandized presentation of a type of physical anomaly important in the history of the freak show that we have not yet discussed: people with extra limbs and other body parts. Her condition resulted from a process similar to that which produces fused twins, only in her case the separation of the two parts of the split fertilized egg was less complete and in other ways flawed.[12] Sometimes, as in the case of Lentini, the famous three-legged man whose prosperous low aggrandized career lasted fifty years, an extra limb is the result. In others, such as Betty Williams, a famous twentieth-century exhibit, a poorly formed parasitic twin is the result. Myrtle Corbin fell somewhere in between, having two small extra legs dangling between her normal lower appendages as well as other organs in duplicate.

Myrtle Corbin was born in Tennessee in 1868 and became an exhibit when she was thirteen. In typical fashion for aggrandized presentations, she is described in her first promotional pamphlet (*Biography of Myrtle Corbin* 1881) as being as "gentle of disposition as the summer sunshine and as happy as the day is long." Her literature, as well as the pictures she sold when she was older (they are of her with her husband and child), provides a classic illustration of a respectable aggrandized presentation.

But another aspect of Myrtle Corbin's exhibition is of special interest, for it clearly reveals the relationship between freak exhibits and medical science. Myrtle lived at the height of interest in teratology, and she was the focus of considerable attention from physicians. Joseph Jones, M.D., followed her case from her infancy. In the *Journal of the American Medical Association* in 1888 he discussed her case extensively while summarizing the field of teratology (Jones 1888). The birth of her first child was cause for Brooks H. Wells, M.D., to write about this "female, belonging to the monocephalic, ileadelphic class of monsters by fusion" in the *American Journal of Obstetrics* (Wells 1888, 1265). Dr. Whaley, who attended the birth of Corbin's first child, provided details of the case to the *British Medical Journal*, following an earlier account in the *Atlanta Medical and Surgical Journal* ("Case of Pregnancy" 1889). The fodder for publicity that these medical reports created made other showmen jealous enough to create gaffs. A number of phony four-legged women were exhibited both during and after Myrtle Corbin's career.

The last profile in this chapter represents a type of exhibit having a long history in the American sideshow but to which we have paid little attention: people who are unusually thin, or, in amusement world jargon, "Human Skeletons."[13] J.W. Coffey started his career in 1884 in the dime museums of Chicago, appearing as "The Ohio Skeleton." At first, while he was finding work in circuses and dime museums, he appeared in a low aggrandized mode wearing tights made from thin cloth. But his lean body was poorly protected from the cold midwestern winters, and soon he hit on an innovation that not only improved his comfort but also launched a career which surpassed his "Ohio Skeleton" presentation. As "The Skeleton Dude" he played a dapper gentleman complete with tight-fitting formal tailed dress, a monocle, makeup, a cane, cigarettes, and a valet (Fig. 69). He pranced about the stage talking about the follies of the day and flirting with the women in the audience (*Theoretical Child* c. 1902). Dr. J.W. Coffey, as he took to calling himself, was considerably warmer as the Skeleton Dude—and financially better off as well. (Other thin men, such as Eddie Masker, copied Coffey's presentation to a tee, even using the epithet "Skeleton Dude" in their presentations.) Playing the swank bachelor, the original Skeleton Dude joked about marriage by saying, "Most women don't like their Coffey thin."

This humorous aggrandized presentation became more serious when, in the late 1890s, he married and became the father of what he described in his 1902 "true life" pamphlet as a beautiful, "remarkably well developed child." In fact, for reasons not explained in the text but obvious to those familiar with the scientific stirrings at the time, Coffey used this booklet to defend the idea that imperfect people, people like himself, could produce perfect offspring. His defense against the eugenics onslaught was to illustrate, with his own child, that people with "inferior" human physical variations—such as, in his case, emaciation—could, by providing an ideal loving and caring environment, overcome genetics. Respectability could prevail.

We have come to the end of profiles of low-aggrandized-mode presentations. The theme of this chapter was the making of respectable freaks. Starting with Chang and Eng, the original Siamese twins, through limbless wonders and bearded ladies, and ending with Dr. Coffey, the Skeleton Dude, we have seen how showmen used the idea of normalcy to forge exhibits.

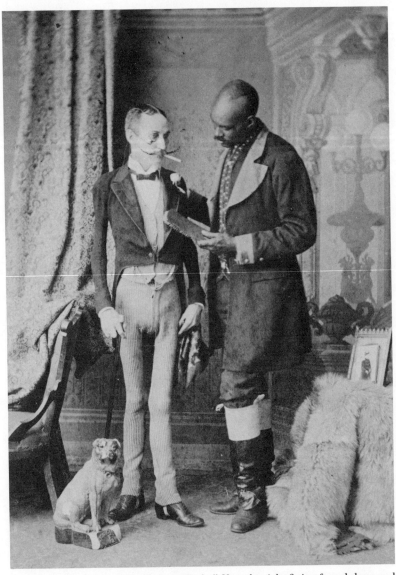

Fig. 69. J. W. Coffey, "The Skeleton Dude." Note the tight-fitting formal dress and formal background. The other man is posing as Coffey's valet. Photo by Charles Eisenmann, c. 1890. (Becker Coll., Syracuse University.)

Although the physical anomaly was the starting point for building these exhibits, here, unlike the exotic-mode presentation of people with real anomalies, exhibits were not presented as alien from respectable society. Quite the opposite, showmen turned around any disposition there might have been to think of people who are physically different as strange. They parlayed pedestrian feats into amazing achievements. By juxtaposing physical differences with normal accomplishments they created human wonders. Showmen, full-time promoters, and exhibits alike orchestrated weddings, capitalized on spouses and children, played up religious and organizational affiliations, and showed how, despite physical differences, freaks could cook, sew, and write—in general, be competent. In the process of making freaks, showmen, by suggesting that superior character traits were behind the exhibits' achievements, produced moral heroes. They milked the adage "You can't keep a good man down."

The success of this mode of presentation was predicated on the assumption that these accomplishments were beyond what should be expected of people with such anomalies. A question that was not publicly raised, at least in the documents available for study, but might have been on patron's minds was: "If the people on the platform are so normal and competent, why do they resort to making a living by exhibiting themselves?" Freak shows were perfectly respectable entertainment, but traveling about the country as an amusement world exhibit was not considered a preferred occupational choice. Could they not make a substantial living and a respectable life settling down in a typical American community? (Some in fact did, and when they came out of retirement to return to the amusement world, they flaunted their other, more normal life.) At the height of freak show popularity the answer to the question was quite obvious. The large salaries and the fame made up for the drawbacks of such an unusual life-style. Indeed, as part of the promotion, showmen exaggerated the salaries that exhibits received. Yet although this logic, to some extent, probably did apply to premier exhibits in the high-status shows, it did not hold up for those in the less prestigious lower rungs of the amusement industry. In addition, as the freak show moved through the twentieth century and met the assault of critics who claimed that exhibits were not just curiosities but that they were ill, the negative connotation of being a freak must have undercut explanations centering on the financial rewards of the whole enterprise.

9

Self-Made Freaks

LEW GRAHAM, late-nineteenth- and early-twentieth-century legendary manager and outside lecturer for the Barnum and Bailey Sideshow, Ringling Brothers Sideshow, and finally the Ringling Brothers, Barnum and Bailey Sideshow, was asked, "What are the key attributes of a premier attraction?" First on his list was "an abnormality"—a remarkable and, if possible, unique abnormality (Bradna and Hartzell 1952, 236).

All freaks were creations of the amusement world: the freak show and the presentation made people exhibits, not their physiology. But as the "Wild Men of Borneo," the Hilton Sisters, Eli Bowen, and Lew Graham's comment point out, many of the greats had demonstrable physical and mental differences. Be it a very small head, a very small body, or a flesh connection holding twins together, the anomaly was the starting point for the exhibit's construction. The success of freak shows depended on the availability of people with uncommon conditions. Yet as we discussed in Part One, at the height of freak show popularity, despite rigorous recruitment at home and abroad, there was a shortage of born freaks.

One did not have to be born with an abnormality to be a popular or even outstanding exotic or aggrandized freak. While it was more difficult for other than born freaks to reach the height of their profession, many exhibits were completely normal except in the way they were presented. Others acquired their physical oddity for the purposes of exhibition. Still others learned to do unusual acts to make them eligible for the freak show.

In this chapter we look at self-made freaks. (My use of this term is slightly different from that of amusement world people; for them novelty acts are a separate category.) Interestingly, although showmen would acknowledge that the freaks discussed here were completely made up for the purpose of exhibition, they did not consider them "gaffs." That word was reserved for fakes who pretended to be born with anomalies. The freaks here are "authentic" fabrications—people who worked within legitimate freak roles with a long history in the amusement industry.

This chapter traces the history of two varieties of exotic self-made exhibits, "Circassian Beauties" and tattooed people. Other attractions such as sword swallowers and snake charmers are considered briefly as well. We will see how showmen took advantage of the stories of lust and barbarism in Asia Minor and other parts of the non-Western world to fabricate exotic and erotic freaks. As in Chapter 5, we will explore the patterns in the construction of standard exhibits, looking at the characters involved, the science behind the stories, and the forces that shaped the constructions.

Self-made freaks had been around throughout the history of the freak show, but during the height of its popularity they played a special role. One dimension of their creation, which is evident in the narrative that follows, is that the number of self-made freaks could easily expand as demand for freak exhibits increased. Because a physical or mental anomaly did not serve as the basis of their freak role, there were not the same limits to the supply as there were for the born freaks. Hence, when the demand for freaks was the greatest, more self-made freaks worked the platforms. In addition, as the exhibiting of people with physical and mental differences became offensive, self-made freaks began increasingly to fill out the list of exhibits. But as we will see, the popularity, the interest, of a freak is tied to his or her uniqueness. Thus, the self-made freak, as a genre, had a built-in problem: the more the ranks expanded, the less attractive certain types of exhibits of this ilk became. We will see how this tendency affected the nature of presentations and the history of particular types of exhibits.

Circassian Beauties

Patrons of any 1880 freak show were likely to encounter on exhibit a woman with puffy, Middle Eastern–style, three-quarter-length pants and flowing garments, topped by a teased-out mound of frizzled, bushy, dark hair. She might also have a water pipe on stage and tell you of her life in a Turkish harem. Whether she called herself Zana Zanobia, Zalumma Agra (Fig. 70), Zoe Meleke, Millie Zulu, Zula Zeleke, Zoberdie Luti,[1] or another exotic-sounding name, the rest of

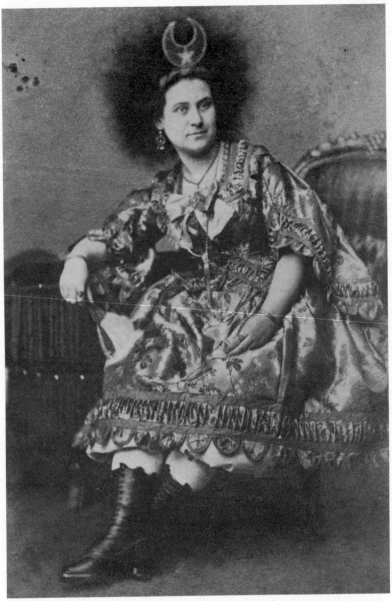

Fig. 70. Circassian Beauty. Zalumma Agra, "The Star of the East." Photo by Doane, c. 1875. (Becker Coll., Syracuse University.)

PORTRAITS OF PRESENTATION

her introduction would state that she was from the purest stock of Caucasian in the world: she was a genuine "Circassian Beauty."

These Circassians were introduced as a novelty into the expanding freak show market in the mid 1860s, and by the late 1870s almost every dime museum and circus sideshow had one to fill out its freak exhibit roster. By the turn of the century, however, the popularity of this variety of exhibit was in precipitous decline. The genre and its rise and fall provide one illustration of how the forces of supply and demand shape the evolution of exhibits.

There was nothing very unusual about the women who were exhibited as Circassians. One of the only requirements was that they be physically attractive—by Victorian standards. These "Circassians" were, in fact, indistinguishable from thousands of other nineteenth-century women, and they existed in unlimited supply. All there really was was the presentation, a creation that wove the history of science together with tales of erotic intrigue from Asia Minor, current events, and a good portion of showman hype.

The "science" behind Circassians goes back to Johann Friedrich Blumenbach, the great German comparative anatomist and first physical anthropologist. In 1775 Blumenback undertook a major revision of Linnaeus's human classification scheme through examination of skulls. He introduced the persistent but misleading term *Caucasian* when he found a strong resemblance between a skull in his collection that came from the Caucasus (Gossett 1963, 38) and the skulls of Germans. Convinced that all human beings had one common origin, he conjectured that the Caucasus was the origin not only of Europeans, the Caucasian type, but of all humans (W. Jordan 1968, 222–223).

According to monogenist thought, God formed humans in their pure form. As they spread out over the globe, they degenerated in appearance. Blumenbach's and other monogenists' ideas led to the widely held conclusion that the purest and most beautiful whites were the Circassians, one tribe of the Caucasian region of Russia, a mountainous area on the Black Sea close to Turkey, then the Ottoman Empire.

The Crimean War, a mid-nineteenth-century conflict between the Russians and the Turks, was in part a land dispute. French and British support of the sultan against Russia focused Americans' attention on Asia Minor. Tales of bloodshed, atrocities, and the abuse of minority groups, as well as of veiled women and harems, were part of the intrigue surrounding the area that is now Turkey. It was alleged that

Circassian women were stolen during Turkish raids and sold in the white slave markets of Constantinople, where they were bought for service in barbaric Turkish and Persian harems. The story of the Circassian concubines was well known to mid-nineteenth-century Americans. Starting in the 1850s and lasting through World War II, Asia Minor was a prime source of images and plots for showmen's exotic freak show constructions.

The story of the incorporation of Circassians into the membership book of standard freak show attractions is more intriguing than the exhibit itself. In the spring of 1864 P. T. Barnum, always interested in staying ahead of the competition, was looking for new attractions to add variety to his American Museum Hall of Human Curiosities. The showman sent his employee John Greenwood, Jr., on a freak hunt with the specific assignment of finding the "horned woman" that Barnum had heard lived in the Middle East (Barnum 1871, 579). Greenwood found the woman, but she had nothing more than a pronounced cyst, hardly enough to justify bringing her to the United States for exhibition.

Barnum wrote Greenwood and told him to stop in Constantinople and buy a "beautiful Circassian girl" (Saxon 1983, 125). Barnum's account (1871, 580) of the outcome, which was published in his autobiography, is evasive. Shortly after Greenwood's return, and with great fanfare, a Circassian Beauty went on exhibit at the American Museum. She was presented as Greenwood's quarry, obtained by him in the disguise of a Turk in the dangerous and provocative slave market (Saxon 1983).

But there is an alternative chronicle of the events leading to the introduction of Circassians into the American freak show (Dingess c. 1899, 923–926). According to an unpublished version by John Dingess, a contemporary of Barnum, Greenwood returned from his trip empty handed. A few weeks after his return a young woman came to the museum looking for work. She had bushy hair but nothing remarkable enough to make her a museum attraction. Disappointed by Greenwood's lack of success, but still bent on getting a Circassian, Barnum saw in her the possibility of creating his own Circassian, and he hired her. A Turk, residing in New York, was consulted as to appropriate dress and name, and in a short time the girl appeared at the museum in her silks as a full-fledged Circassian. The lecturer related details of the perils that attended Mr. Greenwood's exertions and how he finally had to resort to high-priced bribery to ensure success and keep himself out of prison.

If we were not familiar with Barnum's antics we might not know which tale to believe. Barnum's own evasiveness in his autobiography over Greenwood's success lends credibility to Dingess's version. In addition, there is reason to believe that all the other Circassian Beauties exhibited at Barnum's American Museum were in fact local women.

One of Barnum's most popular Circassians was Zoe Meleke. Barnum invented a story, which was sold in pamphlet form as "Biographical Sketch of the Circassian Girl," in conjunction with her appearence, to veil the fact that Zoe was really a native-born American. Whereas others might have shrunk from the disparity between the Circassian imagery and the fact that Zoe spoke perfect American English and knew nothing of the land of her birth, Barnum dismissed the potential embarrassment by telling the patrons, in brazen showmen style:

> Being of a very tender age at the time of her exodus from
> the land of her nativity, her recollections of Circassia
> are of course very imperfect and obscure; the associations
> of her far off country seem to her an imperfect and con-
> fused dream, rather than a reality; and from her long sev-
> erance from the people of her kind, she has partially, if
> not entirely, lost remembrance of her native tongue; and
> yet, as has been stated elsewhere in this little sketch, she
> speaks the language of her adopted land with an ease and
> fluency that would puzzle the most cunning linguist that
> was not otherwise informed to discover that she was not a
> native of America. (*Zoe Meleke* c. 1880)

With the introduction of the Circassian Beauty in the 1860s, Barnum launched the prototype of a self-made freak. In a short time there were a score of imitations of the "original," and by the late 1870s the formula for constructing a Circassian Beauty had become standard-ized. It is doubtful that the frizzled Afro-like hair, which became the exhibits' trademark, had anything to do with the appearance of real Circassians. Those who became "beauties" had to engage in the un-appealing task of washing their hair in beer without rinsing it, then teasing it to take on the appearance of the original fraud.

In the 1890s Dingess observed, "More than thirty years have elapsed, and probably not one of the dozen or more 'Circassian Girls' now being exhibited at Dime Museums and in sideshows, is near that many years old, yet 'the lecturer' when introducing his curiosities almost invariably announces 'She was brought to this country by John Greenwood for Barnum's American Museum'" (Dingess 1899, 925). Late-1890s presentations often referred back to the "orginal," but, as with many self-made freaks, the "orginal" had been so often copied and become so banal that the Circassian Beauty had lost her appeal as a major freak attraction.

As with other varieties of freak exhibits, showmen fought the trivialization of Circassians by innovation. In an attempt to save the exhibit's appeal they altered the Circassians' stories and appearance. Because the original exhibits were women, they tried, with almost no success, to exhibit males. Another, slightly more successful attempt to rouse interest in the genre involved multioddity attractions. That is, although the exhibits' major claim to fame was that they represented the purest form of humans, they also became second-rate snake charmers, sword swallowers, mind readers, jugglers, bird tamers, and the like. To add an exotic dimension to second-rate novelty performers' presentations, some exhibits—sword swallowers, for example—borrowed the title "Circassian" to elevate interest in their stage show. Anything gained from such innovations was short lived and in the long run undermined the genre's appeal by diluting the unique form, making the type even more common.

Another attempt to revive the Circassian presentation and to pump up a class of "born freak" of minor interest was the casting of albino Caucasians in the role of Circassians. This innovation apparently met with some success in the late 1880s and 1890s. The extreme white skin of the albino fit nicely with the idea of purity of race; some albino "harem escapees" let their hair grow, dyed it dark and soaked it in stale beer (Durant and Durant 1957, 121).

By 1910 Circassians had lost their appeal and were dropped as a standard freak show feature. Interestingly, the fascination that Americans had with teased bushy hair lasted longer than the Circassians who introduced it. "Moss-Haired Women" and other bushy-headed freaks remained as occasional exhibits after the Circassians left the scene.

Circassian Beauties were cast in the exotic mode. But unlike mentally retarded exotics and others we will meet later, emphasis was not on their inferiority or primitiveness. In fact, the exotic was combined with the aggrandized to create an attractive, intelligent, and sensual woman. The appeal was the exotic mystery of the Near East and the reputation of the Circassians' captors, the Turks. The juxtaposition of the fair Circassian beauty and dark barbaric Turk provided an erotic twist that appealed to nineteenth-century Americans.

In summing up the history of Circassian exhibits in the American sideshow, famed circus press agent Dexter Fellows put it well when he said that there had been over forty years of exotic intrigue, and "Zuleika, The Circassian Sultana, Favorite of the Harem, was really an Irish immigrant from Jersey City" (Fellows and Freeman 1936, 293).

Tattooed Exotics

Our chronicle of tattooed exhibits starts earlier and in very different parts of the world than did that of the Circassians. This genre evolved over a longer period as well, lasting through the 1930s. Further, with tattooed exhibits different forces influence the history of the form and the nature of presentations. The technology of tattooing itself plays an important role in determining the supply and form of exhibits.

As we saw in Chapter 7, as Westerners continued to explore the world in the eighteenth and nineteenth centuries they encountered peoples whose strange customs and appearance shocked them. Many peoples from the Far East, the South Sea Islands, South America, and the American West practiced the art of permanently marking their bodies with designs through the long and painful process of puncturing the skin with needlelike implements and applying dye (Hambly 1925; Burchett 1958). Naturalists and early anthropologists saw the practice of tattooing as the ultimate sign of primitiveness, revealing a lack of sensitivity to pain and unabashed paganism.[2] This perspective, which the general population shared, made tattooed "aborigines" good exhibits. Well into the nineteenth century, tattooed natives were moneymakers, first in Europe and then in America.[3]

In the early 1800s Europeans began taking up the occupation of "tattooed men." They were seamen who, rather than getting a small tattoo on their arm, had their bodies extensively decorated by native tattooers. When they discovered that people would pay to view such skin art, a new type of freak was created.

At first their presentations were straightforward: they said they had paid to be tattooed by an indigenous practitioner.[4] Without doubt, extensively tattooed whites had exotic appeal, even without an embellished presentation. But from a showman's point of view the unexaggerated exotic appeal of tattoo exhibits was not enough—or at least not when the competition increased. As more such attractions appeared, their presentations became embellished.

In 1828 Britons were fascinated by an account of John Rutherford, a mariner who had returned from New Zealand with tattoos that covered most of his body. Rutherford declared he had been captured by the Maoris who held him prisoner for six years; he had been compelled to marry the chief's thirteen-year-old daughter, had had three children, and was forcibly tattooed. His story aroused sympathy and publicity, on which he capitalized by becoming a successful exhibit. It is unknown how the leaking of the true story affected his career, but it was eventually established, undoubtedly to the dismay of his English wife and children, that Rutherford had actually jumped ship, taken up life with a native woman, and chosen to be tattooed (Burchett 1958, 24; Ebensten 1953, 16). As the practice of exhibiting "tattooed" whites came to the United States, and probably with no compensation to him, variations of Rutherford's presentation were copied, amplified, and exploited.

The first record of a tattooed white being exhibited in the United States dates from 1840. James O'Connell was first shown at the American Museum just prior to Barnum's takeover (Odell 1928, 4:512). O'Connell had tattoos on his left hand, both arms, legs, thighs, back and abdomen, right breast, and left shoulder. The tattoos were engaging, especially to people who had not seen tattoos before, but even more engrossing was the elaborate and titillating story of how he had obtained them. The full fabrication is found in *The Life and Adventures of James F. O'Connell, the Tattooed Man, During a Residence of Eleven Years in New Holland and Caroline Islands* (1846), a thirty-one-page pamphlet he sold to his patrons. The booklet takes the reader through whaling adventures, shipwrecks, narrow escapes from cannibals, cavorting romps with women criminals, false arrests, and finally to his life among the local people of an island in Micronesia. On that island he is forced to undergo tattooing at the hands of indigenous maidens. On completing the ordeal he learns that the last young lady who imprinted him is, by custom, his wife.

We do not know enough about O'Connell to establish how much of the fabrication is grounded in any real experiences he had. Part of the appeal of O'Connell's story, and those of other tattooed exhibits that followed, was the fuzzy line between the true rakehell life of the person being exhibited and the elaborate exotic tales of the sideshow presentation. O'Connell's tattoos were real, even if the story was not, and that is more than can be said for some of his twentieth-century successors.

Compared to the standards set by exhibits that followed, O'Connell's tattoos were inferior and not as extensive. But at the time, the competition was minimal. A few decades later his story and paltry designs would not qualify him for any respectable freak show platform, but in the late 1840s he was quite a success. The last record of him is with Dan Rice's circus troop in 1852 (Parry 1933, 59).

Following O'Connell was a long line of tattooed people who made a living by exhibiting themselves in freak shows. The quality and extent of tattoos on successful exhibits increased markedly as competition raised the standards. The stories of the origin of the body work became more elaborate and fanciful too.

Captain Costentenus came along soon after O'Connell. An Albanian Greek named Alexandrinos—also known as Djordgi Konstantinus or Georgius Constantine, then Captain Constantinus, and later Prince Costentenus—he was the most flamboyant and best known of all tattooed men. This large, bearlike man was covered from head to toe with elaborate tattoos.

Costentenus's decorations were multicolored oriental designs. So plentiful and intricate were they that it looked like he was covered by a close-fitting, finely crocheted shawl. There were tattoos under his hair and on his scalp; even his eyelids and the interior of his ears were adorned. His body was covered by 388 animal and floral designs, all carefully executed with elaborate detail and color.[5] As he once said, "Only the palms of my hands, the soles of my feet, and a few square inches of my face were left as Nature made them" (*Life and Adventures of Capt. Costentenus* 1881, 22). It is hard to imagine how any person could compete with him for the title of outstanding tatooed body of all time.

There was also oriental writing on his skin; the words written between his fingers, he proudly said, branded him as "the greatest rascal and thief in the world" (Parry 1933, 61). And judging from the concocted—and dubious—tale he told of his tattooing, that sentence characterized him accurately.

The whole story, or at least one version of it (for another version, see Sherwood 1926, 148), was found in a booklet he sold, *The Life and Adventures of Capt. Costentenus, the Tattooed Greek Prince* (1881).

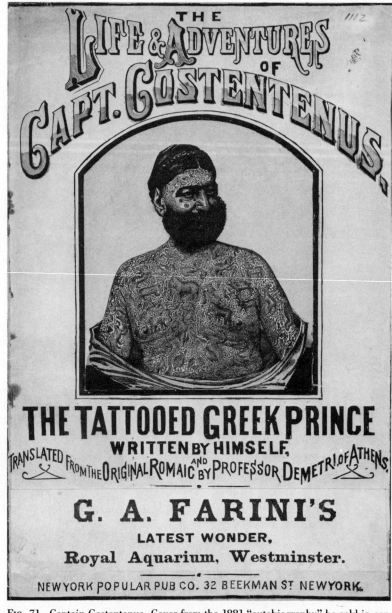

FIG. 71. Captain Costentenus. Cover from the 1881 "autobiography" he sold in conjunction with his appearances. Costentenus is shown in the center lithograph with his elaborate tattoo designs. (Becker Coll., Syracuse University.)

With a beautiful color drawing of him on the cover (Fig. 71), this pamphlet contained twenty-three fine-print pages, with sketches and detail that rivaled his tattoos for intricacy.

As the tale goes, he was born in 1836 to a Christian family from Greek nobility living in the Turkish province of Albania. His family was killed and his town destroyed by a pagan Turkish despot who adopted him as his son. He was raised first in his captor's harem and then, after the despot's death, in a harem in Egypt. Life is described as exotic and erotic: "The women of the harem petted and indulged me to my heart's content" (p. 4). They were fond of dressing him like a girl, and for a time he passed as a female with the name of Fatima.[6]

Costentenus appeared in the freak show at about the same time that Circassians were reaching the height of their popularity. Attesting to showmen's ingenuity and their pre–social science understanding of triangulation, his promoters built Circassians into his "true life" story. The head of the Egyptian harem where he allegedly stayed as a child shared her name, Princess Zuleika, with a well-known American Circassian freak (Fellows and Freeman 1936).

At the age of twelve he finds himself in "full fellowship . . . with a band of the most ruthless pirates that ever roamed the seas." He kills a pirate, is shipwrecked, and then takes up residence in a Persian harem where he meets a Circassian slave, Leila, or Queen of the Zenanah, who helps him escape. Then on across the East, and into conflicts with various groups involved in the Crimean War. Then into the service of Yakoob Beg, Khan of Kashagar, at a copper mine in China. He and two companions organize an uprising of the mine workers against the khan, but the uprising backfires, and Costentenus and two companions, one British, the other Spanish, are caught. They are told they have a choice of punishments: "You may be starved to death, stung to death by wasps, killed by tigers, cut to pieces—beginning at the toes—impaled on spears, burned to death, or tattooed. If you survive the last the Khan will give you your liberty" (*Life and Adventures of Capt. Costentenus* 1881, 19). Not knowing what they were getting into, they chose tattooing.

The "true life" booklet continues with a detailed description of the tortuous three months of continuous tattooing in which Costentenus's companions die. He, however, suffers through the ordeal, fights and kills one of the khan's men, is sold to a Turk, and finally is bought in a slave bazaar by "an American of great wealth, gained in the show business. . . . Heaven bless that generous American."

This version of the story differs from earlier accounts, although the general drift is the same—that the tattooing was a torture for having been involved in an uprising. The most important difference in the contradictory versions concerns who reportedly did the tattooing. Earlier versions of Costentenus's story (from the 1870s) use Burmese tattooists, but in later versions this detail is changed (Fig. 72). An 1881 booklet explains the discrepancies between early versions and the pamphlet version thus:

> So long as Yakoob Beg lived and was accessible to an increase of power, I forbore to publish the facts of my life. The publicity given to his name would have pleased that savage potentate, and I did not care to let him have such an advantage.
>
> Therefore neither in Europe nor America did the name of Yakoob Beg ever cross my lips. I let all sort of absurd stories pass current about me, but I never told any one how I was tattooed or by who.
>
> Since the death of Yakoob Beg, in 1877, the reason for my silence has been removed. The bloody tyrant has gone to his long rest. (*Life and Adventures of Capt. Costentenus* 1881, 23)

More likely the story changed because those who examined his tattoos questioned their origins. In later versions the work was alleged to have been done by two old seamen, one Italian and one Spanish, who were working under the command of the khan. This shift in the tale, much like Barnum's explanation of Zoe Meleke's American accent, illustrates the showmen's creativity in modifying stories to fit new circumstances and stay ahead of the rubes. While the exact origin of the captain's tattoos remain a mystery, a letter from the "Reverend J. C." (Harvard Coll.) reports an interview with Costentenus in which the Reverend was told that the markings had been acquired for the purpose of exhibition and that the "human gallery" was Italian, not Greek.

Costentenus began his career as an exhibit in the early 1870s.[7] He was a smash at the Vienna World Exposition in 1873 (Burchett 1958, 104), where scholars inspected him as an example of oriental art and speculated about the origin of his markings. A Viennese dermatologist, Professor Ferdinand Hebra, showed Costentenus to his students, wrote about him in learned journals, and even included his picture in his dermatological atlas (Parry 1933, 62). For physicians, his interest lay in the fact that he was the most extensively tattooed person in exis-

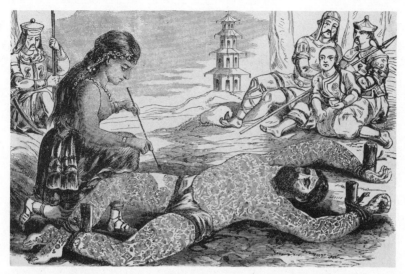

FIG. 72. *Harper's Weekly* advertisement for Costentenus. This May 26, 1877, adver-tisement depicts the earlier version of the tattooing story. (Becker Coll., Syracuse University.)

tence, and they marveled that he could have endured the tattooing without his glands and perspiration being affected.

There are conflicting stories concerning which showmen managed Costentenus and when and where he first appeared in the United States. The 1881 pamphlet states that G. A. Farini, a flamboyant Ca-nadian who managed a number of freakshow greats, including Krao, "The Missing Link," was his first and only agent and that Costentenus was first exhibited in the United States at G. B. Bunnell's Dime Mu-seum. Others say that Barnum brought him to the country in 1873, gave him the title Captain Prince, and advertised him as "The Living Picture-Gallery," a term that became standard amusement world lingo for tattooed exhibits (Parry 1933, 62).

In his trip across the sea his appearance changed in a way that highlighted his exotic presentation (Fig. 73). While abroad he wore his hair and beard natural fashion, but after coming to the United States they were braided and curled and fastened to the top of his head. This style, combined with his loincloth and his burly frame, made for quite a presence. As a touch of contrast, he wore a large diamond ring on the same hand in which he held the cigarettes he chain-smoked. With that getup and the tattoos, he could hardly miss.

American physicians knew about him before he arrived. Dr. P. A.

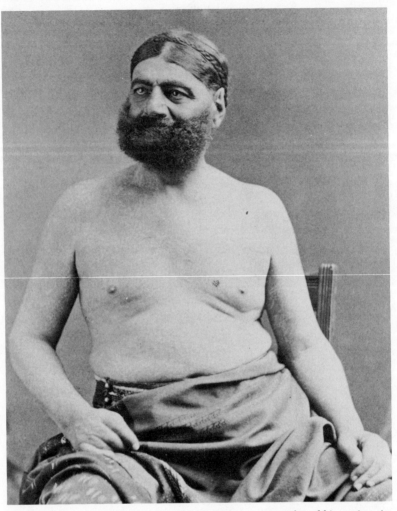

FIG. 73. Costentenus in person. Most of the publicity pictures he sold in conjunction with his appearances were printed drawings like the portrait on the pamphlet in Fig. 71. This rare photograph was taken by one of the premier theatrical New York photographers, Mora, in about 1883. Unfortunately, his tattoos are faint in the aged photo. (Harvard Theater Collection, Cambridge, Massachusetts.)

O'Connell had seen Costentenus in Austria, and he wrote a description of him which was published in the *Boston Medical and Surgical Journal* (O'Connell 1871). when Costentenus appeared in Philadelphia someone questioned the authenticity of his markings. His manager, in typical showman form, invited physicians and the press to a private demonstration at the Continental Hotel. "In a very short

PORTRAITS OF PRESENTATION

time the most stubborn disbelievers were convinced their 'impossibility' was a fixed fact" (*Life and Adventures of Capt. Costentenus* 1881, 23).

In the 1880s Costentenus was a huge draw at dime museums and in circus sideshows. Later in his career, with his exotic story firmly established, there were slight changes in his presentation. Increasingly, the lecturer emphasized the debauched life he had led, and his involvement in murder and crime and with women. The lecturer would end his talk with the words: "And this wild tattooed man is always much admired by all ladies." The erotic, criminal ambience to the presentation reflected changes in the meaning of and expanded interest in tattooing in the scientific community.

Physicians were now linking tattooing with syphilis, and such designs became associated with sexual permissiveness. More important, a new branch of science, "criminal anthropology," began to explore the links between body markings and crime. Cesare Lombroso, an Italian scientist who was widely read in the United States (Parmelee 1912; Savitz 1972, xvii) and whom some consider the father of the scientific study of crime, stated flat out that tattooing was a sign of criminality—or, more accurately, that tattoos were the stigmata of a distinct different physical form of human, the "criminal man" (Lombroso 1887, 1896; Lombroso-Ferrero 1972). The popularity of Lombroso's theories grew out of the impact of Charles Darwin's *The Origin of Species* (1859) and *The Descent of Man* (1871). In *The Descent of Man*, Darwin suggested that some forms of humans were closer to their primitive ancestors than others. This belief was central to Lombroso's writings. According to him and his scientific followers, the practice of permanently marking the body was an atavistic revision, evidence of an individual's regression to a more aggressive, antisocial form of being. As he put it, "Tattooing is, in fact, one of the essential characteristics of primitive man, and of men who still live in the savage state" (Lombroso 1896, 800).

What became of the bad Captain Costentenus is lost to us. While he was a difficult example to live up to, his influence lived on. He personifies the statement that it is not necessary that one be a born freak to have a brilliant career as one. Costentenus was a showman, and along with his manager he playfully responded to controversy and changing times by slightly redoing the presentation. It was never altered too much, however, for that would have undermined the credibility of the exhibit that was to become a legend.

The captain's success as an exhibition stimulated the market for tattooed exhibits. John Hayes followed soon after. He was presented as having been born in Connecticut in 1864 and, at fourteen, joining the army as a drummer boy to fight the Indians in the Far West. Separated from his fellow soldiers, he was captured by Apache braves. Among the Apaches was one white man, a former sailor who, said Hayes, placed the 780 tattoo designs on his body (Parry 1933, 66). This tale allowed, as did Costentenus's earlier fabrication, for the exotic kidnapping or capture of a Caucasian by "savage" people, while at the same time explaining the presence of tattoos that did not have an authentic native look. Explanations such as these were required in the construction of tattooed exhibits. Increasingly, American-born and -trained tattoo artists were using their own designs and doing the handiwork needed to transform a plain-skinned person into a "human art gallery."

Martin Hilderbrant, a German immigrant, is credited with being the first professional American tattooist.[8] Between 1861 and 1865 he tattooed soldiers on both sides of the Civil War (Burchett 1958, 26). But it was not until later in the century that domestic tattooers became generally available and tattoo parlors sprang up in major cities. These resources provided the handiwork both for aspiring freak show exhibits and for ordinary citizens who wanted a few designs on their pale skin. "Professor" Charlie Wagner (Johnston 1934b, 29) saw Costentenus in a New York dime museum in the late 1880s and was so impressed that he got himself tattooed and began studying the art of skin design in earnest (Parry 1933, 63), thus launching his fifty-year career in which he worked on more than fifty freak show attractions.

With the advent of the electric tattooing tool (the first electric tattooing machine was patented by Tom Riley in December 1891 [Ebensten 1953, 19]) and improved technique, tattooing became a common and painless activity (Fig. 74).[9] This fact significantly changed not only the competition but also the nature of tattooed exhibits.[10] Now, extensively tattooed exhibits sought out masters to complete the job. People looking for a new and easy occupation had simply to raise the money to pay the tattoo artist and they could become a "human art gallery." While in the late 1880s and early 1890s exhibits could command large salaries, this situation changed quickly.

Because of the freak show's popularity and the corresponding high demand for exhibits, people desiring an amusement world career were

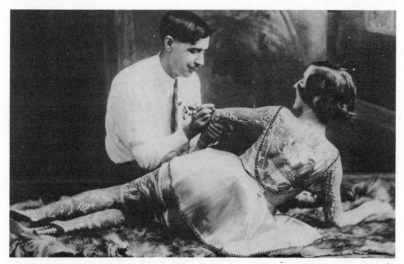

Fig. 74. Tattoo artist using electric tattoo tool on "Stella." Postcard, c. 1910. (Becker Coll., Syracuse University.)

choosing tattooing as their method, even before the new tattooing technology became available. Thus, as with the Circassians, competition increased and the large number of exhibits began to undermine the appeal. And again, showmen tried innovation to keep up interest.

The introduction of male Circassians flopped as a fashion, but a similar tack with "human art galleries" changed the history of tattooed exhibits. In the 1880s tattooed women arrived on the scene, upstaging men completely. One reason for their appeal was that in order to show their tattoos, they had to expose parts of their bodies—their legs and thighs—which under any other circumstances would have been lewd if not illegal. This gave showmen a way of sliding a little bawdiness into the freak show tent, an act that both paralleled and facilitated the incorporation of hoochy koochy shows into the popular amusement industry.

A second appeal of the women exhibits was the contrast between what women were supposed to be—chaste, docile, and inconspicuous—and what the tattoos had come to stand for—criminality, flamboyance, and decadence. Although some women exhibits used the standard exotic stories that had been handed down through Costentenus (forced tattooing by savage captors), other exotic stories evolved as well. La Belle Irene, who Ebensten (1953) claims was the first completely covered tattooed lady in America,[11] explained her tattooing as required protection she obtained in the Wild West of Texas to escape the attentions of the hostile Red Indians. Nora Hildebrandt, who first went on exhibit in 1882, reported that her 365 designs were crafted by her father, operating under the threat of death from his captor, Sitting Bull (*Tattooed Lady* c. 1890). As more women appeared with distinct American designs, increasingly their tattoos were explained as the result of domestic criminal cruelty.[12]

The idea that a woman would permanently mark her whole body with tattoos in order to become an exhibit was difficult to believe.[13] In fact, some women had themselves tattooed in less permanent ways; these india-inked imitations sparked accusations as well as jokes (Alden 1896). Most female human art galleries, however, did have genuine extensive tattooing all over their bodies, with the exception of their hands, necks, and heads. Thus, if they wore a long-sleeved blouse with the top buttoned, their tattooing would not show. This not only allowed them to hide their art work when not working, but it also gave them some chance of an alternative career if the tattooed lady market fell through, which eventually it did.

Annie Howard and Frank Howard were successful tattooed exhibits with Barnum and Bailey's show in the early 1900s. The novelty of their being brother and sister and the quality of their tattooing helped them to eke out a living in the increasingly competitive tattooed exhibit market. While they said they had been shipwrecked and rescued by South Sea savages who forcibly tattooed them, many of Annie's tattoos were actually done by her brother. In the twentieth century it became common for exhibits to be tattoo artists as well. Howard Frank, for instance, left the sideshow to run the biggest tattoo shop in America.

By the early twentieth century the life of tattooed exhibits had fallen on hard times. Whereas at one time they had demanded substantial salaries,[14] by 1910 many were paid little. In fact, in some cases circus and dime museum owners made the exhibits pay for the right to be in the show, their income deriving solely from the sale of pictures and fees collected from tattooing patrons.

Tattooers attributed the slide in salaries and popularity to a New York dime museum's advertisement at the turn of the century for a "Congress of Tattooed Men"—If a whole "congress" could be assembled, the tattooers pointed out, how could patrons think they were rare enough to be worth seeing? That particular event, of course, does not account for the decline of the genre, but an overabundance of exhibits does.

Because tattooed people could be easily produced—the tattooing machine made attractive designs quickly, cheaply, and with little pain—the supply was greater than, and soon undermined, the demand. Human galleries were passé. Efforts were made to increase interest by offering not only tattooed men and women, but also tattooed families, including young children (Webb 1976). One family even introduced a tattooed Fido as part of their exhibit—and others quickly followed suit. Epitomizing how far the tattoo war went was the exhibition at Coney Island of a tattooed cow (Parry 1933, 67).

Tattoo competition became so intense that a merely tattooed person could not get a job. The Circassians' fate was met on tattooed exhibits, but to even greater extremes. Tattooed dwarfs appeared, as well as tattooed fat ladies, and, to illustrate how far people went in the pursuit of novelty, Edward S. Willie was exhibited as the tattooed half man. Willie, a legless man, was tattooed extensively over his chest, arms, and back (Ringling Coll.). To add a touch of the exotic to their performances, amusement world acts were tattooed as well. Frank and Emma Caldwell, with the John Robinson show, tried to beat the competition by appearing as a tattooed knife-throwing couple (Fig. 75).

Although they were no longer featured attractions, tattooed people continued to work in freak shows through the thirties. Attractive women with exotic and erotic stories who were willing to exhibit their anatomy remained viable. Their presentations involved tales of sexual betrayal and their designs changed from foreign themes to patriotic eagles, flags, and the Statue of Liberty. Large religious pieces such as *Madonna and Child* and reproductions of Leonardo da Vinci's *Last Supper* were also popular.[15]

Tattooed men had a more difficult time making it. An article in the *Providence Sunday Journal* of February 21, 1931, reported the plight of James Filbert, a tattooed man who was forced out of the circus and was scrubbing floors and washing dishes because he could not find freak show work. Tattooed men and their decorators had to come up with strikingly original designs and presentations to withstand the competition.[16]

In 1927 a tall, well-built, handsome man called on "Professor" George Burchett, "King of Tattooists," in his London studio with a direct request. The man whom Burchett calls "Major R.," and who went on to be exhibited as "The Great Omi, The Zebra Man" (Fig.

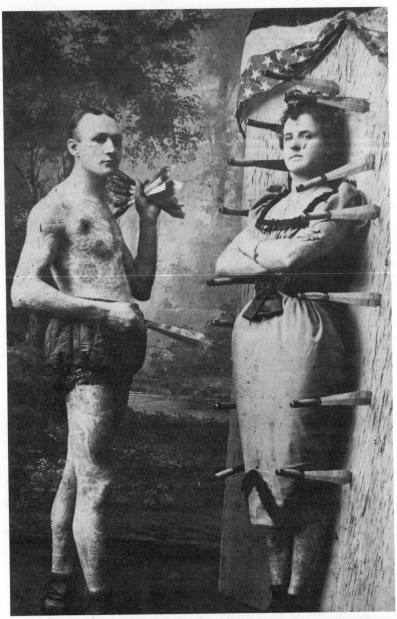

FIG. 75. Tattooed knife-throwing act. Frank and Emma Caldwell. Photo by Frank Wendt, 1899. (Becker Coll., Syracuse University.)

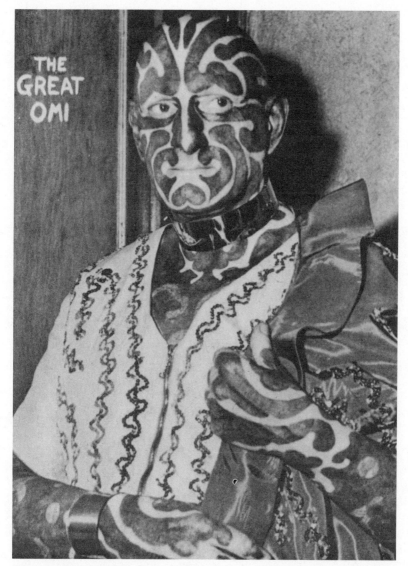

THE
GREAT
OMI

FIG. 76. "The Great Omi, The Zebra Man." Photographer unknown, c. 1939. (Richards Coll., Worcester, Massachusetts.)

76), wanted to become "one of the great human oddities" (Burchett 1958, 164). He brought his own design: he wanted Burchett to tattoo him all over, including his face, with broad dark blue or black zebra stripes. The Great Omi went through as many as five hundred sittings before his aim was achieved. The curved stripes, one to two inches wide, masked most of his previous tattoos. His chest and back were covered altogether, with black dye that turned cobalt blue when inserted under the epidermis.

When he went on exhibit he boasted that he had had to pay $10,000 to have himself tattooed ("Circus Means Animals" 1938), but Burchett said that the entire job ran about $3,000—still a considerable amount in the 1920s. The indelible markings and the money were a heavy investment to make on the speculation that he could break into the freak show market as a major exhibit, but it paid off—the Zebra Man was one of the few tattooed men to make it in the 1930s freak show. In 1938 he went to the United States, where he joined a Ripley's Believe It or Not Show. He spent twenty-six weeks at the Odditorium on Broadway, toured with Ringling Brothers, Barnum and Bailey Circus, and appeared at Madison Square Garden. He traveled from coast to coast, drawing large crowds wherever he went (Burchett 1958, 170; "Circus Means Animals" 1938).

Some tattooed men resorted to bizarre performances to make themselves more marketable on the highly competitive freak market. One 1930s example was Rasmus Nielson. Echoing early exotic stories, he claimed that he had been captured, tattooed, and tortured in the South Sea Islands. He had an additional tidbit to share concerning his torture: the "savages" had implanted rings in the skin of his chest and suspended him with ropes from trees. Part of his presentation involved lifting an anvil—by the torture rings that were still lodged in his chest.

Tattooed men came to the realization that there were better vocational choices.

Serpent Queens

Snake charming was another specialty that moved from being an almost exclusively male occupation to domination by women. In fact, as snake charming and handling moved into the twentieth century it became almost exclusively a female calling (Fig. 77).

Large exotic snakes were exhibited in early museums, and the 1876 and 1893 world fairs imported male snake charmers as part of native villages. During the last two decades of the nineteenth century, when demand for freaks was so high, people, especially partially clad and exotic-looking women,[17] handling or "charming" boas, anacondas, rattlers, cobras, and other serpents became common freak show fare.

Snake charmers—or serpent enchantresses, as they were also

PORTRAITS OF PRESENTATION

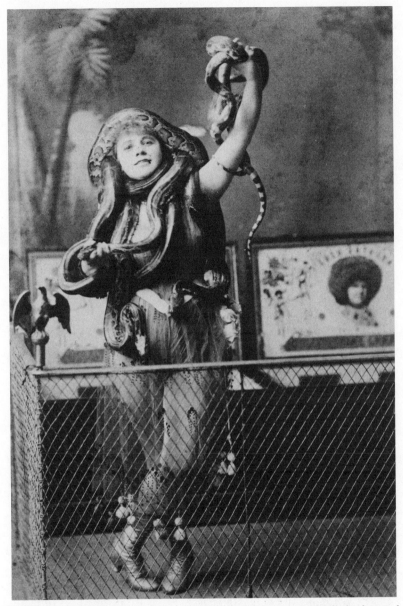

FIG. 77. Lulu Lataska, snake charmer. Her dress and the posters in the background suggest that Lulu presented herself as a Circassian too. Photo by Charles Eisenmann, c. 1885. (Becker Coll., Syracuse University.)

called—were, like tattooed persons and Circassians, easy to come by. Although there were tricks to make large snakes lethargic and poisonous snakes benign, some acts contained a distinct element of danger. For the most part, however, snake charming involved little skill and, aside from the ability to master repulsion and fear, few personal qualifications. There was a seemingly unending supply of charmers— more charmers than snakes by far.[18] Indeed, the cost and supply of snakes was a bigger factor in controlling the number of acts than the number of applicants. While charmers became commonplace and never demanded the high salaries of featured attractions, there was always a place for them on the platform. Audiences continued to squirm in delighted disgust year after year, and, as with human art galleries, innovation provided a continuous element of novelty. After Circassians became commonplace, there were Circassian snake charmers. In search of novelty, one man wrestled pythons in a five-hundred-gallon tank (FitzGerald 1897a). Although the types and numbers of snakes the charmer worked with provided some variety as well, the most important element of the exhibit was the presentation.

There were snake charmers and serpent queens who claimed to be from the East, having learned their skill through apprenticeship to mystics.[19] Others claimed to be born with serpent power. Even though a few who practiced the art probably were from India and other far-off places, most were homegrown Americans. In fact, snake charming was something wives of other freak show employees often took up in order to travel with their husbands, for accommodations were not provided for unemployed tagalongs.[20] "Miss Susan," the wife of Clyde Ingalls, who managed the Ringling Brothers, Barnum and Bailey Sideshow in the 1920s and 1930s, was a snake charmer.

Whether a domestic exotic or an import, one's story and stage presence were important elements of success. The difference between a fill-in and an attraction was ingenuity and flair. But most snake charmers were minor attractions, and we know very little about the women around whom the snakes wrapped themselves. A few, however, like Amy Arlington who was with Barnum and Bailey in the 1890s, left many photo portraits of themselves entwined by serpents. Some "true life" booklets are preserved, and, although less elaborate and sophisticated than those of featured stars, they do provide a glimpse of their presentation—a presentation in the high exotic mode.

Hedjaanta, "The Serpent Queen from the Philippine Islands," played dime museums and sideshows in the United States and En-

PORTRAITS OF PRESENTATION

gland around the turn of the century. Her manager was Count Orloff, a freak exhibit himself—"The Only Living Transparent and Ossified Man"—turned sideshow entrepreneur.[21] All we know about her comes from the pamphlet she sold in conjunction with her exhibition. It, of course, tells us more about conventions of presentation than about the person who played Hedjaanta.

Hedjaanta, according to the booklet, was born in the Philippine Islands. Her birth caused considerable debate within her tribe, as they were very dark skinned people with straight black hair, while she had very light hair and fair skin. Some feared she was an evil spirit, but others said she was sent to watch over them in times of war. After the tribe's first defeat following her birth, she fled on a raft. She was picked up by a sailing vessel on its way to Key West, where she was placed under the care of Dr. James Lewis, a young physician. Lewis adopted the girl, and soon he noticed his adopted daughter's fondness for snakes. She had many "slimy pets," among them some of the most poisonous of serpents. Dr. Lewis "passed over to the silent majority. . . . Like most Americans, wide awake and full of energy, she began to look around for some employment to fill her purse, instead of sitting down to spend the few dollars left her. She at last decided to become a professional Snake Charmer, not caring to part with her pets" (*Life of Hedjaanta* c. 1898).

This outlandish story conveniently explained why Hedjaanta, who was most likely an American-born Caucasian, did not have the appearance of a native from the Philippines. The Philippine backdrop and the story of her escape, combined with the claim of her natural way with serpents, make the potentially mundane activity of handling snakes exotic. Her affiliation with a respected doctor, and the flaunting of her American virtues of energy, independence, and motivation for success, add an aggrandized twist to this tale. (See also *Life of Naomi: Arizonian Snake Charmer* c. 1901.)

With snake charmers like the ones described—or, more to the point, with snake stories like that—we would expect that snake charmers would have gone the way of the Circassians. But they endured to the end of the freak show. They, after all, had serpents to fall back on.

Wild Men, Wild Women, and Geeks

In Chapter 5 we met exhibits with the condition we now call mental retardation who were presented as "wild men." Others cast as "wild men," too, had a real physical disability.[22] But starting in the first half of the nineteenth century, and increasingly toward the end of the century, there were hundreds of others hailed as wild men and women who had no anomalies. Like the Circassian Beauties, these wild men were one hundred percent presentation. They could readily be created to fill the demand.

The archival files contain pictures of these untamed brutes. Some are chained; some have false, tusklike incisor teeth; some are scantily dressed in animal skins. All have straggly long hair and look like the character in their presentation, a person who grew up in the wilds, eating wild game, living in caves, and being raised by some wild animal, most often a wolf.

With exhibits of this kind only the most feeble attempts were made at a scientific wrapping. Statements claiming that the specimen had been examined by physicians and natural scientists were as far as the appeal to science went. Most exhibits were cast as having been found in the wilderness of America or the mountains of Mexico, although later in the nineteenth century more distant locales came to be cited.

Wild men and wild women were so common and so indistinguishable that it is almost impossible to name, much less probe into the background of, individual exhibits. One wild man who left more than most was George Stall.[23] An 1890s exhibit billed as "George, the Mexican Wildman," he is pictured sitting on boulders dressed in typical wild-man style (Fig. 78). But most people who played the freak role of wild man or wild woman were so transient that they changed from month to month.

The circus owner and extraordinary showman W. C. Coup tells a story in his memoir that gives an idea of the nature of wild men presentations as well as illustrates their transient ways. Coup visited a dime museum with a large crowd that had been attracted by an enormous banner depicting the feature attraction, a savage-looking wild man. This creature was described as having been captured deep in the caves of Kentucky and was displayed in a prisonlike cell, chained to an iron grating. His skin was tawny yellow, his body was covered with hair, and he ravenously snapped at and ate lumps of raw beef which an attendant threw to him. Coup recognized the man as a person who had been exhibited in his own sideshow using a different presentation. "For his new job he had dyed his skin yellow and his whiskers and his hair black. After being a wild man for awhile he

PORTRAITS OF PRESENTATION

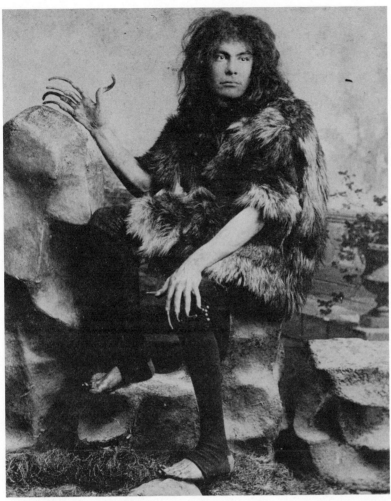

Fig. 78. George Stall, "The Mexican Wild Man." Photo by Charles Eisenmann, c. 1891. (Becker Coll., Syracuse University.)

resumed his former employment as 'Ivanovitch, the hairy man'"
(Coup 1901, 45).

Whereas snakes were the main attraction in the presentation of serpent queens and snake charmers, in the case of wild men and wild
women they were often just part of the background. John Norman, in
an article telling of his experiences as a boy in 1908 working in a traveling show, gives a picture of life behind the scenes of a wild-woman

snake show. The owner and spieler for the show was "Doc." His pitch told the crowds that inside the tent they would see "That strange wild woman—surrounded by thousands of poisonous reptiles—where you or I could not live for a single minute" (Norman 1933, 2). The so-called wild woman was actually a young man equipped with a dirty matted wig and red makeup on his face and hands. Doc would tell the patrons how she had been examined by medical authorities who concluded that she was immune and in fact addicted to the snake venom (the snakes were all harmless, some because they were nonpoisonous, others because they had been defanged). For five years Norman and Doc exhibited many "wild women" to countless thousands in scores of cities and villages from Chicago to the Pacific coast.

Like most wild men and women shows, Doc's was a pitshow. People entered a tent with an eight- to ten-foot-diameter enclosure in the center which they could walk around. Down in the pit would be the wild person, moaning and snarling at the spectators. If there were snakes in the pit the wild person might poke at them to provoke hissing sounds.

There was an endless supply of wild men and women to draw on to fill the demand for freak exhibits. Although sometimes they acted as fillers on the freak show platform, more often they were exhibited in pitshows or during the blowoff.

Wild men were never really in great competition with each other. What made the pitshow a success was the manipulation of the set and the exhibit's acting. One modifiable element that seems related to competition was the exhibit's level of grossness. While it is difficult to place the start of "gloaming geeks" (Boles 1967, 29), this variation on the wild man or wild woman show seems to have originated at the height of the freak show shortage. In present teenage vernacular, "geek" means a strange person, a person who does not have the proper social graces. In the amusement world, a "gloaming geek" was a wild man who, as part of his presentation, would bite the heads off of rats, chickens, and snakes.[24] Often this form of geek was a down-and-out alcoholic who performed in exchange for booze and a place to stay. Second- and third-rung amusement organizations who had a difficult time getting the better-drawing exhibits often resorted to geeks in order to get an audience.

Wild man and woman shows were the bottom rung of the freak show exhibits, and the geek show was the bottom of the bottom. Only the lower-order amusement establishments would carry them, and some municipalities banned them entirely. It was this type of coarse exhibition that helped earn carnivals reputations for being sleazy and morally reprehensible.

Human Ostriches, Sword Swallowers, and Other Ingestors

One of the first sword swallowers in the United States was Sena Sama, who appeared before the mid-nineteenth century (Odell 1927). Sword swallowing was like snake charming: little talent or skill was needed for the average act. (Carrington 1913). As with most novelty acts, the feat looked much more difficult than it in fact was. One could, for example, learn to control the throat muscles and slide a sword down the throat in only a few days. Soon, however, some acts became more complicated, with larger objects and more than one object at a time, and in these more skill was needed. Competition pushed performances to larger and more difficult swallowing. After the invention of the neon light bulb many of the more daring sword swallowers incorporated those into their acts. The finale often consisted of swallowing a long tube, turning off the house lights, and turning on the ingested bulb.

Many sword swallowers were women who worked in skimpy outfits and were presented in a low exotic mode. They were said to be from the Middle East or some other mysterious land. Medical explanations and physicians' endorsements often accompanied the demonstration and exaggerated the difficulty of the feat and the unique physiology of the performer.

There were other exhibits whose claim to fame was ingesting foreign objects. While each had his own favorite, coal, coke, nails, broken glass, sawdust, coins, Ping-Pong balls, watches, and other such objects were common on the menu. Competition called forth ever greater variety in appetite.

Perhaps the most famous of turn-of-the-century ingestors was Alfonso, "The Human Ostrich" (*Life and History of Alfonso* c. 1903). He started his career in Kohl and Middleton's dime museums, then moved to Barnum and Bailey's Greatest Show on Earth, and finally to Buffalo Bill's Wild West Show. Although he claimed to be from Barbados, and his exhibitions of swallowing poisoned beans, cork, glass, cotton, wool, and paraffin were exotic, this black man was not presented in a high exotic mode. He wore a suit, and his carriage and presentation were as much aggrandized as savage. Another human ostrich was Monsieur Antoine Menier, "The Great Human Ostrich." His performance was similar to Alfonso's, but his attire included "war paint," a nose ring, and outlandish exotic dress (FitzGerald 1897b). Although his presentation was exotic, it was more humorous than straight (*Antoine Menier* c. 1899).

A talented ingestor of the 1930s who obtained some fame was "The Great Waldo." Originally from Germany, he could gobble objects of unusual size such as lemons. What made his act incredible was his ability to regurgitate the objects he devoured. In the late thirties he traveled with one of the Ripley Believe It or Not shows. The highlight of his act was swallowing a live mouse and then bringing it back up. Believe it or not, his performance was cast in the aggrandized mode, with Waldo decked out in a tuxedo.

Perhaps the most novel of the swallowers was a fellow from Britain who billed himself as "English Jack, Live Frog Eater." His Eisenmann portrait, in which he is standing beside a ten-gallon aquarium that contains his partners, can be found in the Harvard Theater Collection.

Other Novelty Performers

Ingestors were just one type of novelty performance that proliferated at the end of the nineteenth century and start of the twentieth to fill the ranks of the popular freak show. (For a full and colorful discussion, see Jay 1986.) Some of the acts required special training, skill, practice, talent, and even physical adeptness, but others involved nothing more than bravado, hoopla, and trickery. And other animals beside snakes were included as well—performing fleas, birds, and monkeys, for example, are on record. Fire eaters, hot-coal walkers, anatomical wonders, mind readers, knife throwers, and contortionists tended to be cast as exotic performers; human calculators, child prodigies, and magicians were often presented in the aggrandized mode—but many acts could go either way. With presentations of novelty acts, there was much room for experimentation and mixing of modes.

The careers of people who worked in the novelty act genre were often divided between vaudeville and the freak show. Thus as their ranks expanded there was room for them to move out to other audiences. Those whose talent was limited to a one- or two-item act fit the format of the sideshow and the dime museum better. At the end of the nineteenth century the line that divided vaudeville from dime museum displays was not always easy to draw, and various establishments competed with each other by imitation.

The finale of this chapter is a list and short description of a few of novelty acts from the 1890s:[25]

—William Le Roy, "The Human Claw-Hammer," who, among other similar feats, used his teeth to extract large spikes driven through a two-inch plank

—Charles Baldwin, "The Weeping Wonder," who gave emotional exhibitions of tearful sobbing

—"Marinelli, The Man Snake," a contortionist who dragged his body slowly along the stage disguised as a serpent

—Moung-Toon, "The Burmese Juggler," who never touched with his hands the things he juggled

—"Little Zeretto, The Champion Child High Kicker," who demonstrated how she could kick to a height well above her head

—F. C. Bostock, "The Man with the Largest Mouth in America," who proved it by swallowing his whole fist on stage

—Madame Rice, "The Most Diminutive Lady Samson in the World," who displayed the strength of her small frame with barbells

—Cinatus, "The Upside-down Dancer," who did the jig standing on his hands.

The exotic self-made freaks discussed in this chapter illustrate the showmen's ingenuity in creating and promoting exhibits in a time of great freak show expansion. Toward the end of the nineteenth century and into the twentieth, not only were there more freak shows than ever before, but each show increased the number of attractions offered as the competition became more intense. Self-made freaks served a handy function. Because some acts needed no special talent and were not dependent on a deformity or aberration, there was a ready supply of people to fill the platforms. In addition, variety was not limited by nature as was the case with people who were truly disabled. With creativity new freak acts could be invented and promoted. In many cases, starting with nothing more than an idea and an ordinary person, showmen created an exhibit that would attract patrons. As standard exhibits became commonplace, they innovated with old forms and added new varieties. Some, like the Circassians, died out; others, like the tattooed exhibits, survived by adaptation.

Thus, at the height of freak show interest, freaks such as the ones discussed here, self-made and presented as novelty acts, increased in number. And more and more, these acts were incorporated into the sideshow, making it less a display of scientific species and more a variety entertainment event. Jugglers, mind readers, fire eaters, knife throwers, human dynamos, and a huge assortment of other acts gave the freak show a totally different flavor.

10

Conclusion: Freak Encounter
Notes on the Sociology of Deviance and Disability

JACK EARLE was the tall Texan whom Clyde Ingalls recruited to be a giant. Earle, along with Barney and Hiram Davis ("The Wildmen of Borneo"), Tom Thumb ("The Diminutive General"), Zoe Meleke ("The Circassian Beauty"), Captain Costentenus ("The Tattooed Prince"), Eli Bowen ("The Legless Wonder") and Clicko ("The Dancing Bushman"), was a freak. No specific attribute made them freaks. A freak was defined not by the possession of any particular quality but by a set of practices, a way of thinking about and presenting people with major, minor, and fabricated physical, mental, and behavioral differences.

In the United States the patterns that became the freak show coalesced in the first half of the nineteenth century, rose to prominence in the second half, and experienced a slow decline in this century. The rise of complex organizations, changes in science and medicine, exploration of the world, urbanization, the development of the amusement world, the dynamics of supply and demand, changes in technology, and other factors both societal and internal to the institution itself helped shape the freak show and the showmen's presentations. With some exceptions, namely certain non-Westerners and people we would now call mentally retarded, exhibits were showmen. They actively participated in the construction of their freak creation.

Although many people on the freak show platforms had no physical or mental disabilities, numerous freak roles did require the incumbent to have what we now call congenital malformations, hormonal dysfunctions, and chronic disorders. Some roles merely required cultural and phylogenetic differences. Today many people meet one or another of these rquirements, but, with the exception of a few sleazy remnants, the freak show no longer exists. The concept of "freak" no longer sustains careers.

267

Human differences are framed in different modes and by different institutions.

Ward Hall is one of the last practicing freak show managers. When I wrote to him seeking firsthand information on the history of these shows, he replied generously. His letter ended with a retort that anticipated a critical assessment of his profession in my writing: "I exhibited freaks and exploited them for years. Now you are going to exploit them. The difference between authors and the news media, and the freak show operators is that we paid these people." His use of the word *exploit* was playful. He does not think he exploited them. He had a business relationship, complete with contract, with his troupe of human oddities. His livelihood depended on them, as theirs did on him. He had no pretensions of doing good, and the exhibits knew this. Together they shared the amusement world. Hall did not have to profess motives manufactured from higher ideals—curing, protecting, and serving—ideals that made the person with the physical or mental difference unsure of where he or she stood.

In many ways, the concept of "freak," as we have traced its history, is an anomaly in current social scientific thinking about demonstrable human variation. During its prime the freak show was a place where human deviance was valuable, and in that sense valued. Modern social scientists advocate a view of people with physical, mental, and behavioral anomalies as stigmatized, rejected, and devalued. While this viewpoint may reveal part of the story of people who were exhibited, it leaves out a great deal. Some were exploited, it is true, but in the culture of the amusement world most human oddities were accepted as showmen. They were congratulated for parlaying into an occupation what, in another context, might have been a burden.

The freak show reminds us that there is money to be made on human variation. This was at one time so true that people feigned disability in order to qualify for freak roles. Abnormality was a meal ticket, not only to the exhibits themselves but to a host of other showmen who understood the money-making potential. Because of their dubious luck at having been born demonstrably different, exhibits with disabilities had an advantage. In the best of times, the more popular and competent exhibits took control in negotiating the conditions of their contract. As Ward Hall knows, their work was not predicated on the charity of their employers or patrons. In this way some achieved an element of independence.

Not only is the freak show as an institution an anomaly in current social scientific thinking about deviance, but many of the personal stories of the individuals who undertook freak show roles break with social scientists' understanding of what such people should have met with. Because the freak show thrust common people into the limelight, we have records of the offstage lives of people with unusual physical and mental differences that otherwise might have passed unrecorded. Many exhibits, because they were, in some way, out of the ordinary, charted a life course which those whose specialty is understanding human differentness neither document nor explain. These unusual strangers confront our most taken-for-granted assumptions and institutions. The study of what they made of their situations and what others made of them provides fertile ground to enlarge our understanding of human variation.

Many exhibits lived the miserable lives one might expect given current social scientific thinking about deviance with its emphasis on labeling and exclusion. But some did what current theory would suggest was impossible. Chang and Eng, the original Siamese twins, for example, in spite of a blatant physical difference and the fact that they were of a different race and culture, settled down to become respectable citizens in a rural town in the South. Captain Bates and Anna Swan, the couple whose claim to fame was their enormous height, married and became citizens of Seville, Ohio. Al Tomaini, a former sideshow giant, and his wife, Jeanie, a legless wonder, retired to the motel business in Florida.[1] Outside the boundaries of the freak show, many so-called human oddities had neighbors and family; they loved and were loved, were accommodating and accommodated, were respectful and respected. In addition, while freak show participants were not on the highest rung of the amusement world's own stratification system, they were a welcomed and taken-for-granted part of that culture. Indeed, from the life histories of freak show exhibits we might learn more about how blatantly different human beings are included into the human community, which knowledge could, if taken to heart, call forth a new direction in the study of human difference: a sociology of acceptance. The process by which demonstrable physical and mental differences become normalized, taken for granted, needs to be understood. The study of human oddities as individual persons is a fruitful starting point.

Begging for study as well are puzzles posed by exhibits with particular physical and mental abnormalities. Joined twins, for example, had an identical genetic heritage and were raised in as similar social environments as is possible. Yet, according to most accounts, these siblings had strikingly different personalities. They offer challenging cases for investigators who try to explain human variation and argue about the contribution of nature and nurture to the formation of human character.[2]

In another realm, many people who were exhibits and who had blatant physiological differences had normal children, children who reached adulthood and became well-adjusted citizens who loved and honored their parents. Further, unusual exhibits often married normal peers. Even exhibits with the strangest appearance and body configuration, or with subnormal mental functioning, found affection and lifelong bonds both in and out of the amusement world. Those who suggest a deep, rudimentary, and lasting psychic fear of particular types of human abnormality need to account for these apparent aberrations.

Throughout the pages of this book the emphasis has not been on the freak as person—on the personal dimensions and life chances of exhibits. Rather, we focused on the institution of the freak show, the manufacture of freaks, and the modes of presenting exhibits. But the book abounds in illustrations drawn from flesh-and-blood exhibits who climbed onto the platform day after day. In the end only they, and the stories of their freak show involvement, can bring the freak show and its history to life and make it understandable. It is the intersection of their lives and the history of their culture that allows us to see the freak show as it was.

Revolt of the Freaks

In April of 1903 the *New York World* published a letter signed by representatives of the Barnum and Bailey Sideshow lodging a complaint with their employer, James A. Bailey. Other papers picked up the story ("Prodigies in Conference" 1903; "Circus Nearly Over" 1903; "'Freaks,' a Word of Bitter Grief" 1903). The essence of the protest was captured in a paragraph from the statement:

> We the undersigned members of the Prodigy Department,
> at an informal meeting held on April 5 were selected as a
> committee to draft you a letter expressing our respectful
> though emphatic protest against the action of some person
> in your employ in placing in our hall a sign bearing the,

to us, objectionable word "Freak," and permitting another
person to call aloud, "This way to the Freaks," and beg
you to remedy both these matters as soon as possible.
("Forget 'Freak,' Prodigies Pray" 1903)

Post–freak show authors (Drimmer 1973; Fiedler 1978) have taken
this uprising, and a similar one staged earlier, as a serious matter for
the exhibits. After all, their assertions affirm some of our modern notions about the ugly and demeaning connotation of the term *freak*;
their protest strikes a familiar note in all of us who live in the age of
disability rights and collective action. This historical tidbit, at first
glance, seems to be a pertinent, little-known moment in the origins of
that movement.

In fact, however, the press release is a prime example of the razzle-
dazzle art of circus publicity as practiced by Bailey's public relations
expert, Tody Hamilton. As he had done in London four years before,
Hamilton deliberately initiated and orchestrated the "revolt of the
freaks" (Lentz 1977).

But did exhibits really not care about what they were called? They
did, but not the way our present sentimentality would have us think.
A few might have been sensitive to such words as *freak*. Those presented in the high aggrandized mode, for example, sometimes sought
more theatrical designations as their calling cards, thus helping them
dissociate from the run-of-the-mill freak show. As the eugenics movement clouded the scene and human differences became medicalized,
the status of human oddities declined, and some exhibits began to re-
sent what they were called. As we shall see, Robert Wadlow, an extremely tall young man who lived in the 1920s and 1930s, avoided
being associated with the word *freak*. But other than a few isolated
cases, there is no evidence that exhibits took the nouns used to refer
to them seriously. The word *freak* remained the preferred title through
the 1930s (Johnston 1934c, 70).

Why didn't they care? Simply put, the "self-made" freak, the novelty act, and even those exhibits with demonstrable physical differences did not take what they were called personally. Words like *freak*
did not have the deep stigmatizing and discrediting meaning that they
have today. The great majority of exhibits were troupers, amusement
world showmen, and in that world the outsider was held in contempt
(Lewis 1970, 74). Life was about tricking the rube, and making

money. The exotic and aggrandized presentations of the freak show were abundantly fraudulent. The most important criterion for judging the appropriateness of the word *freak* was, most likely, whether it was good for business. Any phrase that kept the dimes flowing in would do. The trumped-up debate over what to call the exhibits generated by the "revolt of the freaks" must have given them and the other showmen a good laugh. What they were called is an issue for us; it was not one for them.

As freaks sat on the platform, most looked down on the audience with contempt—not because they felt angry at being gawked at or at being called freaks, but simply because the amusement world looked down on "rubes" in general. Their contempt was that of insiders toward the uninitiated. For those in the amusement world it was the sucker who was on the outside, not the exhibit.

Robert Wadlow

We recall the eight foot eleven inch Robert Wadlow from Chapter 1, where the citizens of Alton, Illinois, his hometown, were erecting a statue in his honor. Robert Wadlow died in 1940 at the age of twenty-two. During his brief life he remained vigilant against being cast as a freak (Fig. 79).

The watch was started by his parents when Robert was a young boy. It had become evident that their son was destined to be unusually tall, but they vowed not to accept the many offers from showmen to put their son on exhibit. They understood that for him to have a career as a human oddity would further distort his relationship with other human beings. The Wadlows saw that Robert's friends and relatives, through regular and sustained contact, were able to forget his size and to treat him as they would any other person. This is what they wanted for Robert and, eventually, what he wanted for himself (Fadner 1944). For the Wadlows, to subject the boy to a life in which his height would be the focus of his livelihood seemed detrimental to his happiness.

Although Robert Wadlow was a good student and, from all accounts, a well-adjusted and likable human being, he began to realize that his plans to be a lawyer were impractical. As much as he and his parents tried to avoid the problem, his height restricted his future. His monumental stature dominated his relations with strangers. Chairs, cars, and all the objects made for people of normal size created barriers to living as an ordinary person might. And so Robert,

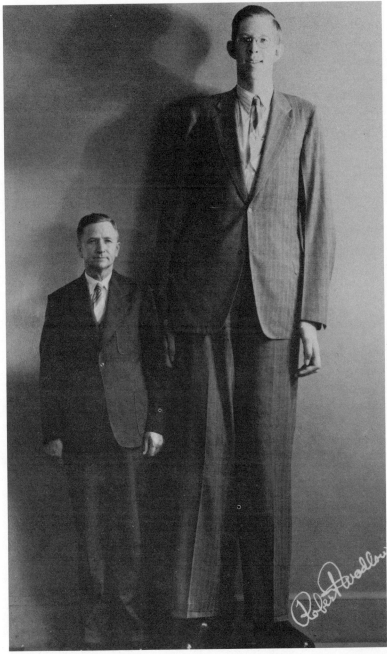

FIG. 79. Robert Wadlow with his father. Photographer unknown, c. 1939. (Raymond Coll., Baltimore, Maryland.)

more so than earlier exhibits and exhibits who were less limited by their differentness, was pushed, not pulled, toward the freak show.

In his teens he began traveling, promoting shoes. In his appearances at department and shoe stores, Robert's height was exploited to draw crowds. Yet he deemphasized this aspect of his work, choosing to think of himself not as an exhibit, but as being in the advertising business. In 1937, when Robert Wadlow was nineteen, he received a letter from a representative of the Ringling organization asking him to appear in the circus. When circus and carnival showmen had made such offers to him in the past the answer had always been an emphatic "no." But Robert was having problems with his health, and the salary offer was so enticing that he agreed. He stipulated in his contract that he would appear only at the engagements at Madison Square Garden and the Boston Garden, that his exhibition would be two times a day for three minutes each, and that he would not appear in the sideshow but in the center ring.

In all the appearances Robert made, be it for Ringling or while promoting shoes, he always dressed in a plain business suit. He refused to wear high-heeled shoes, a high hat, or any of the other showmen's devices that Jack Earle wore and that had become standard amusement world fare for getting a few extra inches out of giants. He even objected strenuously to attempts by photographers to create the illusion of greater height by shooting at angles that exaggerated his size.[3] When the manager of the Ringling circus suggested that he wear a formal dress suit with tails and a high silk hat, he refused to cooperate (Fadner 1944, 96). Robert attacked overdrawn press accounts—one widely circulated story stated that he ate four times the amount of a normal person—as "deliberate falsehoods" (Fadner 1944, 118). Thus Robert Wadlow, despite his potential to be an outstanding sideshow attraction, never succeeded as a major exhibit. Although very tall, he was not a giant. And he resisted playing the role of freak with the script that had been written over the more than hundred years of the freak show's history.

In the late 1930s Wadlow turned his back on the beckoning freak show. By that time the meaning of being different had changed in American society. Scientific medicine had undermined the mystery of certain forms of human variation, and the exotic and aggrandized modes had lost their flamboyant attractiveness. People who were different had diseases and were now in the province of physicians, not the general public.

Showmen hounded Wadlow, but physicians did as well. In the biography of his son, his father reveals that Robert was more concerned about how physicians would present him than he was by his treatment at the hands of any showman (Fadner 1944). In June 1936, prior to his circus appearances, Charles D. Humberd, M.D., had made an unannounced visit to the Wadlow household, requesting to see the tall boy. Robert, disheveled by a rainstorm, was surprised to find Humberd sitting in the living room when he arrived home. The doctor became disgruntled when the family refused to cooperate fully with his requests to perform a physical examination. Humberd left after a very short visit.

The next February, an article by Dr. Humberd appeared in the *Journal of the American Medical Association* which provoked anger and shame in Robert Wadlow and his family. Entitled "Giantism: Report of a Case" (Humberd 1937), the article produced a deluge of phone calls to the family and other unwanted attentions. Although the article did not mention Robert by name, it stated that the "case" was of a young man from Alton, Illinois, with the initials R.W. He was referred to as a specimen of "preacromegalic giant." Robert and his family felt violated because, as they put it, they had not realized that any person in the name "of science had a right to come into a home, make whatever cursory observations he could, and then broadcast these observations to the world" (Fadner 1944, 151). Not only did Wadlow resist being cast as a freak, but he also fought being presented as "sick." He wanted to be seen as a normal person, with the same concerns, feelings, and aspirations as his Alton neighbors.

While physicians did not have license to burst into people's homes, and no one would defend the rudeness and inaccuracy of Humberd's observations today, by the 1930s the medical profession had gained the authority to present people with physical and mental differences to the public in the terms of their choosing, and these were the terms of pathology.

Robert was mortified and sorely grieved to find himself described in the following way:

> His expression is surly and indifferent, and he is definitely inattentive, apathetic and disinterested, unfriendly and antagonistic. . . . His defective attention and slow responses hold for all sensory stimuli, both familiar and unexpected, but he does manifest a rapid interest in seeing any memoranda made by a questioner. All func-

tions that we attribute to the highest centers in the frontal
lobes are languid and blurred. (Humberd 1937, 545)

Not only were these remarks insulting and humiliating, but from descriptions of Robert's personality and intellectual talents given by his teachers and others who knew him well, they were also grossly inaccurate. At best, they were impressionistic of Robert under the worst circumstances; at worst, they were a vindictive assault by a egotistical physician who had been offended by Wadlow's unwillingness to cooperate. More likely the description was the manifestation of the stereotypes fostered by clinical descriptions of other "preacromegalic giants" and applied by a professional who believed he could, and had the right to, capture a person's essence after only a short observation and with medical jargon.

The Wadlows filed suit against Humberd and the American Medical Association. Of course, they could not bring suit against them for casting Robert in the medical model; their complaint had to focus on the article's libelous inaccuracies. Robert did not seek a large financial settlement. He wanted merely to be vindicated from the published presentation. In the first round of the legal battle, the case against the author was heard in Humberd's home state of Missouri. The American Medical Association supported Humberd with legal assistance from two of their attorneys. Witnesses verified that the description of Wadlow as published was a blatant distortion of his general condition. But Wadlow lost the case on a technicality: the judge ruled that the description was a case study and that the portrait painted of Robert might have been accurate on the day he was examined. The action against the American Medical Association never came to trial. After three years of maneuvers it was dismissed, after Robert died.

Humberd and the American Medical Association had not dressed Robert in an exotic jungle outfit and said he was the last of the Amazon giant warriors. Nor had they put an aggrandizing top hat and tails on him and said he was born to royalty. But they had "presented" him nonetheless. Even if what Humberd had said was accurate, it would still have been a presentation—a carefully constructed description that emphasized particular aspects of the person, directed toward fostering a particular impression in the audience. Humberd did not cast Wadlow as a freak. He was a medical man, not a showman. He presented Wadlow in the medical model, in terms of pathology. The

276   PORTRAITS OF PRESENTATION

medical model of presentation does not involve bannerlines, outside lecturers, or platforms, but it does have its standardized elements. The person is not a person but a diagnosis. When under the direct supervision of the medical profession, patients wear standardized garments—gowns and other institutional accoutrements. The "true life" stories are one-sided clinical descriptions, and the photos are posed straight on, with blank expressions, as if the person were only the carrier of the diagnosis. The pictures are not in family albums but in medical atlases.[4] Sterility is presented as synonymous with objectivity. If we were to study these presentations carefully, as we have studied freak show presentations, we might see the variety, the different modes of presenting human beings within the medical model.

By seeing human variation as valuable and people with differences as presentations, we can begin to understand how images of disability could be manufactured and managed for profit (Liazos 1972). Well into the twentieth century, freak shows were an accepted part of American popular culture. As we have seen, the way exhibits were presented—through the exotic mode, exploiting the public's interest in the "races of man," and the aggrandized mode, capitalizing on the public's status concerns—was not offensive to nineteenth- and early-twentieth-century citizens. There are a few isolated examples of attractions promoted in a way designed to work on the sympathies and compassion of the audience for the plight of the "freak," but these are rare. "Pity" as a mode of presentation was absent. Promoters capitalizing on pity would have developed presentations emphasizing how difficult life was for the poor exhibits, how unhappy they were; they would have explained how the admission charge would help pay the exhibits' expenses, relieve their suffering, and even lead to a cure for their affliction. That approach, however, did not draw or please crowds. Pity did not fit in with the world of amusement, where people used their leisure and spent their money to have fun, not to confront human suffering.

Using pity as a presentation mode for people with physical, mental, and behavioral differences fits better the modern conception of human differences, that is, as pathological. In the nineteenth century, whereas natural scientists, teratologists, and other professionals examined freaks, they did not approach them as patients. Science and medicine had not gained control over human deviation. People with physical and mental anomalies were still in the public domain—curiosities. Later, in the twentieth century, however, as the power of professions increased, people with physical and mental anomalies came under the purview of professionals. Many were secluded from the public. Their conditions were to be treated, and possibly cured, behind closed doors. They were to be pitied and, from a eugenics perspective, feared. They needed to be locked away for the protection of society. This trend was followed by the growth of organized charities, the rise of professional fund-raising, and the invention of the poster child, with "pity" used as the dominant mode of presenting human differences. It is through this imagery that we look back on freak shows and find them repulsive.

Of course, the earlier imagery of the freak show did not enhance the well-being of the disabled any more than did more modern renderings. The exotic mode presented people in ways that offend current taste and go against present ideas of the capabilities of people with physical and mental differences. Steeped in racism, imperialism, and handicapism (Bogdan and Biklen 1977), this mode emphasized the inferiority of the "human curiosity." This negative imagery paralleled natural-scientific visions of the time by casting the exhibits as specimens, inferior and contemptible. The association of various human differences with danger, their depiction as something subhuman, animalistic, and inferior, was developed as well as perpetuated by these exhibits. The association of disability with danger, so prominent in later horror, adventure, and gangster movies (Bogdan et. al. 1982) had the freak show as its predecessor and, as Wolfensberger (1975) suggests, can perhaps be linked to the unprecedented building of massive custodial warehouses designed for control, not care.

What of the aggrandized imagery? What did it contribute to our vision of people with human differences? The analysis here is more complicated. At first glance the imagery was positive. Exhibits were lauded for what they could accomplish, for their achievements, and, aside from their particular physical anomalies, for their normalcy, if not superiority. Because freak shows made visible people with fairly unusual conditions, presenting some in a quite positive way, the practice might have led to or revealed the acceptance of human variation. There is, however, another side to the argument. As discussed in Chapter 8, a question must have been in the mind of the audience: "If they are so competent, why do they live by having others look at them?" Although to some extent the imagery of the aggrandized mode was positive, and freak show careers truly benefited participants, the exhibits' mere presence on stage and as part of the amusement world, a world which became tainted in the public view, suggested that they belonged with their own kind and were not competent to prosper in the larger world. In addition, by flaunting normal accomplishments as extraordinary, and by hailing people with disabilities as human wonders, aggrandized presentations probably taught the lesson that achievement for people with differences was unusual rather than common.

Whenever we study deviance we must look at those who are in charge—whether self-appointed or officially—of telling us who the deviant people are and what they are like. Their versions of reality are presentations of people filtered through stories and worldviews. For sideshow participants, the worldview was that of show business, and the images were fabricated to sell the person as an attraction. In the hands of professional organizations, the images created will be designed to reach their organization's aim most effectively. In the professions and the human services, success often comes to be defined as survival and expansion, which is possibly only with a proper cash flow, through charitable contributions and public support. In the end, the freak show has much in common with human service agencies. The imagery may be different, but the relation between presentation and profit is similar. The job of those who want to serve people known as disabled should be to get behind the scenes, to know them as they are, not as they are presented. Presentations are artifacts of changing social institutions, of the formation of organizations and worldviews. To understand the presentations, to become dislodged from their hold on our reality, we have to trace their origins and understand their place in the world as it is presently constructed.

Return to Otis the Frog Man

It was the summer of 1984. I arrived at Sutton's Sideshow, where Otis Jordan, "The Frog Man," was working, just as the morning paper arrived carrying the story of his forced exile from exhibition (see Chapter 1). He was cooking brunch—two boiled hot dogs—on a single-unit hot plate in his small, crudely furnished, makeshift, rundown trailer. I interviewed him and watched him prepare his food using his arms with greater agility than he revealed when I saw him do his act on the freak show platform. The bannerline, the picture he sold, and other aspects of the show contained some of the elements of the old days, but the extravagantly embellished presentation was gone as was the splendor of the grand days of the freak show.

Otis's performance consisted of rolling, lighting, and smoking a cigarette exclusively with his lips. This trick was one that Randian, "The Human Caterpillar," had made famous much earlier in the century. When I asked Jordan if he had ever heard of Randian, he showed no recognition of the name. In fact, as I queried him I discovered that he knew nothing of the rich history of the freak show. He got into the business in 1963, too late to see it in its prime, too late to know of the businesses greats.

But Mel Burkhart, "The Anatomical Wonder," a co-worker on the Sutton show, remembered. Burkhart, who does various novelty acts—pounding a spike up his nose, contorting his body—reminisced about his days with the Ringling show and Ripley's Odditorium back in the thirties. He had been on the platform with some of the best: with Clicko, "The Wild Dancing Bushman"; with Jack Earle, "The Texas Giant"; and with the Snow Sister "Pinheads." Burkhart is one of the last of those who remember firsthand the final days of the freak show's greatness.

Otis did not share my interest in Mel's stories. For him the issue at hand was his livelihood. Born in 1926, he was raised in Barnesville, Georgia, not exactly the land of opportunity for a black man with a disability. He spent his first twenty-eight years doing a variety of things, including selling pencils and powder from a goat-drawn wagon which he rode around town. Then one day the carnival showed up. On a dare, Otis showed a showman his cigarette-rolling trick—and that was it. He was on the road. According to him, it was the best thing that ever happened. He likes to travel and meet people and his new profession enabled him to buy a small house back home which he lives in when the show winters. He has no complaints except one. He thought the woman who was complaining about his being exploited ought to talk to *him* about it. He would tell her there "wasn't anybody forcing him to do anything." As he put it, "I can't understand it. How can she say I'm being taken advantage of? Hell, what does she want for me—to be on welfare?"

Barbara Baskin, the woman who sought to ban the freak show from the New York State Fair, sees it quite differently. She too knows nothing of the history of the freak show. She grants that she has never met Mr. Jordan, and regrets that he is personally hurt by her action. But for her, Jordan's exhibition is symbolic of the degradation disabled people have experienced in this society. The freak show is to disabled people as the striptease show is to women, as "Amos 'n' Andy" is to blacks. Individuals who exhibit themselves on the sideshow platform present a message to the world that disabled people are freaks, freaks in the most pejorative sense of the word. Their exhibition presents the disabled as so different that they have to be set apart, so incapable that exhibiting is the only way they can make a living. That is not the situation of people with blatant disabilities today, she reminds us. Jordan could do better for himself. To end freak shows is a symbolic struggle closely tied to the very transformation of America that disability activists seek.

Otis's view, however, is that of a showman. The issue as he sees it is his right to make a living, to live a particular life-style, not the negative imagery or the harm that might be done to future generations of disabled people by the symbolism of the freak show platform. Otis has his own life to get on with; he is not interested in, and in fact does not identify with, disability rights. He may be unaware of the rich history of his profession, but he still sees himself as a showman: independent and proud.

Abbreviations

Baraboo Coll.	Circus World Museum, State Historical Society of Wisconsin, Baraboo, Wisconsin
Becker Coll.	Ron Becker Collection, George Arents Library, Bird Library, Syracuse University, Syracuse, New York
CNYC Coll.	Theater Collection, Museum of the City of New York, New York City
Flint Coll.	Richard Flint Collection, Baltimore, Maryland
Goldman Coll.	Karla L. Goldman Collection, Baltimore, Maryland
Harvard Coll.	Harvard Theater Collection, Harvard College Library, Cambridge, Massachusetts
Hertzberg Coll.	Hertzberg Collection, San Antonio Public Library, San Antonio, Texas
Koste Coll.	Craig Koste Collection, Plattsburgh, New York
Lib. Cong.	Picture Collection, Library of Congress, Washington, D.C.
Meserve Coll.	Meserve Collection, National Portrait Gallery, Smithsonian Institution, Washington, D.C.
NYPL Coll.	New York Public Library, Lincoln Center, New York City
Pfening Coll.	Pfening Archives, Columbus, Ohio
Raymond Coll.	Warren A. Raymond Collection, Baltimore, Maryland
Richards Coll.	Ron Richards, Worcester, Massachusetts

Ringling Coll.   Ringling Museum of the Circus, Sarasota,
                        Florida
Westervelt Coll.   Westervelt Circus Collection, New York
                        Historical Society, New York City

Notes

Chapter 1

1. The controversy occurred in August 1984. The next year the restrictions were dropped. Although the word *freak* did not appear on the advertisement banners, a banner depicting Otis Jordan as "The Frog Man" was displayed in a prominent place, and Jordan was the leading attraction. In 1986 there was no human freak show at the fair. Rather than being dropped because of official action, however, it was discontinued primarily because it was not profitable.

Barbara Baskin was the disability rights activist who led the fight to ban the sideshow. She wanted "this anachronism permanently abolished" (personal correspondence, 1983). For court rulings regarding the right of people with disabilities to display themselves for profit, see Lewis (1970, chap. 21); *Gaylon v. Municipal Court of San Bernardino* (1964); *World Fair Freaks and Attractions, Inc. v. Hodges* (1972); and Shipley (n.d.).

2. Most notable is Diane Arbus (Arbus 1972; Bosworth 1984). See also Levenson and Gray (1982); Fiedler (1978); Price and Price (1981); and Steinbrunner and Goldblatt (1972).

3. This phrase was used by Douglas Biklen of the Center on Human Policy, Syracuse University, Syracuse, New York.

4. Five were estimated to be still in operation during the 1985 season (Ward Hall, personal correspondence, 1985).

5. The only sociologists who have dealt with circuses, carnivals, and sideshows are Truzzi (1968a, 1968b, 1973, 1979) and Easto (Easto and Truzzi 1972, 1974).

6. Earle's real name was Jacob Ehrlich. Prior to joining the circus he had a number of minor film roles. He was actually seven feet seven inches tall, but was promoted as being eight feet seven inches—"the tallest man in the world." See Johnston (1934c, 72–73) and Lee (1970).

7. I approach the subject relying on the theoretical assumptions of the sociological theory of symbolic interaction (Blumer 1969). Also see Berger and Luckmann (1967); Spector and Kitsuse (1977); and Conrad and Schneider (1980). To the extent I am also interested in the taken-for-granted aspects of the freak show world and the structure of that world, I draw on ethnomethodology (Garfinkel 1967). In my emphasis on "presentation" I draw from Goffman (1959). With regard to the social context of freak shows, their rise and fall, some ideas of structural functionist analysis are employed. My analysis has been inductive (Bogdan and Taylor 1982; Glaser and Strauss 1967).

8. For a discussion, see Drimmer (1973) and Fiedler (1978). Later in the book I will discuss the controversy surrounding the "Revolt of the Freaks," which was supposedly precipitated by Barnum and Bailey exhibits not wanting the word *freak* used to refer to them. As we shall see, this was a publicity stunt, not an issue or an action initiated by those on display (Lentz 1977; Latzke 1903).

9. The word *monster* derives either from *moneo*, meaning to warn, or *monstro*, meaning to show forth. In both cases the origin reveals ancient beliefs that abnormal births were an evil sign. See Fiedler (1978).

10. See Ringling Collection for a photo of a phony four-legged girl.

11. I use the word *organization* here in the sociological sense of the "formal organization."

12. Memoirs reviewed include Barnum (1855, 1872); Bradna and Hartzell (1952); Coup (1901); Dadswell (1946); Dufour and Kirby (1977); Fadner (1944); Fellows and Freeman (1936); Hall (1981); Holtman (1968); Kelly (1982); Robinson (1925); and Middleton (1913). See Chapter 4 notes for a fuller listing.

13. In the big circuses the profit was split between exhibit and management. The details of the arrangements can be found in contracts between attractions and owners (Pfening Coll.).

14. The original glass negatives are in the Meserve Collection.

15. In some cases the photos were supplied, and thereby were chosen by the owner of the establishment that the exhibit worked for. This was most often the case when exhibits worked for organizations such as the circus, where they signed up for the season. (See contracts in Pfening Coll.).

16. Ron Becker pointed this out to me when I was reviewing his extensive collection of freak portraits.

17. The list includes Harrie Rose Studio in Indianapolis; Sword Brothers in York, Pennsylvania; Burrell in Providence, Rhode Island; Star Photo Gallery in Detroit; Johnson's in Kansas City; Grier Brothers in Philadelphia; Pugg Studio in Minneapolis; Hall Studio in Lowell, Massachusetts; Stuart in Buffalo; Gardner in Atlanta; Potter and Roberts in Cleveland; Wilker in Baltimore; Landi in Cincinnati; Herschel in Chicago; Baker in Columbus, Ohio; Hughes in St. Louis; Lonma in Eastport, Maine; Chickerney in Boston; Morris in Pittsburgh; and Rulofon in San Francisco— to name only a few.

18. Kern, Wood, Obermuller, Mora, Wendt, Chapman, Bogardus, O'Brien, Edward, Pachmann, Feinberg, Oliver, Sherman, McHugh, and Falk are but a few of the names that appear in decorative letters on the bottom or back of 1880, 1890, and 1900 cabinet photos taken in New York. See "Artists of the Bowery" (1885) for a description of the Bowery photographic scene.

19. Eisenmann was born in Germany in 1850 and immigrated to the United States in his teens. He went into business as a photographer in 1876, moving to his shop at 229 Bowery in about 1879. The two-story building, which remains intact today, served as both his business and his home. He, his wife, who assisted him in his work, and their daughter lived in these cramped quarters for seven years. The business prospered, and by 1884 he had opened a branch studio on 14th Street and moved his family to a house in the northern suburbs of Manhattan.

For fifteen years, Eisenmann was the most popular and prolific photographer in the freak show world. He produced thousands of negatives and countless prints. Most freaks passed through the Bowery during their careers, and the best came to him for their pictures. Even the aging Barnum sat for Eisenmann in 1885. Frank Wendt was his partner and eventually took over the business.

20. Booklets go back as far as 1834. The largest collection of these booklets is in the Hertzberg Collection, San Antonio Public Library, San Antonio, Texas.

Chapter 2

1. There were many such fairs but none as raucous and wildly popular as the Bartholomew Fair. The exhibition of human oddities goes back to the start of recorded history. For information and discussion about this early history, see Clair (1968); Thompson (1968); Frost (1971); and Fiedler (1978).

2. The record of the "female from Guinea" reported here was found in a newspaper clipping in the Harvard Collection. The first entry in Vail's (1956) chronicle of freaks is August 21, 1771.

3. Authors disagree about the dates of arrival and exhibition of the various animals. Vail (1938) states that the first lion arrived in 1716. In his famous 1956 publication, however, he says that the first lion arrived in 1720.

4. The word *scientist* was uncommon in the American vocabulary until the closing years of the nineteenth century (Miller 1970, vii).

5. When I first saw these words used I thought that they were meant as insults. Apparently this was not the case (Sellers 1980, 206).

6. The distinction of human oddities as being either examples of unknown races or "freaks of nature" was evident in the publicity promoters used and in newspaper reports in the first half of the nineteenth century. Despite this distinction, however, not all exhibits were neatly categorized as either "nondescripts" or "monsters." Dwarfs and giants born in this country, for example, whose physiological peculiarity was not evident at birth, did not lend themselves as easily to these categories, although some observers suggested that they were atavistic throwbacks to earlier forms of humans.

7. See Daniels (1968), esp. chap. 5, for a discussion of the goals of eighteenth- and nineteenth-century science. For works in teratology that capture the thinking about causes, see G. Gould and Pyle (1896); Jones (1888); Terry (1869); Ellis (1871); and Fisher (1866).

8. See Odell's multivolume history (1927, 1928, 1931) of the New York stage to trace the incorporation of exhibits into the museums.

9. At this time certain exhibits began associating with particular museums.

10. The information here all comes from Odell's *Annals of the New York Stage* (1927, 1928, 1931) and Vail (1956). These works contain quotations from many of the early freak advertisements. Original material of that sort can be found in the Ringling, Hertzberg and Harvard collections.

11. Middleton (1913, 68) claims to have started the first dime museum in the United States in New York in 1880. But dime museums were in existence long before then. It was typical of showmen to claim to have the first, the biggest, and the best of every conceivable thing. Middleton's claim is more in this spirit than a serious statement of fact. Old-style museums gradually evolved into dime museums, leaving the matter of which was the "first" dime museum a matter of opinion. In my opinion, the American Museum was the first.

12. Barnum became the owner on December 27, 1841. He didn't open for business until January 1842.

13. There are many accounts of the 1880s–1890s Bowery and its dime museum. M. Mitchell provides the best summary in his book *Monsters of the Gilded Age* (1979), which focuses on Charles Eisenmann, the popular photographer of freaks. Other sources include Harlow (1931); Campbell (1896); Isman (1924); Allen (1980); and McCardell (1925).

14. While fifty is most likely an exaggeration, there were many dime museums from the Bowery to Broadway to Brooklyn. Some of the better-known establishments were the Globe, Wonderland, the New York Museum, the Chatham Square Museum, the Apollo, the Grand, Huber's, Doris's, Alexander's, and Worth's.

15. The list above comes from photographs sold by exhibits. Also see M. Mitchell (1979, 11).

16. The list of Chicago establishments includes the West Side Museum, Whit John's Museum, the Arthur Putney Museum, the West Side Dime Museum and Theatre, Wonderland Compound, the Congress Museum, and the London Dime Museum. See Jackson (1931, 583) for a discussion of Philadelphia dime museums. For a full discussion of the Boston Museum, see Ryan 1915.

17. Barnum and Bailey introduced three rings under the big top in 1881. See Truzzi (1968a) for more details and other references.

18. Truzzi (1968a) says the Golden Age was from 1871 to 1915.

19. After the American Museum disbanded—and for that matter, during its operation—Barnum was in the practice of renting his name to various amusement establishments.

20. For lists of terms and discussion concerning amusement world language, see Dadswell (1946); Bradna and Hartzell (1952); Maurer (1931); and McKennon (1980).

21. Social scientists and historians writing about the circus sometimes do not even include the sideshow in their definitions. Truzzi (1968a), the only sociologist to write about the circus, defines the circus this way (p. 315): "A circus is a traveling and organized display of animals and skilled performances within one or more circular stages known as 'rings' before an audience encircling these activities." In this sense, the wild west shows were "circuses." This definition, however, does not capture the evolving form of the circus. According to it, the circuses that are on television are not strictly speaking circuses.

22. Robert Parkinson of the Baraboo Circus World Museum told me that, of their 6,400 posters, only 10 advertise freaks.

23. See Holley (1893) for a description of the beauty show.

24. Middleton ran a dime museum which catered to the fair crowd. W. C. Coup and Frank Uffner ran the Great Chicago Museum for the 1893–1894 season.

25. The most minor contribution is the word *ballyhoo* or *bally* to the amusement world vocabulary (McKennon 1972).

26. Barnum featured "ethnological" exhibits prior to this time. The Barnum and London Circus of 1884, for example, featured an "Ethnological Congress of Savage Tribes" (Courier, 1884, Ringling Circus Museum, Sarasota, Florida).

27. See Chapter 9 for a discussion of the Ringling Brothers, Barnum and Bailey exhibition of the "Ubangi Saucer Lipped Savages."

28. Robert L. Ripley had been drawing cartoons for the sports page of the *New York Globe* when, one day in 1921, he drew a cartoon depicting an unusual sporting feat. He captioned the cartoon "Believe It or Not!" The cartoon brought much favorable comment from the readers, and the editor suggested that he do another. Before long the "Believe It or Not!" became a feature branching out to cover all sorts of strange facts and oddities, what Ripley called "queeriosities," including reports of "human oddities" or freaks. The cartoon and text, which became part of the feature, were soon syndicated and delighted a national audience (Ripley 1929). Before long, showmen picked up on the idea. Some bought permission, but others pirated the title or facts of Ripley's feature, and many contrived deceptively similar titles as a device to promote their freak shows. World's fairs had their odditoriums, and traveling dime museums had their Believe It or Not shows. See Pfening (1983); "Throngs View Wonders of Hercules Odditorium" (1933); and "Ripley's Freaks on Way to D.C." (1934).

29. These shows are all listed in 1937 and 1938 issues of *Billboard*. There is a photograph taken by Marion Post Wolcott, in the Farm Security Administration Collection at the Library of Congress, of the "World's Fair Show, International Congress of Oddities, Believe It or Not" playing in Granville, West Virginia, in 1938.

30. Luna Park featured one of the strangest exhibits we have encountered. This exhibit, Dr. Martin Arthur Couney's "Incubator Babies," seems bizarre in that we so clearly divorce serious medical practice from the sideshow, but apparently the exhibit fits easily with the pseudoscientific trappings of early exhibits.

Although Barnum held "smallest baby" contests at the American Museum, Couney's exhibit had no predecessor. (Ironically, the heirs of such shows are the high-technology neonatal units that have engendered so much controversy in regard to the rights of disabled infants.) The "Incubator Babies" display, moreover, was one of the longest running exhibitions in Coney Island history. Couney was an authentic medical doctor and very serious about providing care for his exhibits, premature babies—patients to whom hospitals and medical practitioners were indifferent at the time. He developed the incubator and a system of care that claimed a high success rate. His exhibits were the children of the poor who, without Couney's intervention, would have died. The exhibit was decked out like a hospital, with all those in attendance wearing hospital uniforms. Dr. Couney lectured and minimized the carnival atmosphere that was part of Coney Island by demanding proper medical decorum of his staff. Parents were given free tokens for visits. Couney's show was extremely popular. When Dreamland opened, he moved there. His exhibit was featured at Coney Island and a number of world's fairs until 1943 (D. McCullough 1983; Silverman 1979).

31. The article was wrong in its "diagnosis" of Waino and Plutano. The author's conclusion that the "wild men of Borneo" were "negroes" gathered from our "Southern plantations" suggests that he never saw the brothers.

32. In 1914 an article appeared in *Billboard*, the popular show world publication, which suggests that the showmen were exposed to such views of human variation also (Stanley 1914).

Chapter 3
1. McKennon (1972, 76) mentions the famous Francis Lentini, "The Three Legged Man," as an owner. Count Orloff, a so-called Ossified Man, was in the freak booking business.

2. As we see in the chapter dealing with the exhibition of people with the condition we now call mental retardation, many of those exhibits were not willing participants. Similarly, many people recruited from the non-Western world never became "showmen."

3. McKennon (1972) has a section on carnival women in his book. The women mentioned are not owners or managers. In fact, most are discussed as spouses of carnival men. The only woman circus owner I came across in my research was a Mrs. Lake (Robinson 1925, 126). She became a successful owner/manager by taking over her husband's circus after he was shot in 1869 by a man trying to see the show without paying.

4. There was some overlap with other parts of show business, most notably vaudeville, and with commercial sports, boxing for example.

5. See Truzzi (1979) and McKennon (1972) for examples.

6. McKennon (1980, 49) reserves the term *hopscotching* for "jumping from one place, or show to another to make a season's work."

7. See McKennon (1972) for profiles of managers and their carnival careers.

8. The Ringling management was "circus," but even here, John Ringling North dabbled in other amusement enterprises, including the 1939 New York World's Fair (R. Taylor 1956, 40–41). John Robinson's career seems to have been strictly with the circus (Robinson 1925).

9. In the twentieth century, some showmen even formed communities to winter in. These later doubled as retirement retreats. The most famous is Gibtown, outside of Tampa, Florida.

10. Joe McKennon made this point in a conversation I had with him in 1985. McKennon explains his own movement into the carnival this way.

11. I was told by one circus old-timer that the clowns in some shows were low status because many were gay, a sexual preference that was tolerated but not held in high esteem in the amusement world.

12. An example of the brutality exhibited by towners is the case of William Lake, owner and manager of a popular tent show. In 1869 he was shot through the head and killed in Granby, Montana, by a local bully named Jake Killian. Lake refused Killian admission because Killian had no ticket, whereupon he was shot in cold blood at the main entrance. Killian's penalty was three years in the penitentiary (Robinson 1925, 127).

13. McKennon (1980, 46) claims that the term "Hey, rube!" is used more by writers than by circus or carnival people. He says that he never heard it used in his twenty-five years traveling with large circuses and carnivals. They got into plenty of fights with towners, but they did not yell, "Hey, rube!"

14. If all this hostility was not enough for them, showmen had other problems. In the nineteenth century, traveling popular amusement organizations played on the frontier and in rural areas where they were under constant danger of attack from outlaws. The roads were rough, almost impassable in foul weather, and accommodations were often poor and in many cases nonexistent.

15. Amusement organizations engaged in campaigns to combat their poor image. Some owners insisted that ticket sellers and others who had direct contact with

customers be well dressed and washed. Others made serious efforts to curtail some of the practices that outsiders pointed to as offensive, to the extent of hiring Pinkerton guards.

One approach that almost all used to combat their poor reputation was to include in their advertisements blatant repudiations of any allegation of impropriety that traveling shows might have been accused of. Barnum's pledge to his patrons of the American Museum in 1860 illustrates this promotional thrust: "I therefore gladly renew my pledge to families and the better portion of the community to keep the Museum always free from every objectionable feature, to permit no intoxicating drinks within its halls, no vulgar or profane allusions on the stage, no improper visitors of either sex, and to use the same precaution to protect any visitors while in the Museum that I would my own family, so that any lady or child shall be as safe here as in their own house" (*Barnum's American Museum Catalogue* 1860).

This form of propaganda continued through the twentieth century. The 1920s letterhead of M. E. Polhill's Beacon Shows Carnival read: "One of the cleanest aggregations of amusements in America. Absolutely no girls shows or gambling devices" (McKennon 1972, 203).

16. Horace Greeley publicly pronounced his distaste for such exhibits back in the early days of the American Museum. His utterances were not for the good of the exhibits, nor was it suggested that they should be discontinued. He just preferred not to see certain ones.

17. These words are standard in the amusement world vocabulary. E. Smith (1922) uses "monkey" also, but this word did not appear to be as common.

18. On October 16, 1903, an article in a Nashville, Tennessee, paper reports on the extensive pickpocketing at the circus (Ringling Coll.). The following articles on pickpocketing were found in the Syracuse, New York, *Standard:* "Pickpockets Fared Well at the Circus" (June 14, 1858); "A Gang of Thieves and Pickpockets Follow Howe's Circus" (June 16, 1871); "Fraudulent Practices Associated with the Circus" (July 20, 1884).

19. See Inciardi and Peterson (1973) for an extensive and perceptive discussion of the changes in grifting patterns.

20. For a similar analysis of other subcultures, see Sykes and Matza (1957); Scott and Lyman (1968); Lofland (1969); Hong and Duff (1977); and S. Taylor and Bogdan (1980).

Chapter 4

1. For stories of gaffs, see Norman (1933); Hall (1981); Coup (1901, chap. 3); Marcosson (1929); Middleton (1913, 69); Dadswell (1946, 211); Metcalf (1906); Holtman (1968); and Robinson (1925). For instruction on how to set up a gaff, see Boles (1967).

2. Circus and dime museum publicity campaigns were the forerunners of modern advertising (Presbrey 1929, chap. 25).

3. Showmen did not use these expressions. Whether they consciously thought in terms of them is not clear, but their actions suggest that they were part of the showman's perspective.

4. Scientists and laypeople alike thought this to be true during the nineteenth century and into the twentieth (Oppenheimer 1968, 147).

5. In some cases, such as the "ossified man," they were presented as "sick" even in the 1880s.

6. A favorite form of juxtaposition in the exaggerated aggrandized mode was arranged marriages between incongruent freaks, such as the fat lady and the human skeleton. See Chapter 8.

7. Further into the twentieth century, some freak show promoters incorporated into their presentations information about genetics, glands, and biological causes. As a ploy to make the show more inviting, the audience would be told that advances in medical treatment and prevention would eliminate freaks. But even in the 1930s, the freak as someone to be pitied was never established as a mode. Indeed, the elements of pity in twentieth-century freak shows signaled their decline.

Chapter 5

1. A picture of them was published in McCulloch (1981, 36), but it is mislabeled as "Pinhead the Monkey Man and Friend." Other pictures are in the Hertzberg Collection and the Harvard Collection.

2. Ironically, professionals and scholars in the field of mental retardation have totally neglected the freak show. Scheerenberger (1983, 156) is the only historian in the field of mental retardation who devotes any space to the topic, and his discussion consists of only one paragraph with information derived from one secondary source, Fiedler (1978).

3. What I present are the most accurate and complete biographies I could construct given the limited source material. Some of what is included contradicts earlier renderings. Such situations are explained in footnotes.

4. Secondary sources (Durant and Durant 1957, 102; M. Mitchell 1979, 78) say Barney was born in England and Hiram in New York. This would mean their parents crossed the Atlantic three times, once with one infant and another time with two. Since the Davises were of modest means, and considering the hardships of such a journey, this seems unlikely. More likely, Hiram was born in England and Barney in the United States, and after one writer switched the boys around, others copied the mistake.

5. Reports about their height are contradictory. A reporter visiting Plutaino in 1906 said he was three feet tall. Another report lists their height as four and one-half feet. Their aunt remembered them as being a little over three feet tall (see "Wild Men of Borneo Were Ohio Fakes" 1973; Randall 1937; "Wild Man of Borneo" 1906).

6. Various sources spell "Hanford" differently. The variations include Hansford (Roth and Cromie 1980), Hannaford (M. Mitchell 1979), and Hanaford (Durant and Durant 1957). Randall (1937) refers to a M. E. Warner as the brothers' manager. He may be Hanford's brother, although there is no indication that Hanford had a brother. Pictures of M. E. Warner and Hanford A. Warner look like the same person.

7. From the *New York Journal of Commerce*, as quoted in *The Life of the Living Aztec Children* (1860).

8. A dealer in old postcards recently sent me three German cards, c. 1915, with pictures of the aged Maximo and Bartola. The pair might have spent the latter part of their lives in Europe.

9. *Freaks* was a Tod Browning film made by MGM and released on February 20, 1932.

10. Some report that Johnson was born in Bridgeport, Connecticut (Lindfors 1984). A plaque in Bound Brook, however, indicates that he was born there. Arthur Saxon (personal conversation) said that he saw Johnson's grave in Bound Brook and his date of birth was given as 1857. In the "Zip" file at the Circus World Museum in Baraboo, Wisconsin, is a newspaper article from April 19, 1926 ("Zip, Circus Freak Dies" 1926), from a local Bound Brook paper saying that Johnson was a Bound Brook citizen and telling about the plaque. ("Circus Freak Buried Here" 1926) quotes a women who says she was Johnson's sister as saying he was born in Liberty, New Jersey.

11. In his photos he appears taller than the four feet he was reported to be in an earlier press release. This disparity supports the idea that the "What Is It?" shown by Barnum in 1860 may not have been Johnson. But of course, 1860 advertisements were notorious distorters of reality. The first picture available of Barnum's "What Is It?" was taken by Mathew Brady. The person in that picture (c. 1863) appears to be the same as the person in later pictures. The Brady glass negative print is in the Meserve Collection.

12. Lindfors is the only writer who suggests that Johnson was not mentally retarded (Lindfors 1984, 1983). Lindfors seems to be saying that Johnson was intelligent enough to go along with his front and therefore was not "retarded." Yet many people diagnosed as mentally retarded would be capable of doing that. Lindfors relies on the comment that Johnson was alleged to have made before his death—"Well, we fooled them a long time" (Bradna and Hartzell 1952, 242)—as evidence of normal intelligence. People who knew him describe Johnson as cheerful and kind, but never in any way that would suggest he was not mentally retarded (Fellows and Freeman 1936, 309). I showed pictures of Johnson to three people whose clinical field is mental retardation. Although assessment by photograph has its limitations, all three agreed that Johnson had a condition we would now call microcephaly, which is almost always associated with mental retardation.

13. One story asserts that Barnum and Johnson met in Bridgeport while Johnson was working in the kitchen for another showman (Lindfors 1983a). Teel (c. 1930) says that Johnson was first exhibited in 1864 and prior to joining Barnum worked at Bunnell's Museum.

14. A story repeated in accounts of Johnson has it that Dickens gave him the name "What Is It?" when visiting the American Museum accompanied by Barnum (Fellows and Freeman 1936, 308; Teel c. 1930, 13; Bradna and Hartzell 1952, 242; Leech 1926). The phrase "What Is It?" had been around long before the American Museum, and as the Barnum letter indicates, Barnum had named Johnson early in his career.

15. In the 1870s a popular play with the title of "Zip" played in New York.

16. Some sources say that Johnson had a sister, Mrs. Sarah Van Dyne, who lived in Bound Brook, New Jersey, who was with him at his death and at the funeral (Fellows and Freeman 1936, 309). Others do not mention her. One report mentions Johnson having both a sister and a brother, Theodore ("Many Circus Folks at Zip's Funeral" 1926). Another report claims that he had six siblings ("Circus Freak Buried Here" 1926). There was also a report of Johnson's father visiting him at the sideshow,

but this is unsubstantiated. For newspaper articles on the funeral, see "Many Circus Folks at Zip's Funeral" (1926) and "Fellow Freaks Mourn" (1926).

17. This information comes from the back of a publicity photograph found in "Freak Picture Box" at the Baraboo Collection. Also, a picture taken of the "Human Freak Side Show" at the 1941 Vermont State Fair by Jack Delano has a banner for Zip and Pip (Lib. Cong.).

18. "Zippy the Pinhead" T-shirts are popular on campuses. I was told some dormitories even have Zippy floors.

19. At the 1893 Chicago Columbian Exposition, Barnum exhibited a "What Is It Couple" who had microcephaly. In this century Ringling Brothers Circus exhibited a man and a woman as brother and sister "pinheads," "Gondio and Apexia, the Famous Sweeks-Sere People of Lower Burmah, B. E., India." They also exhibited a man and woman (dressed in leopard skins and sporting shaved heads with a tuft of hair) in the late 1920s as "Kiko and Sula, Pinheads from Zanzibar." Two people with microcephaly were exhibited at the World Circus Sideshow, Coney Island, New York, in the 1930s as "Pip and Flit." In the 1940s Gresham (1948) reports a boy with microcephaly, Julius Graubart, who toured in sideshows. Allegedly he was the son of a tailor and his pay was sent home to his family.

20. I assume that the prevalence of microcephaly is not because of an identification or sampling problem on my part. I believe this assumption is warranted. In the over two thousand pictures of freaks I reviewed, I saw no one with Down's syndrome. "Pinheads" were mentioned in memoirs as being mentally subnormal. Two brothers, Iko and Eko, were "black" albinos exhibited in the 1920s and 1930s. They were referred to as "having a low grade of intelligence" (Robeson 1935, 277).

21. George E. Shuttleworth's paper "Some of the Cranial Characteristics of Idiocy," read at the International Medical Congress, London, in 1881, and William W. Ireland's paper "On the Diagnosis and Prognosis of Idiocy and Imbecility," which were published in the *Edinburgh Medical Journal* (June 1882), are reprinted in Rosen, Clark, and Kivitz (1976).

Chapter 6

1. For a full description, see *Sketch of the Life, Personal Appearance, Character, and Manners of Charles S. Stratton* (1854).

2. It is not clear whether it was Colonel Wood or his son. See Saxon (1979).

3. Lavinia was originally hired for a European tour but actually was exhibited in the United States (Saxon 1979).

4. Warren uses the word *levee* in her autobiography. It means a formal reception, usually held by a high-ranking person such as a monarch.

5. It is unclear just at what point in Lavinia and Tom's career the hoax was perpetrated. It may even have happened twice, for, in addition to the 1863 birth, Desmond (1954, 215) reports that when the couple was traveling with the Barnum and London Circus in 1881 they were exhibited with a baby.

6. One fear of midget performers is that, as often does occur, in later life they will grow. In these cases the height they attain puts them between that of a typical adult and a successful attraction—the worst of two worlds (Dadswell 1946).

7. There is no evidence to show that the man exhibited was not a Russian

prince, but hundreds of examples of other such stories were showmen's creations. My guess would be that at best Nicholi was a commoner Russian immigrant. He might, however, have been a product of New York City.

8. Examples of misproportioned dwarfs cast in the aggrandized mode do exist; they are just not as common.

9. Truzzi (1968b) estimates that in 1934 there were three thousand midgets in the whole world, or about one-millionth of the earth's population. Dwarfs, in contrast, are more numerous.

10. A note on the back of a postcard freak portrait of the sisters dated 1953 states that they were then being managed by Essar Productions, a Cincinnati, Ohio, company.

11. The Hilton Sisters are among the last in a long line of Siamese twins who were displayed in this country. The only ones presented in the exotic mode were the male "Korean Twins" who appeared with Barnum and Bailey's show in the early 1900s ("The Korean Twins" 1903; "The Life of a Xiphopagis" 1902), and the female "Orissa Twins" from India, who were with the same circus in 1897; otherwise, all Siamese twins exhibited in this country were presented, as the Hilton Sisters' career personifies, in the aggrandized mode.

Two other sets appeared at approximately the same time as the Hilton Sisters. One set, Simplicio and Lucio Godino, come the closest to equaling the Hilton Sisters in high aggrandized style. (*The Only Boy Siamese Twins* c. 1928).

12. In fact, some midgets, Tom Thumb being the prime example, became adults prematurely as showmen pushed them into freak careers when they were mere children and at their smallest.

Chapter 7

1. See Lindfors (1983a, 1983b, 1984) for the African story.

2. The spelling in the "true life" pamphlet is Thokambau. In Thomson (1908) and in Williams and Clavert (1859) it is spelled Thakombau.

3. Apparently they were some of the last of Brady's customers in his New York studio, which, as a result of Brady's debts and the financial disaster of 1873, he was forced to sell. See Meredith (1970).

4. The picture is a contact print made from the original glass-plate negative found in the Meserve Collection.

5. Barnum was not the principal producer and manager of this show. W. C. Coup and Dan Castello were. Barnum did handle the publicity and press releases, however.

6. Other pictures are in the Harvard Collection and the Becker Collection.

7. From a newspaper article taped to the back of the Hertzberg Collection photograph.

8. For a more complete account of Bushmen in England, see Altick (1978).

9. The description is at the back of *Life of the Living Aztec Children* (1860).

10. A copy of the photograph can be found in the Baraboo Collection. Information concerning the exhibit is handwritten on the back.

11. See a postcard in the Ringling Collection with that title.

12. In none of the material I have reviewed is it suggested that Clicko was

anything but a South African. Promoters claimed that there was a replica of him in the Museum of Natural History in New York.

13. Dufour (1977) reports that he imported them himself and then transferred the contract to Ringling.

14. Bradna reports these numbers. According to Tucker (1973), however, eight women and five men came to the United States. Fellows and Freeman (1936) give the same figure as Tucker.

15. Although Lewiston, Eagle, and Dufour worked together, the details of their accounts are not the same. All three were flamboyant egotists and undoubtedly exaggerated the extent of their own participation. Yet despite contradictions in the accounts, the fraud portrayed is constant across the three men's stories. In telling this tale, then, I am selecting material from each account, not knowing for certain what is accurate. I do this because I wish to lay out the pervasiveness of the fraud, which all the tales illustrate admirably, and it is impossible to get to the bottom of the details given that we are dealing with pervasive liars.

Chapter 8

1. Chang and Eng were two of the nineteenth century's most studied human beings. Almost from the moment they stepped off the boat in Boston they were probed, pinched, pictured, and pondered by physicians and other scientists representing the spectrum of learned associations. Starting in 1829 and ending with their autopsy report in 1874, they were a favorite subject of medical journals and scientific speculation. Joined twins were one of the principal types of human monsters in teratologists' typologies (Fisher 1866; Ellis 1871; Jacobi 1895; Jones 1888; G. Gould and Pyle 1896) and everyone with interest in the field wanted to get a look at the brothers. As we have seen, showmen regularly used physicians to confirm the authenticity of exhibits; but in the case of these Siamese twins, phrenologists used them to confirm their own theories ("Phrenological Character of Chang and Eng" 1846). But the interest was not limited to phrenologists and teratologists. The twins' managers, as well as Chang and Eng themselves, used medical reports and other "scientific" literature in effect to generate free publicity.

2. M. Mitchell (1979) gives Chauncey's year of birth as 1869; FitzGerald (1897c) says 1872.

3. Although we cannot be sure of their exact height, she was reported to be 7'11" but advertised as 8'1". He was a few inches shorter than she (Lee 1970, 79).

4. Another strange couple presentation, one in which the exotic mode was mixed with the aggrandized, was that of "Percilla the Monkey Girl" and "Emmitt the Alligator-Skinned Boy." They appeared in freak shows from the 1930s into the 1970s. Her body was covered with silky hair and his skin was extremely scaly.

5. Other twentieth-century exhibits of people exhibited as legless wonders were the stylish and bejeweled Mademoiselle Gabriele, "The Half Lady" (Rusid 1973), Harry Williams, and Alvina Gibbs.

6. Information on Nellis reported here, unless otherwise indicated, is taken from a magazine clipping, c. 1840, found at the New York Public Library.

7. Her name is spelled in various ways, including Anna Leake. I am using the version that appears in her 1871 pamphlet, *The Autobiography of Miss Ann E. Leak*.

8. Her father's lodge provided one of the endorsements of her exhibition in her "true life" pamphlet.

9. See *Personal Facts Regarding Percilla the Monkey Girl* (c. 1940) and *Krao, the Missing Link* (c. 1884) for examples.

10. Annie's "true life" story, sold when she appeared with Barnum's Great Traveling Museum, Menagerie, Caravan and Hippodrome in 1872, was published in the same pamphlet with Admiral Dot's (see *Admiral Dot: The Smallest Man in the World* (1872).

11. Two of the most famous ossified men were Count Orloff and Jonathan Bass. The only ossifed women I came across was Dolly Regan (Mannix 1976, 30).

12. Extra fingers is sometimes an inherited condition.

13. These human skeletons include D. J. Major, "The Living Skeleton," who was one of the earliest (*Life of D. J. Major* 1859); Harry V. Lewis, "Shadow Harry" (*Biography of Shadow Harry* c. 1930); and I. Sprague, who was one of the best known (*Life of Isaac W. Sprague* c. 1885). Women exhibits include Emma Schiller (*Biography of Emma Schiller* 1890).

Chapter 9

1. Pictures of Zula and Zoberdie can be seen, along with other unnamed Circassians, in the theater collection at the Harvard Collection. Zoe and others can be seen at the Hertzberg Collection. Barnum's Circassians were photographed by Brady; the original glass negatives are in the Meserve Collection. A picture of Za-lumma Agra is included in Saxon (1983, 126), the plate for which is in the Meserve Collection.

2. According to Hambly (1925), the word *tattoo*, derived from the Tahitian word *tatau*, meaning "to mark" (Ebensten 1953, 14), was not adopted into the English language until the late eighteenth century. Burchett (1958), however, says that Captain Cook introduced the word much earlier; he also gives a slightly different version of its origin. Burchett's discussion of the background of the term as well as the history of the practice is extensive.

3. The first record of an extensively tattooed person shown publicly in England was a Prince Giolo, "The Painted Prince." Burchett (1958, 20–21) provides a long account of this attraction, as well as copy from an advertisement for his show. This South Sea Islander was brought to Europe in 1691. The famous Captain James Cook brought Omai, another South Sea Islander, back from a 1774 voyage. Omai exhibited his designed body all over England before sailing back home in 1776 (Ebensten 1953, 16; Burchett 1958, 22).

4. Joseph Cabri, a Frenchman tattooed while in the South Seas, returned to Europe where he was first studied by physicians and members of learned societies and then exhibited to any spectator who paid the price of admission. He made a living as an oddity for a number of years before his death in 1818 (Parry 1933, 58).

5. See Parry (1933, 6) for more details on Costentenus's decorations.

6. Fatima became a common name in the amusement world. One of the first belly dancers from the streets of Cairo at the Columbia Exposition was named Fatima.

7. This is what his "true life" story claims. Others, too, place the date of

Costentenus's first exhibition in Europe in the early 1870s. Burchett (1958, 104), however, contends that Barnum exhibited him in the 1860s.

8. Burchett (1958) uses the word *tattooist*, although he acknowledges that *tattooer* is the more accepted term in general. Many tattooers, however, prefer *tattooist* because they see themselves as artists.

9. See Parry (1933) for the history of the profession of tattooing in America and for a discussion of the tattoo machine.

10. See Jennings (1882, chap. 44) for an account of how domestic tattooing was arranged in the early 1880s.

11. Irene was supposed to have had her feet and the space between her toes covered, to go one better than her famous male predecessor. Pictures of Mary Brooks and Nora Hildebrandt (M. Mitchell 1979) suggest that there were tattooed women before Irene.

12. In a 1985 show in Texas, Ward Hall was showing an elderly tattooed woman whom he presented as having been forced by her crazed husband to undergo tattooing.

13. At the turn of the century small tattoos became a fad among upper-class English women. Some scientists, including Lombroso, were incredulous.

14. Most reported salaries are part of the hype of sideshow publicity. I am very reluctant to use any figures except those of contracts and other official documents.

15. A large collection of photos of tattooed people is housed at the Circus World Museum, Baraboo, Wisconsin. Levenson and Gray (1892) contains an excellent image of an aged tattooed woman, Anna "Artoria" Gibbons, with religious and patriotic designs. She was tattooed in 1921 by her husband. In 1976 she was with the Hall and Christ Sideshow in Lincoln, Nebraska.

16. One exhibit had Christ's head in a crown of thorns tattooed to his bald head. Kobel's collection of tattooed people is extensive (Kobel c. 1968).

17. FitzGerald (1897b, 415) says that nine out of ten snake charmers were women.

18. See Vail (1956) and the early volumes of Odell's *Annals of the New York Stage* (1927) for the introduction of snakes as exhibits.

19. FitzGerald (1897b) profiles an Indian woman "serpent queen" allegedly named Saidor A. Isoha. She was supposed to include six Indian pythons, three boa constrictors, and three African pythons, all between eight and twelve feet long, in her act.

20. Husbands could work as managers, ticket collectors, or manual laborers. Apparently women were restricted from these tasks; they either had to be built into the act or not travel. Omi, the tattooed man discussed in this chapter, did travel with his wife, who introduced his act.

21. He had a company called Count Orloff's International Agency, which specialized in human oddities and novelty acts.

22. There is a photograph in the Pfening Collection of a person exhibited as Nona (her real name was Amanda Crepton) who had deformed legs and arms. She wore false tusks and was presented as half human and half animal—a wild woman.

23. Pictures of Stall are in the Hertzberg Collection, the Ringling Circus Museum, and the Baraboo Collection.

24. See Levenson and Gray (1982) for a picture of a more modern geek. The Picture Collection of the Library of Congress contains a photo taken by Russell Lee of a snake eater at the South Louisiana State Fair.

25. Most of the acts listed are described in the FitzGerald (1897) articles.

Chapter 10

1. While many ex–freak show stars retired to live in communities where they were the only people with such a background, others formed communities with "their own kind"—that is, other showmen. See Gresham (1948) for descriptions of Gibtown.

2. Dave Smith of Lynchburg College is writing a book on Siamese twins which explores this question.

3. Wadlow did sell thousands of pictures of himself, though, and seemed to enjoy autographing them. On a trip of appearances after his short stand in the circus he sold seven hundred in one day.

4. The pictures chosen for display often exhibit the condition in its most blatant form. See D. Fox and James (1978) for a discussion of medical photographs of patients.

References

Aaron Moore: The coloured giant. C. 1899 (Hertzberg Coll.)

Ablon, Joan. 1984. *Little people in America.* New York: Praeger.

Admiral Dot: The smallest man in the world. 1872. (Pfening Coll.)

Advance courier of P. T. Barnum's greatest show on earth. 1881. (Ringling Coll.)

The adventures of an Australian traveler (Captain J. Reid) in search of the marvelous, wild Australian children. 1872. Buffalo: Warren, Johnson. (NYPL Coll.)

Adventures of the three Australian travelers in search of the marvelous, wild Australian children. 1864. New York: Booth. (Flint Coll.)

Alden, W. L. 1896. *Among the freaks.* New York: Longmans, Green.

Allen, Robert C. 1980. B. F. Keith and the origins of American vaudeville. *Theatre Survey* 21(November): 105–15.

Altick, Richard. 1978. *Shows of London.* Cambridge, Mass.: Belknap Press.

American Sunday School Union. C. 1840. *The circus.* Philadelphia: Sunday School Union (Baraboo Coll.)

Amusements at the abnormal. 1908. *Nation* 86:254–55.

Antoine Menier: The human ostrich. C. 1899. (Hertzberg Coll.)

Appelbaum, Stanley. 1980. *The Chicago World's Fair of 1893.* New York: Dover.

Arbus, Diane. 1972. *Diane Arbus.* New York: Aperture.

Are you a freak? 1907. *New York Globe*, January 21.

Around New York with a cannibal girl. 1895. *New York Sunday World*, April 21.

Artists of the Bowery. 1885. *New York Times*, April 12, 14.

Autobiography of Miss Ann E. Leak, born without arms. 1871. New York. (Flint Coll.)

The Aztec children. C. 1851. *Journal of the Fine Arts.* (Harvard Coll.)

The Aztecs at the society library. 1931. *Circus Scrapbook*, April 17.

Barnum, P. T. 1855. *The life of P. T. Barnum.* New York: Redfield.

———. 1871. *Struggles and triumphs.* New York: American News Company.

———. 1872. *Struggles and triumphs.* Buffalo: Warren, Johnson.

Barnum and Bailey courier. 1903. (Ringling Coll.)

Barnum and Bailey route book. 1888. (Ringling Coll.)

Barnum's American museum catalogue or guidebook. 1860 (Becker Coll.)

Barnum's museum fire. 1864. *New York World*, March 4.

Barnum's wild men of Borneo were Ohioians. 1937. *Cleveland Plain Dealer*, July 18.

Barr, Martin. 1896. Some studies in heredity. *Journal of Psycho-Asthenics* 1 (1).

———. 1904. Classification of mental defectives. *Journal of Psycho-Asthenics* 9 (2).

Barry, Richard. 1901. *The grandeurs of the exposition: Pan American exposition, 1901*. Buffalo: Robert Allen Reid.

Bassham, Ben L. 1978. *The theatrical photographs of Napoleon Sarony*. Kent, Ohio: Kent State University Press.

Bates, Ralph S. 1965. *Scientific societies in the U.S.* Cambridge: MIT Press.

Beal, George B. 1938. *Through the back door of the circus*. Springfield, Mass.: McLoughlin.

Bearded lady dead. 1902. [Brocton, Mass.] *Times*.

Becker, Howard. 1963. *Outsiders*. New York: Free Press.

Behrens, L. H., and D. P. Barr. 1932. Hyperpituitarism beginning in infancy. *Endocrinology* 16 (120).

Bell, Whitfield J., Jr., ed. 1967. *A cabinet of curiosities*. Charlottesville: University Press of Virginia.

Benedict, Burton. 1983. *The anthropology of world's fairs*. Berkeley, Calif: Scolar Press.

Berger, Peter, and Thomas Luckmann. 1967. *The social construction of reality*. Garden City, N.Y.: Doubleday.

Bernard, Charles. 1932. A giant story. *Circus Scrapbook*, January 12–18.

Bernstein, Charles. 1922. Microcephic people sometimes called 'pinheads.' *Journal of Heredity* 13:30–39.

Betts, John R. 1959. P. T. Barnum and the popularization of natural history. *Journal of the History of Ideas* 20:353–68.

Biography of Emma Schiller, the greatest of all living skeletons. 1880. (Pfening Coll.)

Biography, medical description and songs of Miss Millie Christine, the two headed nightingale. 1883. New York: Rooney and Otten. (Hertzberg Coll.)

Biography of Myrtle Corbin: The four legged girl. 1881. New York: Popular Press. (Hertzberg Coll.)

Biography of Shadow Harry. C. 1930. (Hertzberg Coll.)

Blumer, Herbert. 1969. *Symbolic interactionism*. Englewood Cliffs, N.J.: Prentice-Hall.

Bodin, Walter, and Burnet Hershey. 1934. *The world of midgets*. New York: Coward-McCann.

Bogdan, Robert. 1972. Learning to sell door to door. *American Behavioral Scientist*, September/October, 55–64.

Bogdan, Robert, and Douglas Biklen. 1977. Handicapism. *Social Policy*, March/April, 14–19.

Bogan, Robert, and Steven Taylor. 1982. *Inside Out*. Toronto: University of Toronto Press.

Bogdan, Robert, Douglas Biklen, Arthur Shapiro, and David Spelkoman. 1982. The disabled: Media's monster. *Social Policy*, Fall.

Boles, Don. 1967. *The midway showman*. Atlanta: Pinchpenny Press.

Bosworth, Patricia. 1984. *Diane Arbus: A biography*. New York: Alfred A. Knopf.

Bouvé, Thomas. 1880. *Anniversary memoirs of the Boston Society of Natural History*. Boston: Society of Natural History.

Braden, Frank. 1922. The wonders of a circus sideshow. *Illustrated World* 36: 673–76.

Fox, Daniel M., and Terry James. 1978. Photography and the self image of American physicians. *Bulletin of the History of Medicine* 52 (3): 435–58.

Freak hunting through India. 1894. *New York Herald*, April 1.

Freaks touch elbows. 1888. *New York Morning Journal*, March.

"Freaks," a word of bitter grief. 1903. *New York World*, April 12.

Frost, Thomas. 1971. *The old showmen and the old London fairs*. Ann Arbor, Mich.: Gryphon Books.

Funnell, Charles. 1975. *By the beautiful sea*. New York: Alfred A. Knopf.

Garfinkel, Harold. 1967. *Studies in ethnomethodology*. Englewood Cliffs, N.J.: Prentice-Hall.

Gaylon v. Municipal Court of San Bernardino Judicial District. 1964. 229 Cal. App. 2d 667, 40 Cal. Rptr. 446.

George, Wadsworth M. 1938. Forty-one years of York fair coverage. *Billboard*, April 9, 56.

The giants' wedding. 1871. *Harper's Bazaar*, July 29.

Gilliams, E. Leslie. 1922. Side-show freaks as seen by science. *Illustrated World* 38:213–15.

Glaser, Barney, and Anslem Strauss. 1967. *The discovery of grounded theory*. Chicago: Aldine.

Goffman, Erving. 1959. *Presentation of self in everyday life*. Garden City, N.Y.: Doubleday/Anchor.

———. 1963. *Stigma*. Englewood Cliffs, N.J.: Prentice-Hall.

Gorham, Maurice. 1951. *Showmen and suckers*. London: Percival Marshall.

Gossett, Thomas F. 1963. *Race*. Dallas: Southern Methodist University Press.

Gould, George M., and Walter Pyle. 1896. *Anomalies and curiosities of medicine*. New York: Bell.

Gould, Stephen Jay. 1981. *The mismeasure of man*. New York: W. W. Norton.

———. 1985. *The flamingo's smile*. New York: W. W. Norton.

Greene, John C. 1959. *The death of adam*. Ames: Iowa University Press.

Gresham, William L. 1948. *Monster midway*. New York: Rinehart.

Grifting isn't so good. 1924. *Saturday Evening Post*, May 17.

Grossman, Herbert J. 1983. *Manual on terminology and classification in mental retardation*. Baltimore: American Association of Mental Deficiency.

Hall, Ward. 1981. *Struggles and triumphs of a modern day showman*. Sarasota, Fla.: Carnival.

Haller, Mark H. 1963. *Eugenics*. New Brunswick, N.J.: Rutgers University Press.

Hambly, Wilfrid D. 1925. *The history of tattooing and its significance*. London: H. F. and G. Witherby.

Hannah Battersby. 1930. *Circus scrapbook*, April.

Harlow, Alvin. 1931. *Old Bowery days*. New York: Appleton.

Harmetz, Aljean. 1977. *The making of the Wizard of Oz*. New York: Alfred A. Knopf.

Harris, Neil. 1973. *Humbug*. Chicago: University of Chicago Press.

Hartt, Rollin. 1909. *The people at play*. New York: Houghton Mifflin.

Havig, Alan. 1982. The commercial amusement audience in 20th century American cities. *Journal of American Culture* 5:1–19.

Hewitt, William J. 1937. Three hundred carnivals to tour. *Billboard*, April 10.

High social set in freakdom. 1914. *New York Sun*, March 3.

Hilton, Daisy, and Violet Hilton. C. 1942. *The intimate Hilton sisters: Siamese twins.* (Hertzberg Coll.)

Hilton, Suzanne. 1975. *The way it was: 1876.* Philadelphia: Westminster.

Historical and descriptive account of the Siamese twin brothers from actual observation. 1831. New York. (Boston Public Library.)

Historical rings. 1871. *Harper's Bazaar,* January 14, 24.

The history and description of Abomah, the African Amazon giantess. C. 1900. (Hertzberg Coll.)

The history and life of Unzie, the Australian aboriginal beauty. 1893. New York: Dick's. (Becker Coll.)

The history and medical description of the two-headed girl. 1869. Buffalo, N.Y.: Warren and Jones.

History of Miss Annie Jones, Barnum's Esau lady. 1885. New York: Popular Press. (Becker Coll.)

History of P. T. Barnum's Fiji cannibals. 1872. (Harvard Geography Library.)

Hogg, Garry. 1958. *Cannibalism and human sacrifice.* London: Robert Hale.

Holley, Marietta. 1893. *Samantha at the World's Fair.* New York: Funk and Wagnall's.

Holtman, Jerry. 1968. *Freak show man.* Los Angeles: Holloway House.

Hong, Lawrence, and Robert Duff. 1977. Becoming a taxi-dancer. *Sociology of Work and Occupations* 4 (3): 327–43.

Howard, Martin. 1977. *Victorian grotesque.* London: Jupiter.

Huff, O. N. 1889. An ischiopagus monster. *American Journal of Obstetrics* 22: 923–26.

Humberd, Charles D. 1937. Giantism: Report of a case. *Journal of the American Medical Association* 108 (7): 544–46.

Hunter, Kay. 1964. *Duet for life.* New York: Coward-McCann.

Hutchinson, H. N., J. W. Gregory, and R. Lydekker. C. 1895. *Living races of mankind.* London: Hutchinson.

Hutton, Laurence. 1891. *Curiosities of the American stage.* New York: Harper.

An illustrated catalogue and guide book to Barnum's American Museum. 1860. New York. (Becker Coll.)

Inciardi, James A., and David Petersen. 1972. Gaff joints and shell games. *Journal of Popular Culture* 6 (3): 591–606.

Interesting facts and illustrations of the royal Padaung giraffe-neck women from Burma. 1933. (Ringling Coll.)

The intimate Hilton Sisters: Siamese twins. C. 1942. (Hertzberg Coll.)

Irwin, Will. 1909. *Confessions of a con man.* New York: B. W. Huebsch.

Isman, Felix. 1924. *Weber and Fields.* New York: Boni and Liveright.

Jackson, Joseph. 1931. *Encyclopedia of Philadelphia,* vol. 2. Harrisburg, Pa.: National Historical Association.

Jacobi, A. 1895. Dr. S. Tynberg's pygopagus. *Archives of Pediatrics* 12 (10): 721–29.

Jacobs, T. J. 1844. *Scenes in the Pacific Ocean.* New York: Harlem.

James, Theodore, Jr. 1975. Giant wedding of the little people. *White Tops* 48 (1).

Jay, Ricky. 1986. *Learned pigs and fireproof women.* New York: Villard Books.

Jennings, John. 1882. *Theatrical and circus life.* Cincinnati: Forshee.

Jessup, R. B. 1888. Monstrosities and maternal impressions. *Journal of the American Medical Association* 11 (14): 519–20.

Johnston, Alva. 1933. Profiles. *New Yorker*, May 6, 27–29.
———. 1934a. Sideshow people I. *New Yorker*, April 14, 27–30.
———. 1934b. Sideshow people II. *New Yorker*, April 21, 28–34.
———. 1934c. Sideshow people III. *New Yorker*, April 28, 70–77.
Jones, Joseph. 1888. Abstracts of contributions to teratology. *Journal of the American Medical Association* 11 (15): 545–51.
Jordan, Joseph. 1925. "Old Tobey"—king of circus fakers. *New York Evening World*, n.d.
Jordan, Winthrop. 1968. *White over black.* Chapel Hill: University of North Carolina Press.
Kaleina, Georgene. 1984. "Frog man" banned from work. *Syracuse Herald-Journal*, August 31, 9.
Kasson, John F. 1978. *Amusing the million.* New York: Farrar, Straus and Giroux.
Kelly, F. Beverly. 1982. *It was better than work.* Gerald, Mass.: Petrice Press.
———. 1950. Freakshow. *Pageant*, May.
Knox, Thomas W. 1896. Street life. In *Darkness and daylight*, edited by Helen Campbell and T. W. Knox. Hartford: Hartford Press.
Kobel, Bernard. C. 1968. *829 photographs of the wonders Mother Nature has carved on human bodies. . . .* Clearwater, Fla.: Bernard Kobel. Mimeograph.
The Korean twins. 1903. *Scientific American* 88 (April 25): 318.
Krao, the missing link. C. 1884. (Gordon Brown Coll., Edmonton, Alta., Canada.)
Kunhardt, Dorothy M., and Philip B. Kunhardt, Jr. 1977. *Mathew Brady and his world.* Alexandria, Va.: Time-Life Books.
Kyriazi, Gary. 1976. *The great American amusement parks.* Secaucus, N.J.: Citadel Press.
Latham, R. G. 1856. Ethnological remarks upon some of the more remarkable varieties of human species represented by individuals now in London. *Ethnological Society of London Journal* 4:148.
Latzke, Paul. 1903. Fortunes and freaks in advertising. *Saturday Evening Post*, August 22, 4.
Lee, Polly J. 1970. *Giant.* New York: A. S. Barnes.
Leech, Margaret. 1926. Zip, freak belied his description. *New York Evening World*, April 27.
Lees, Hannah. 1937. Side show diagnosis. *Collier's* 99:224.
Lentz, John. 1964. How medical progress has hastened the passing of the sideshow. *Today's Health*, March, 48–51.
———. 1977. The revolt of the freaks. *Bandwagon* 21 (5): 26–29.
Levenson, Randal, and Spalding Gray. 1982. *In search of the monkey girl.* Millerton, N.Y.: Aperture.
Lewis, Arthur. 1970. *Carnival.* New York: Trident.
Liazos, A. 1972. The poverty of the sociology of deviants. *Social Problems* 20: 103–20.
Life and adventures of the Burdett twins. 1881. New York: Popular Press.
The life and adventures of Capt. Costentenus, the tattooed Greek prince. 1881. New York: Popular Press. (Becker Coll.)
The life and adventures of James F. O'Connell, the tattooed man, during a residence of eleven years in New Holland and Caroline Islands. 1846. (Flint Coll.)

The life of Barney Nelson: The armless phenomenon. 1883. New York: Popular Press. (Hertzberg Coll.)

The life of Count Ivan D. Orloff: The only living transparent and ossified man. 1900. Liverpool: Nicol, Kendrick. (Hertzberg Coll.)

The life of D. J. Major. 1859. (Flint Coll.)

The life of Hedjaanta the serpent queen from the Philippine Islands. C. 1898. (Hertzberg Coll.)

The life and history of Alfonso, the human ostrich. C. 1903. N.p.: Buffalo Bill. (Hertzberg Coll.)

The life history of Clicko: The dancing Bushman of Africa. C. 1922. Ivyland, Pa.: n.p. (Hertzberg Coll.)

Life history of Francesco A. Lentini: Three legged wonder. C. 1930. (Hertzberg Coll.)

The life of Isaac W. Sprague, the living skeleton. C. 1885. New York: Popular Press.

Life of the living Aztec children. 1860. New York: American Museum.

The life of Naomi: Arizonian snake charmer. C. 1901. London: Showmen's Printers. (Hertzberg Coll.)

The life story and facts of the San Antonio Siamese twins. C. 1925. (Hertzberg Coll.)

The life story and facts of the San Antonio Siamese twins. 1926. (Hertzberg Coll.)

The life story of Mr. and Mrs. Al Tomaini, the world's strangest married couple, giant and half girl. C. 1939. (Hertzberg Coll.)

The life of a xiphopagis or Siamese twins. 1902. *Scientific America Supplement* 54 (November): 22440.

Lifson, Robert. 1983. *Enter the sideshow.* Bala Cynwyd, Pa.: Mason.

Lindfors, Bernth. 1983a. Circus Africans. *Journal of American Culture* 6 (2): 9–14.

———. 1983b. "The Hottentot Venus" and other African attractions in nineteenth century England. *Australasian Drama Studies* 1 (2): 82–103.

———. 1984. P. T. Barnum and Africa. *Studies in Popular Culture* 7:18–25.

Lofland, John. 1969. *Deviance and identity.* Englewoods Cliffs, N.J.: Prentice-Hall.

Lombroso, Cesare. 1887. *L'homme criminel.* Paris: F. Alcan.

———. 1896. The savage origin of tattooing. *Popular Science Monthly,* April, 793–803.

Lombroso-Ferrero, Gina. 1972. *Criminal man.* Montclair, N.J.: Patterson Smith.

Looney, Robert F. 1976. *Old Philadelphia in early photographs, 1839–1914.* New York: Dover.

The loving Lilliputians. 1863. *New York Times.* February 11, 8.

Ludmerer, Kenneth M. 1972. *Genetics and American society.* Baltimore: Johns Hopkins University Press.

McCabe, James D. 1876. *The illustrated history of the Centennial Exhibition.* Philadelphia: National Publishers.

McCardell, Ray L. 1925. When the Bowery was in bloom. *Saturday Evening Post,* December 19, 36.

McCulloch, Lou W. 1981. *Card photographs: A guide to their history and value.* East Exton, Pa.: Schiffer.

McCullough, David. 1983. *Brooklyn.* New York: Dial Press.

McCullough, Edo. 1957. *Good old Coney Island.* New York: Charles Scribner.

———. 1966. *World's Fair midways.* New York: Exposition Press.

McKennon, Joe. 1972. *A pictorial history of the American carnival*. Sarasota, Fla.: Carnival Publishers.

———. 1980. *Circus lingo*. Sarasota, Fla.: Carnival Publishers.

McNamara, Brooks. 1974. A congress of wonders: The rise and fall of the dime museum. *Emerson Society Quarterly* 20:216–32.

McWhirter, Norris, and Ross McWhirter. 1969. *Guinness book of world records*. New York: Sterling.

Manager of Zip dying from grief. 1926. *New York Times*, June 28.

Mangels, William F. 1952. *The outdoor amusement industry*. New York: Vantage.

Mannix, Daniel. 1976. *We who are not as others*. New York: Pocket Books.

Many circus folk at Zip's funeral. 1926. *New York Times*, April 28.

Marcosson, Issac A. 1929. The earnings of circus people. *Circus Scrapbook* 1 (2).

Maurer, David. 1931. Carnival cant. *American Speech* 6:327–37.

Meredith, Roy. 1970. *The world of Mathew Brady*. Los Angeles: Brooke House.

Metcalf, Francis. 1906. *Sideshow studies*. New York: Outing.

Middleton, George. 1913. *Circus memoirs*. Los Angeles: George Rice.

Miller, Howard. 1970. *Dollars for research*. Seattle: University of Washington Press.

Miss Millie-Christine: The living and only two headed woman. C. 1874. Handbill, Eden Musee (New York). (Hertzberg Coll.)

Mitchell, Joseph. 1943. *McSorley's wonderful saloon*. New York: Duell, Sloan and Pearce.

Mitchell, Michael. 1979. *Monsters of the Gilded Age*. Toronto: Gage.

Mizruchi, Ephraim. 1983. *Regulating society*. New York: Free Press.

Morris, Ramona, and Desmond Morris. 1966. *Men and apes*. London: Sphere.

Night scene in the Bowery. 1881. *Harper's Weekly*, February 26, 135.

Norman, John. 1933. A sideshow man confesses. *Omaha World Herald*, March 26.

The number of colossal organizations on the increase. 1876. *Centennial*. (Baraboo Coll.)

O'Connell, P. A. 1871. Interesting case in Prof. Hebra's lecture room. *Boston Medical and Surgical Journal*, 323–24.

Odell, George. 1927. *Annals of the New York stage*, vols. 1–3. New York: Columbia University Press.

———. 1928. *Annals of the New York stage*, vols. 4 and 5. New York: Columbia University Press.

———. 1931. *Annals of the New York stage*, vol. 6. New York: Columbia University Press.

Official guide book of the fair. 1933. Chicago: Century of Progress.

Offical Programme and book of wonders combined of the Barnum and Bailey greatest show on earth with full descriptions of human abnormalities and rare animals. 1903. (Ringling Coll.)

Official souvenir programme for Hagenbeck's arena and world's museum at the Midway Plaisance World's Columbian Exposition. C. 1893. (Author's Coll.)

The only boy Siamese twins in the world, Simplicio and Lucio Godino. C. 1928. (Hertzberg Coll.)

Oppenheimer, Jane. 1968. Some historical relationships between teratology and experimental embryology. *Bulletin of the History of Medicine* 68: 145–59.

Our summer resorts. 1881. *Harper's Weekly*, August 6.

Parmelee, Maurice F. 1912. *The principles of anthropology and sociology in their relations to criminal procedure*. New York: Macmillan.

Parry, Albert. 1933. *Tattoo*. New York: Simon and Schuster.

Peiss, Kathy. 1986. *Cheap amusements*. Philadelphia: Temple University Press.

Personal facts regarding Percilla the monkey girl. C. 1940.

Pfening, Fred, Jr. 1977. The evolution of the bannerline wagon. *Bandwagon* 21 (5): 21–25.

———. 1983. The flamboyant showman and his six title circus. *Bandwagon* 27 (4): 4–17.

———. 1985. Sideshows and bannerlines. *Bandwagon* 29 (2): 16–22.

Pfening, Fred, III. 1973. A note on giraffes and the American menagerie industry in the 1850's. *Bandwagon* 17 (4): 13–14.

The phrenological character of Chang and Eng. 1846. *American Phrenological Journal*, October 316–17.

Physicians quit lecture to freaks. 1914. *New York Herald*, April 17.

Pilat, Oliver, and Jo Ranson. 1941. *Sodom by the sea*. Garden City, N.Y.: Doubleday.

Plowden, Gene. 1982. *The circus press agent*. Caldwell, Ida.: Caxton.

Polacsek, John. 1973. A history of the giraffe and the circus. *Bandwagon* 17 (1): 14–15.

Predmore, Richard L. 1949. Introduction to J. L. Stephens, *Incidents of travel in Central America, Chiapas, and Yucatan*. New Brunswick, N.J.: Rutgers University Press.

Presbrey, Frank. 1929. *The history of advertising*. Garden City, N.Y.: Doubleday.

Prodigies in conference. 1903. *New York Times*, April 12.

Pygopagus marriage. 1934. *Time*, July 16, 20.

Randall, Edwin. 1937. Barnum's "Wild Men of Borneo" were Ohioans. *Cleveland Plain Dealer*, July 18.

Ripley, Robert L. 1929. *Believe it or not!* New York: Simon and Schuster.

Ripley's freaks on way to D.C. 1934. *Washington Times*, January 4.

Robertson, Archie. 1952. Chang-Eng's American heritage. *Life*, August 11, 70–81.

Robeson, Dave. 1935. *Al G. Barnes, master showman*. Caldwell, Ida.: Caxton.

Robinson, Gil. 1925. *Old wagon show days*. Cincinnati: Brockwell.

Rosen, Marvin, G. Clark, and M. Kivitz. 1976. *The history of mental retardation*. Baltimore: University Park Press.

Roth, Hy and Robert Cromie. 1980. *The little people*. New York: Everest House.

Rusid, Max. 1975. *Sideshow: Photo album of human oddities*. New York: Amjon.

Ryan, Kate. 1915. *Old Boston museum days*. Boston: Little, Brown.

Rydell, Robert. 1984. *All the world's a fair*. Chicago: University of Chicago Press.

Sad news for old circus freaks. 1908. *New York Morning Telegraph*, March 1.

San Antonio's Siamese twins. 1926. (Publicity advance campaign pamphlet; (Hertzberg Coll.)

Sarason, Seymour, and John Doris. 1979. *Educational handicap, public policy, and social history*. New York: Free Press.

Saucer lips, Ubangis savages, French Equatorial Africa, historical sketch, origins, habits and customs. C. 1931. (Baraboo Coll.)

Savage, Thomas, and Jeffries Wyman. 1847. Notice of the external characteristics and habits of *troglodytes gorilla*, a new species of orang from Gaboon River. *Boston Journal of Natural Science* 5 (4): 417–41.

Savitz, Leonard. 1972. Introduction to G. Lombroso-Ferrero, *Criminal man*. Montclair, N.Y.: Patterson Smith.

Saxon, A. H. 1983. *Selected letters of P. T. Barnum*. New York: Columbia University Press.

———, ed. 1979. *The autobiography of Mrs. Tom Thumb*. Hamden, Conn.: Archon Books.

Sayers, Isabelle. 1981. *Annie Oakley and Buffalo Bill's Wild West*. New York: Dover.

Scheerenberger, R. C. 1983. *A history of mental retardation*. Baltimore: Paul H. Brooks.

Schneider, William H. 1982. *An empire for the masses*. Westport, Conn.: Greenwood Press.

Scott, M. B., and S. M. Lyman. 1968. Accounts. *American Sociological Review* 33 (February): 46–62.

Seale, William. 1981. *The tasteful interlude*. Nashville: American Association for State and Local History.

Sellers, Charles. 1980. *Mr. Peale's museum*. New York: W. W. Norton.

Sharpe, Adrian. 1970. Circus grift. *Bandwagon* 14 (6): 31–36.

Sherwood, Robert E. 1926. *Here we are again*. Indianapolis: Bobbs-Merrill.

Shettel, James W. 1929. Death of Barnum's cannibal. *Circus scrapbook* 1 (4): 43.

Shipley, W. E. N.d. Validity and construction of statute or ordinance prohibiting commercial exhibition of malformed or disfigured persons. 62ALR3d1237.

Show family album. 1938. *Billboard*, February 19.

Siamese twins "bondage" trial packed courtroom. 1969. *San Antonio Express*, January 8.

Siamese twins found dead of flu at home. 1969. *San Antonio Evening News*, January 6.

Silverman, William A. 1979. Incubator-baby side show. *Pediatrics* 64 (2): 127–41.

Sketch of the life of General Decker, the smallest man in the world. 1874. Nashville, Tenn.: n.p. (Hertzberg Coll.)

Sketch of the life of General Tom Thumb. 1847. (Becker Coll.)

Sketch of the life, personal appearance, character and manners of Charles S. Stratton, known as General Tom Thumb, and his wife Lavinia Warren Stratton. 1867. New York: Wynkoop and Hallenbeck. (Becker Coll.)

Sketch of the life, personal appearance, character and manners of Charles S. Stratton, the man in miniature, known as General Tom Thumb. 1854. New York: Van Norden. (Becker Coll.)

A sketch of the life of the Russian prince. C. 1900. (Becker Coll.)

Skinner, Otis. 1924. *Footlights and spotlights*. New York: Blue Ribbon Books.

Sloan, William, and Harvey Stevens. 1976. *A century of concern*. Washington, D.C.: American Association of Mental Deficiency.

Smith, Edward H. 1922. Hey, rube! *Collier's*, April 22, 11–12.

Smith, Morton. 1935. Czar of the circus realm. *Jewish Tribune*, April.

Sontag, Susan. 1977. *On photography*. New York: Farrar, Straus and Giroux.

Spector, Malcom, and John Kitsuse. 1977. *Constructing social problems*. Menlo Park, Calif.: Cummings.

Stanley, Frank. 1914. Rare freaks of nature's hand or deviations from the normal? *Billboard*, March 21, 40.

Stanton, William. 1960. *The leopard's spots*. Chicago: University of Chicago Press.

Starr, Fredrick, 1893. Anthropology at the World's Fair. *Popular Science Monthly* 43:621.

Starr, Paul. 1982. *The social transformation of American medicine*. New York: Basic Books.

Steinbrunner, Chris, and Burt Goldblatt. 1972. *Cinema of the fantastic*. New York: Galahad.

Stephens, John L. 1841. *Incidents of travel in Central America, Chiapas, and Yucatan*, vol. 1. New York: Harper.

———. 1843. *Incidents of travel in Yucatan*. New York: Harper.

Strange sights at the circus. 1894. *New York Sunday Mercury*, April 1.

Sweet, Robert, and Robert Habenstein. 1972. Some perspectives on the circus in transition. *Journal of Popular Culture* 6 (3): 583–90.

Sykes, Gresham, and David Matza. 1957. Techniques of neutralization. *American Sociological Review* 22.

Szasz, Thomas. 1961. *The myth of mental illness*. New York: Harper and Row.

Taft, Robert. 1938. *Photography and the American scene*. New York: Macmillan.

The tattooed lady, Miss Nora Hildebrandt. C. 1890. (Flint Coll.)

Taylor, Robert. 1956. *Center ring*. Garden City, N.Y.: Doubleday.

———. 1958a. Talker I. *New Yorker*, April 19.

———. 1958b. Talker II. *New Yorker*, April 26.

Taylor, Steven, and Robert Bogdan. 1980. Defending illusions. *Human Organization* 39 (3): 209–18.

Teel, J. C. 1930. *True facts and pictures*. Asted, W.Va.: Pentland.

Terry, C. C. 1869. Remarks upon some recently reported cases or monstrosity. *American Journal of Obstetrics* 2 (3): 368.

Thayer, Stuart. 1976. The anti-circus laws in Connecticut, 1773–1840. *Bandwagon* 20 (1): 18–20.

———. 1980. Some class distinctions in the early circus audience. *Bandwagon*. 24 (4): 20–21.

———. 1981. Legislating the shows: Vermont, 1824–1933. *Bandwagon* 25 (5).

The theoretical child: A proof of pre-natal influence, as propounded by Dr. J. W. Coffey (skeleton dude of the USA and the Old World). 1902. (Hertzberg Coll.)

Thompson, C. J. 1968. *The mystery and lore of monsters*. New York: Bell.

Thomson, Basil. 1908. *The Fijians*. London: William Heinemann.

Throngs view wonders of Hercules odditorium. 1933. *Boston Record*, December 15.

Toll, Robert. 1976. *On with the show*. New York: Oxford University Press.

Tom Thumb's baby. 1901. *Billboard*, May 4.

Traube, Leonard. 1936. Coney Island. *Billboard*, August 29.

Truzzi, Marcello. 1968a. The decline of the American circus. In *Sociology and everyday life*, edited by M. Truzzi. Englewood Cliffs, N.J.: Prentice-Hall.

———. 1968b. Lilliputians in Gulliver's land. In *Sociology of everyday life*, edited by M. Truzzi. Englewood Cliffs, N.J.: Prentice-Hall.

———. 1973. Circuses, carnivals and fairs in America. *Journal of Popular Culture* 6(3): 529–34.

————. 1979. Circus and sideshows. In *American popular entertainment*, edited by M. Matlaw. Westport, Conn.: Greenwood Press.

Tucker, Albert. 1973. The strangest people on earth. *Sarasota Sentinel*, July 7, 14.

Tully, Jim. 1927. *Circus parade*. New York: Albert and Charles Boni.

Twins were popular. 1969. *San Antonio Light*, January 9.

Uno. Coney Island, New York. *Billboard*, September 10.

Unthan, Carl. 1935. *The armless fiddler: A pediscript being of a vaudeville man*. London: Allen and Unwin.

Vail, R. W. G. 1938. The circus from Noah's ark to New York. *Bulletin, Museum of the City of New York* 1(5): 52–56.

————. 1956. *Random notes on the history of the early American circus*. Barre, Mass.: American Antiquarian.

Wallace, Irving. 1959. *The fabulous showman*. New York: Alfred A. Knopf.

Wallace, Irving, and Amy Wallace. 1978. *The two*. New York: Simon and Schuster.

Warkany, Joseph. 1959. Congenital malformations in the past. *Journal of Chronic Disease* 10(2): 84–96.

Warren, J. Mason. 1851. An account of the two remarkable Indian dwarfs exhibited in Boston under the name of Aztec children. *American Journal of Medical Sciences* 42(April): 285–93.

Webb, Spider. 1976. *Heavily tattooed men and women*. New York: McGraw-Hill.

Weber, A. F. 1965. *The growth of cities in the nineteenth century*. Ithaca, N.Y.: Cornell University Press.

Weedon, Geoff, and R. Ward. 1981. *Fairground art*. London: White Mouse Editions.

Weeping mother puts her Siamese twins in circus. 1951. *Cleveland Plain Dealer*, April 6.

Wells, Brooks. 1888. A unique monstrosity. *American Journal of Obstetrics* 21 (December): 1265–71.

Werner, M. R. 1926. *Barnum*. Garden City, N.Y.: Doublday.

What we know about Waino and Plutano, wild men of Borneo. C. 1878. (Hertzberg Coll.)

The "wild boy" tamed by the "spotted girl." 1903. *Leader*, August.

Wild man of Borneo. 1906. (Newspaper article in "Freak" scrapbook, Circus World Museum, Baraboo.)

Wild men of Borneo were Ohio fakes. 1973. *Cleveland Press*, May 14.

Wiley, E. P. 1931. Side-show freaks and barkers. *Circus Scrap Book* 10(April): 25–30.

Williams, Thomas, and J. Calvert. 1859. *Fiji and the Fijians*. New York: D. Appleton.

Wilmeth, Don. 1982. *Variety entertainment and outdoor amusements: A reference guide*. Westport, Conn.: Greenwood Press.

Wittke, Carl F. 1968. *Tambo and Bones*. Westport, Conn.: Greenwood Press.

Wolfensberger, Wolf. 1975. *The origin and nature of our institutional models*. Syracuse, N.Y.: Human Policy Press.

The wonder of the wide, wide world: A true history of Mr. Eli Bowen. 1880. New York: New York Publisher. (Hertzberg Coll.)

Wood, Edward J. 1868. *Giants and dwarfs*. London: Richard Bentley.

Wood, J. G. 1885. Dime museums. *Atlantic Monthly* 55(January–June): 759–65.

Wood, Warren H. 1980. With Ringling-Barnum in 1935. *Bandwagon* 24(5): 17–19.

World Fair freaks and attractions, Inc. v. Hodges. October 11, 1972. FLA. 267 So. 2d 817.

Yriazi, Gary. 1976. *The great American amusement park.* Secaucus, N.J.: Citadel Press.

Zip back in circus sober and humble. C. 1910. (Hertzberg Coll.)

Zip, circus freak dies. 1926. *Bound Brook News.* April 19.

Zip's manager griefstricken at losing freak. 1926. (Baraboo Coll.)

Zip, pride at B & B Circus, is host of feast of freaks. 1914. *New York Morning Telegraph,* April 6.

Zip the 'What Is It?' plays host to all the circus freaks. 1914. *New York World.* (Ringling Coll.)

Zoe Meleke: Biographical sketch of the Circassian girl. C. 1880. New York: P. T. Barnum's Greatest Show on Earth. (Hertzberg Coll.)

Index

Fiedler, Leslie, 7
Fiji cannibals, 12, 179–87
Filbert, James, 253
Fillmore, Millard, 130
Fisher, Mr. and Mrs., 208
Flora, 187–89
Flower, Mr., 136
Forepaugh, Adam, 71, 205
Freaks: and photography, 11–16; "revolt" of, 270–72; social construction of, 2–10; and "true-life" pamphlets, 17–20. *See also* Freak shows
Freaks (Fiedler), 7
Freaks (film), vii–viii, 62, 66, 134, 142, 146, 172–73, 216, 223, 229
Freak Show Man (Lewiston), 143–44
Freak shows: acceptance of, 1–2; American Museum, 32–35; in amusement parks, 54–58; and amusement world organization, 70–74; in carnivals, 58–60; in circuses, 40–47; decline and demise of, 62–68, 267; defined, 10; in dime museums, 35–39; in early museums, 29–31; emergence of, 25–29; modes of presenting, 94–116; sources for study of, 11–20; terminology of, 3–6; and travel, 74–77; in world's fairs, 47–54; worldview and practices of showmen in, 81–93. *See also* Aggrandized presentations; Amusement parks; Carnivals; Circuses; Dime museums; Exotic presentations; World's fairs

Gaffed freaks, 8, 10, 11, 38, 68, 89, 97, 234–35
Geeks, 262
Genetics, 62–63, 111
Giants, giantism, 6, 7, 287 n.6; construction of, 3, 25; and marriage, 205–8, 210; modes of presenting, 97, 103, 109, 112, 114–15; and photography, 13; Wadlow case, 272–76
Gibbons, Anna "Artorea," 298 n.15
Girlie shows, 88–89
Gloaming geeks, 262
Goshen, Colonel, 41
Graham, Lew, 234
Great Depression, 40–41, 67
Great Ethnological Congress, 50–51, 185
Great Omi, The Zebra Man, 253–56
Great Waldo, 264
Greeley, Horace, 130, 291 n.16
Greenward, Charlotte, 168

Greenwood, John, Jr., 238–40
Griffith, Bill, 142
Grift, 86–93
Gumpertz, Evie, 198
Gumpertz, Samuel W., 56–57, 71–72, 89, 127, 159–60, 190, 197–98

Haggar, Jack, 54
Haight, Mattie, 213
Hall, Ward, 268
Hamilton, Tody, 63–65, 100, 271
Hammond, Hoke, 90–91
Harper, Ella, 15–16
Harper's Bazaar, 206
Hauser, Casper, 31
Hayes, John, 250
Headbinders, 143–44
Healey, W. A., 189
Hebra, Ferdinand, 246
Hedjaanta, 258–59
Hershey, Burnet, 159
Heth, Joice, 31
Hilderbrant, Martin, 250
Hilton, Edith. *See* Meyers, Edith
Hilton, Mary, 166–68
Hilton, Violet and Daisy (Hilton Sisters), 60, 62, 113, 148, 174, 200–202, 234; career of, 166–73
Hollis, A. C., 229
Honeywell, Martha Ann, 28–29
Horvath Midgets, 161
Hottentots, 187
House family, 144
Howard, Annie and Frank, 252
Huber's Dime Museum, 38, 183, 205
Human ostriches, 263–64
Human skeletons, 7, 231
Human trunks, 224
Humberd, Charles D., 275–76
Humboldt, Baron von, 131
Humor, 114, 152, 210
Hybridity theory, 106

Ike, 208
Ilikuluin and Zanbezi, 143
Illustrated London News, 188
Illustrated World, 66
Illy and Zambezi, 143, 195
Incubator Babies, 289 n.30
Ingalls, Clyde, 2–3, 25, 89, 95, 194, 258, 267
Ingalls, H. P., 207